MW00715646

Health Occupations
Exploration and Career Planning

Joan M. Birchenall, RN, MEd
Manager, Bureau of Career Orientation
and Prevocational Programs
Division of Vocational Education
New Jersey Department of Education
Trenton, New Jersey

Mary Eileen Streight, RN, BSN
Instructor, Health Occupations Education
Mercer County Vocational Technical School
Trenton, New Jersey

The C.V. Mosby Company
ST. LOUIS * BALTIMORE * TORONTO * 1989

Library of Congress Cataloging-in-Publication Data

Birchenall, Joan M.
Health occupations.

Includes bibliographies and index.
1. Medical personnel—United States—Vocational guidance. 2. Career development. I. Streight, Mary Eileen. II. Title. [DNLM: 1. Allied Health Personnel. 2. Career Choice. 3. Health Occupations W 21.5 B617h]
R690.B56 1989 610.69 89-3247
ISBN 0-8016-0477-X

Editor-in-chief: David T. Culverwell
Assistant editor: Christi Mangold
Editorial project manager: Lisa G. Cunninghis
Production: The Production House
Cover/interior art: Rhonda Meyers
Index: Blue Pencil, Inc.

Printed in the United States of America

The C.V. Mosby Company
11830 Westline Industrial Drive
St. Louis, Missouri 63146

ISBN 0-8016-0477-X

PH/VH/VH 9 8 7 6 5 4 3 2 1

To our families
for their patience, sacrifice,
understanding, and support

References

Califano, Jr., J.A.: America's health care revolution, New York, 1984, Random House, Inc.

Chabner, D.: The language of medicine, ed. 2, Philadelphia, 1981, W.B. Saunders, Co.

Clayton, et. al.: Squire's basic pharmacology for nurses, ed. 8, St. Louis, 1985, The C.V. Mosby Co.

Eschelman, M.M.: Introductory nutrition and diet therapy, Philadelphia, 1984, J.B. Lippincott, Co.

Health Occupations Students of America: National handbook, sections A, B, C, Dallas, 1985, HOSA.

Kimbrell, Grady, Vineyward, B.S.: Succeeding in the world of work, ed. 4, Encino, 1986, Glencoe Publishing Co.

Kowtaluk, H.: Discovering nutrition, Peoria, 1986, Bennett & McKnight.

O'Connor, J.L. and Goldsmith, E.: Life management skills, Cincinnati, 1987, South-Western Publishing Co.

Perry, A.G. and Potter, P.: Clinical nursing skills and techniques, St. Louis, 1986, The C.V. Mosby Co.

Potter, P. and Perry, A.G.: Fundamentals of nursing, St. Louis, 1986, The C.V. Mosby Co.

Townsend, C.: Nutrition and diet therapy, ed. 4, Albany, 1985, Delmar Publishers, Inc.

Sorrentino, S.A.: Mosby's textbook for nursing assistants, ed. 2, St. Louis, 1987, The C.V. Mosby Co.

Preface

TO THE STUDENT

Many students considering a career in the health field base their choice on a romantic notion about a specific career or on idealized feelings of wanting to help others. Unless they have had some contact with a variety of health workers, they are not aware of the number of career opportunities in this field. Some people still believe that pursuing the traditional careers of medicine, dentistry, and nursing is limited according to one's sex. Doctors and dentists are males; nurses are females. In addition, the media tend to present a distorted picture of health workers, their duties and relationships with colleagues and with the public. These misconceptions, and the idea that *all* health careers require excellent skills in mathematics and the sciences, complicate the student's career decision-making process.

To most people, health careers are associated with hospital employment and involvement in caring for the sick. Many do not know that employment in the health field can take place in a variety of settings outside a health care institution. Health workers are involved, not only in caring for the sick, but also in assisting all of us to maintain our health and to prevent illness.

The purpose of **Health Occupations — Exploration and Career Planning** is to provide reliable and realistic information about health careers. A variety of exploratory learning experiences are suggested to help you make tentative career choices based on fact, not fantasy. The book also provides a basic foundation of knowledge to build upon as you progress to the next step in developing skills in a particular health career.

Part One of the book is devoted to exploring careers. Chapter 1 discusses how the "knowledge explosion" with its technological advances has influenced the growth of health careers and has brought about radical changes in health care through the years. Chapter 2 describes the misconceptions and realities about health careers as well as practical steps to take in the career decision-making process. The next five chapters describe the five major groups of health careers. Related careers in each group are clustered to show the interrelationships between and among them. Careers with similar job responsibilities are grouped together so that you may see how each worker interacts with the others, as members of a team. The narratives in Chapters 3, 4, 5, 6, and 7 describe situations where members of the various career groups work together to meet a common goal.

Part Two, Chapters 8 to 16, lays the foundations for future employment in a variety of health occupations. The chapters include basic information about the computer and its valuable use in the health field. Other topics include communicating effectively with co-workers and clients, medical terminology and abbreviations, and essentials for maintaining a safe environment. A review of nutrition and growth and development is also given.

The last two chapters give important information to help you find and keep a job in the career of your choice. Tips to follow for advancing in your job or selecting the right educational program after high school are included. The privileges and responsibilities as a member of the health occupations family are also discussed.

At the end of each chapter, Student Activities are suggested to help you gain additional experiences. They are offered as ways to increase your understanding of the chapter and to help the book become more "alive."

If **Health Occupations — Exploration and Career Planning** provides a better understanding of careers in health and assists you to develop your career goals, the authors will consider their efforts successful.

ACKNOWLEDGMENTS

The authors wish to express their gratitude to those people who gave invaluable assistance during the preparation of the manuscript. Special thanks is given to: Dr. Michael G. Curran, Jr., Manager, Bureau of Vocational Programs, New Jersey Department of Education, Division of Vocational Education, for his contribution of Chapter 9; Mary Lynn Fracaroli, Business Education Specialist, New Jersey Department of Education, Division of Vocational Education, for contributions to Chapters 15 and 16;

and Shirley Morton, nationally certified career guidance specialist formally with the New Jersey Department of Education, Division of Vocational Education, for her review and suggestions during the development of Part One of the manuscript.

The following persons provided illustrations to enhance the text: Celeste Montgomery, St. Lawrence Rehabilitation Center, Lawrenceville, New Jersey, Ronald J. Czajakowski and Gina Gonzales, New Jersey Hospital Association, Princeton, New Jersey; Maria Barbetta, St. Mary Hospital, Langhorne, Pennsylvania; Betty Moak, Bridgeton Hospital and Bridgeton High School, Bridgeton, New Jersey; Peggy Carroll, Morristown Memorial Hospital, Morristown, New Jersey; Michael Gallagher, Camden County Vocational and Technical Schools, Sicklerville, New Jersey; Captain Albert Petroni, New Jersey National Guard, Trenton, New Jersey; Janice Calaiaro, Visiting Nurse Association of Trenton, New Jersey; Evelyn Hawrylak, Mercer St. Friend's Center, Trenton, New Jersey; and Michael Mancuso, Photographer, Trenton, New Jersey.

The agencies listed below were most generous in permitting us to photograph health workers and clients: Henry J. Austin Health Center, Trenton, New Jersey; Rusling Hose Ambulance Corps and Rescue Squad, Hamilton Township, New Jersey; Division of Health, Emergency Medical Services, Hamilton Township, New Jersey; Yardville Animal Hospital, Yardville, New Jersey; and Division of Water Pollution Control, Hamilton Township, New Jersey.

Ginny Lutkewitte, Marketing Support Representative, Office Business Systems, Inc., Edison, New Jersey, gave her expertise in assisting with technical aspects of manuscript preparation and Mary Ann Ryan assisted in typing the Teacher's Guide. Also, thanks to Margaret B. Birchenall who provided research and review assistance during the preparation of the manuscript.

Finally, the authors wish to thank Doris Smith, Telemarketing Representative, C.V. Mosby Company, for her suggestions and encouragement during the manuscript development.

Contents

Chapter 1

Health Careers in Review

Objectives

After completing this chapter, you should be able to:

- Discuss four factors that have influenced the growth of the health services industry.
- List five places where health workers are employed.
- Discuss how health care has changed to meet the needs of modern society.
- Define 70 percent of the key terms listed for this chapter.

Key Terms

- **aseptic** Sterile; free from living microorganisms
- **community health** The state of health of a particular community
- **diagnostician** One skilled in the use of scientific methods to determine the cause and nature of a sick person's disease

• **monitoring** To check the heartbeat, blood pressure, and body functions by use of electronic devices

• **mortality rate** The death rate; ratio of number of deaths to a given population

• **rehabilitation** The process of restoring to useful life a person who has been ill or who is handicapped

• **stethoscope** Instrument used to listen to sound within the body

• **telemetry** Transmission of information to a distant point by using electronic devices

• **trephination** Surgical removal of a disc of bone from the skull

EARLY CONCEPTS OF HEALTH CARE

Long before there were written records, people cared for their sick. Archaeologists have unearthed prehistoric skulls that show evidence of trephination — the surgical removal of a disc of bone from the skull. Scientists today think that trephining may have been practiced because the ancients thought this would permit evil, disease-producing spirits to escape from the body of a sick person. Was this thought to be treatment for a headache? Other bones excavated by scientists demonstrate the remarkable ability of primitive people to set broken bones so skillfully that fractures healed without deformity.

Prehistoric drawings found on cave walls emphasize certain body parts, such as hands, ears, and sex organs; some drawings depict horses and other animals, as well as human figures and weapons. Scientists have speculated about the meaning and purpose of these drawings and, as you may imagine, many theories have been proposed to explain the drawings. Were the paintings merely decorations? Or were they records of daily life in the caves? Did they have a magical purpose, such as

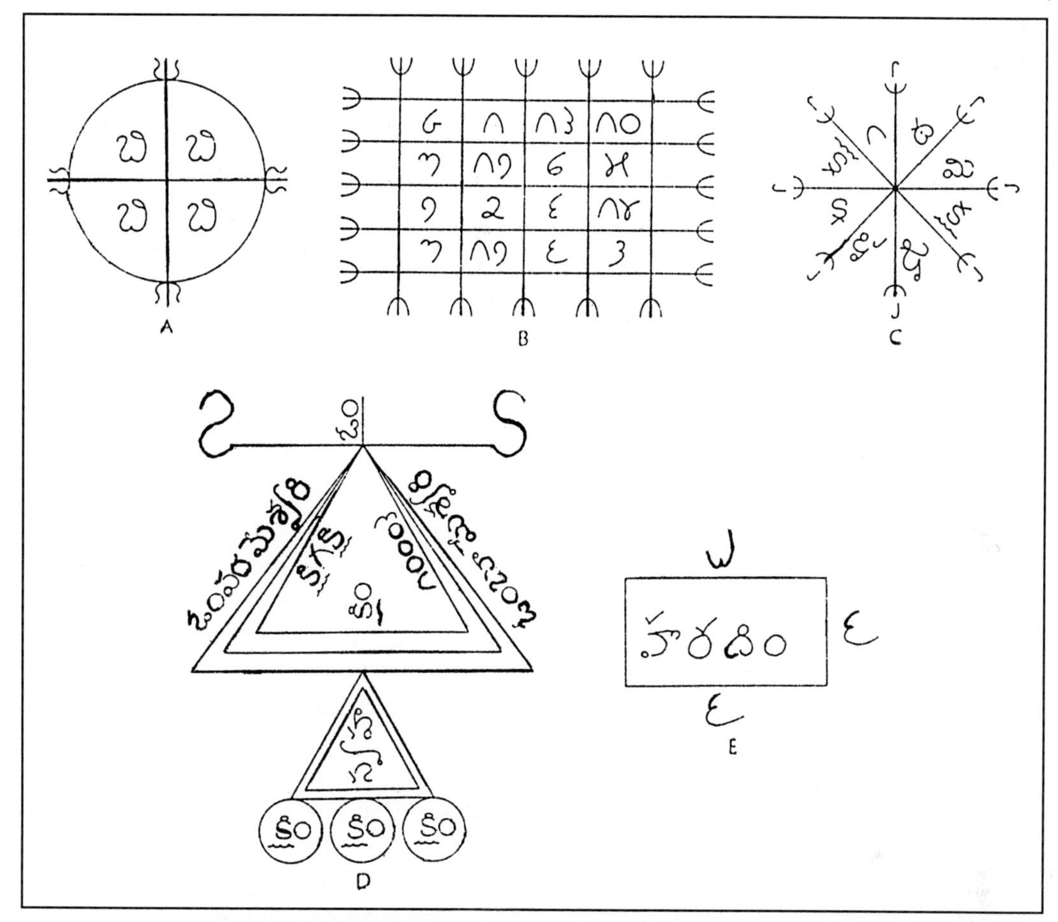

Figure 1–1. Magical charms such as these were believed to produce the desired results. These charms supposedly cured headache, assured conception, and treated malaria. (From *Konduru,* Paul G. Hiebert, University of Minnesota Press, 1971.)

protection from evil spirits that were believed to cause harm and illness? Many scientists accept the "magical" theory, but, unfortunately, there is no way to discover the true answer (**Fig. 1–1**).

We know from examination of ancient bones and fossils that people suffered from a variety of diseases and injuries, such as cancer, arthritis, tooth decay, and fractured bones. Illness was thought to be caused by forces beyond their control, and a variety of unearthly or supernatural treatments were used as cures (among them trephination, as described above). The tribe's medicine man "cured" illnesses through charms, spells, and trances as well as ritual songs and dances. The medicine man administered all of the "treatments," while the patient's family gave personal care.

Modern health care is a far cry from the days of the medicine man. There are now more than 300 different job titles to describe the health workers who help modern people to recover from illness, to maintain health, to promote wellness, and to prevent disease. In many ways, the development of health careers has paralleled the expansion of knowledge. A brief survey of the history of health care and a review of a few of the milestones will help you to further understand how civilization and health careers developed side by side.

The importance of protecting health through hygiene and sanitation was appreciated even thousands of years ago. Ruins of ancient Babylonian sewers and toilets have been found in archaeologic digs. The Bible reveals Moses as an early **sanitarian**; in fact, the Mosaic laws regarding food storage, leprosy, quarantine, and refuse disposal form the basis of modern sanitary science. Remnants of Roman sanitation methods can be seen in the ruins of the aqueducts, sewers, and baths of that period. In cities as large as Rome, Athens, and Alexandria, disease prevention and community health were as essential as they are today.

The first hospitals were established in Rome by the early Christians as their way of carrying out the teachings of Christ. Churchwomen established and staffed these institutions known as hospices, and deaconesses visited the sick and poor. Nursing sisterhoods and brotherhoods were founded to care for the hospitalized sick. During the Dark Ages, hospitals continued to develop, but these were primarily institutions that offered hospitality to the old, disabled, and homeless.

During the Middle Ages, the character of the hospice slowly changed from that of a charity to that of a medical institution. In general, this change occurred as governments (city or state) began to take an active role in the provision of medical and health care.

By the end of the Middle Ages — about A.D. 1450 — the care being given to the sick declined in quality. This was a reflection of the general decline in European society caused by endless wars and great plagues.

Eighteenth century industrialization brought with it widespread unemployment and slums. Illness, crime, and disease flourished. The time was ripe for social changes that would bring with them reforms in the care of the sick. In 1836, the modern deaconess movement was established at Kaiserwerth, Germany. The instruction in nursing provided at Kaiserwerth was so outstanding that the fame of the deaconesses spread throughout Europe. In 1850, Florence Nightingale visited and received training at the school. This upper-class Englishwoman revolutionized the care of sick and wounded British soldiers during the Crimean War, and by her practices of cleanliness, skill, and organization she was able to bring about a significant reduction in the mortality (death) rate.

OF STETHOSCOPES, ANESTHETICS, AND OTHER MILESTONES

In the early 1800s, the world saw tremendous advances in medical knowledge that produced far-reaching effects. The invention of the stethoscope — said to be one of the eight or ten greatest contributions to the science of medicine — revolutionized the diagnosis of disease. Before its discovery, diagnosing disease was done by the "hit or miss" method, otherwise known as "guessing." The invention of the hypodermic needle, the discovery of ether and chloroform, and the aseptic technique introduced by Doctor Joseph Lister, a British surgeon, influenced the development of surgical procedures. Anesthesia permitted pain-free surgery and produced the need for new kinds of health workers. People were needed to administer the anesthetic, to hold the lamp, and to assist in many other ways.

About the time that Lister's antiseptic technique was introduced, Oliver Wendell Holmes, a poet and physician in the United States, and Ignaz Semmelweis, a Hungarian physician, made an important discovery. They observed that the simple measure of handwashing, when performed by attendants between their examinations of women who had just delivered their babies, dramatically reduced the number of deaths due to puerperal (childbed) fever.

By the end of the 1800s, there were further discoveries and inventions: the clinical thermometer, aspirin, rubber gloves for surgical use, and the x-ray machine. Shortly after Dr. Roentgen invented the x-ray machine, a London firm advertised x-ray-proof underwear! Since this new invention was a tool in diagnosis, new workers were needed: to prepare patients, take x-rays, and develop them. The modern hospital radiology department grew out of this modest beginning. Sweeping social changes also occurred during the nineteenth century, and these, in turn, brought their share of change to the health care scene.

MEDICAL PROGRESS IN THE SERVICE OF SOCIETY

When the American frontier pushed westward during the nineteenth century, the need for physicians increased. Railroad companies recruited at least one physician to care for the residents of each town along the railroad line. The frontier physician also acted as the dentist until the traveling dentist arrived. As communities grew, more and more health workers were needed to serve the population. Nurses, pharmacists, dentists, and veterinarians moved into the towns and cities of the West.

Our recent exploration of space involved a small army of health workers representing diverse skills. No longer could the physician accompany the explorers into the unknown and foreign territory. Instead, information about the explorers' state of health (in this case, the astronauts) was relayed from outer space to a receiving station on earth by means of radio signals. The process is called telemetry. The design and development of the system of telemetry required a combination of engineering ability and medical knowledge provided by **biomedical engineers**. These health workers develop the techniques and design for the equipment needed by modern medicine.

Like most concepts that change people's lives, telemetry was considered revolutionary only a few years ago. Today, however, many ambulances are equipped with machines to take **electrocardiograms** (electrical tracings of the heartbeat) and to transmit these to a nearby hospital where a cardiac specialist can make a preliminary diagnosis. The physician can also talk to the ambulance personnel — called emergency medical technicians (EMTs) — and prescribe emergency treatment.

Something as commonplace as the telephone becomes a diagnostic aid when it is connected to a medical computer system. The electrocardiogram can be converted into electronic signals and transmitted by the telephone system to a hospital computer center hundreds of miles away. A diagnosis is made, or a treatment evaluated by the computer at the distant **cardiac** center. This is almost the same as having an expert **cardiac diagnostician** in constant attendance at the patient's bedside.

Of course, medical progress has not been limited to the invention and development of new techniques and equipment (**Figs. 1–2a** and **1–2 b**). To list and describe the drugs and vaccines that have been introduced in recent years would fill many books. Several once-dreaded diseases

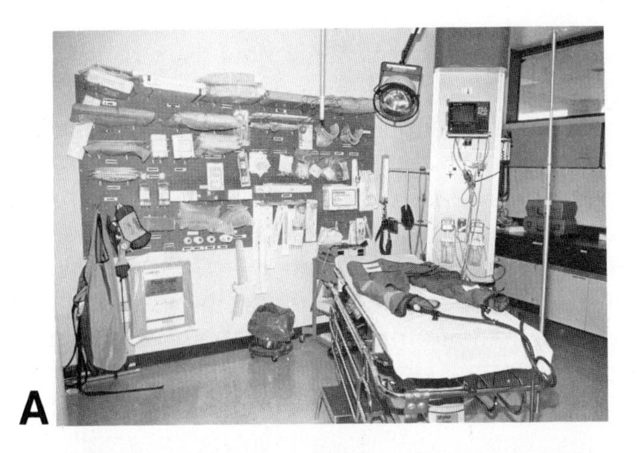

A

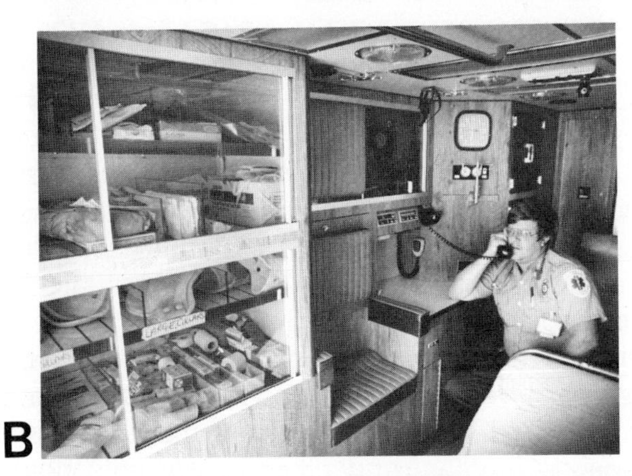

B

Figure 1–2. "High-tech" equipment, shown here in an emergency room (**A**) and mobile intensive care unit (**B**), is just one of the ways in which medical care had progressed. (Photo 1–2A courtesy of St. Mary Hospital. Photo 1–2B by Michael Mancuso. Courtesy of Rusling Hose Ambulance Corps and Rescue Squad, Hamilton Township Dir. of Health, N.J.)

such as measles, mumps, and poliomyelitis — are no longer life-threatening because of preventive vaccines and improved hygiene and nutrition. Drugs have brought **tuberculosis** under control and have made it possible to close sanatariums where patients formerly had to spend many months or years. The discovery of insulin has extended the life span of countless diabetics. Insulin, once obtained only from animal organs, can now be produced in the laboratory. This new form of insulin has several advantages: it does not require the sacrifice of an animal; it eliminates allergies to the animal source; and it ensures an adequate supply.

"Human glue" (scientific name: autologous fibrinogen adhesive) has been developed for use in ear surgery. It is injected into the ear through a thin needle. A clot forms quickly and keeps a broken middle ear bone in position until healing takes place. It is projected that the "glue" will be used in many delicate operations where the use of ordinary sutures is not possible. The adhesive is made from agents which are taken from the patient's own blood supply. Therefore, they cannot spread infectious diseases, for example, acquired immune deficiency syndrome (AIDS) and hepatitis.

THE HEALTH WORKER DURING TIMES OF WAR

Americans have been involved in four wars in the twentieth century, an involvement that has created a need for rehabilitation services to help the wounded and disabled. Thus, more opportunities in the health field opened. Wars have also given rise to critical situations and health workers have had to find ways to meet them.

For example, advances in plastic surgery were a direct result of the needs of wounded soldiers during World War I. Years later, on the home front during World War II, Americans had to make do with many fewer physicians, surgeons, nurses, and other health personnel because so many of these were needed in the war effort. Since hospitals were forced to operate with a minimum of trained personnel, nurses began to instruct others in handling some of their duties. Programs for educating practical nurses and nursing aides were started in local hospitals. The era of "assistants" began in the 1940s because the available health workers could no longer carry the heavy workload.

During the Korean Conflict, Mobile Army Surgical Hospitals (MASH), located a short distance from the battle lines, developed specialized emergency techniques for caring for the injured with multiple life-threatening wounds. Procedures used for emergency airlifting of the wounded from the battlefields of Korea and Vietnam are being used today. Now, helicopters are used as ambulances in the air, transporting victims from the scene of an accident to a medical center equipped to provide care to those with massive, critical injuries. More and more veterans returned from battle with obvious handicaps, including missing or severely damaged limbs. As a result, great improvements were made in the design and manufacture of artificial limbs (prostheses) and new careers in this field emerged.

MYTHS ABOUT HEALTH CAREERS

Many people think there are only three careers in the health services industry — doctor, dentist, and nurse. They tend to assign medicine and dentistry to males and nursing to females. These beliefs are nothing but myths.

First of all, as we mentioned, there are more than 300 titles of health workers today. Out of 100 health workers, less than ten are physicians, and the remainder are in nursing services, dental services, medical services, environmental health, and other kinds of health occupations.

HEALTH CARE WORK PLACES

Though many health workers are employed in large numbers in hospitals, some work in other places. Health personnel may be found in a large medical center in a metropolitan area or in a migrant farm workers' clinic in a rural district. All communities — rural, urban, and suburban — need the services of health workers.

A career in health care can take you to foreign lands. One example is Project HOPE, a worldwide organization that shares medical knowledge and techniques with people of other lands. The health workers of Project HOPE are invited to the host countries where they teach, advise, and assist their professional counterparts. As a result of their new knowledge, the trained host personnel are able to serve their own population better. Project HOPE's health care personnel include doctors, nurses, laboratory technicians, sanitarians, and health educators. Other opportunities for foreign service can be found in the Peace Corps or in the missionary service as a lay worker, minister, priest, or sister.

Many health workers are employed by the federal government. Veterans' hospitals, the Indian Health Service, and the armed forces are typical examples of areas where federal health workers are employed (**Fig. 1–3**). These workers give direct care and provide diagnostic, therapeutic, and restorative services.

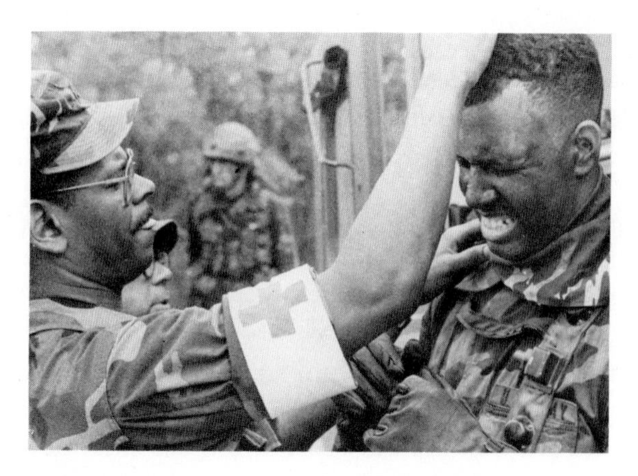

Figure 1–3. The National Guard is a branch of the federal government in which to pursue a health career. (Courtesy of the New Jersey National Guard.)

The federal government also employs veterinarians, sanitarians, environmental health technicians, etc. Their responsibilities range from testing air samples to inspecting meat and poultry for quality.

Some federal health workers act as consultants to state and local health departments. They help to track down the causes of regional health problems that extend beyond state boundaries, such as polluted ocean waters and massive fish kills. Other consultants assist individual states to plan and establish health programs to meet the needs of specific populations such as programs for preschool immunizations, pregnant women, suicide prevention, and nutrition programs for the elderly.

While the federal government provides consulting services and some funding for community health programs, each state carries out its own programs. Therefore, states employ many workers in public health programs, as well as in hospitals, nursing homes, prisons, and clinics. Municipal governments also employ health workers in the same areas.

Neighborhood health centers were developed to serve people who live in concentrated urban localities. These centers are available to all who live within the geographic boundaries that it services. For a nominal fee, patients receive many medical services including immunizations, treatment, health counseling, family planning advice, maternity services, and adult and child care. Neighborhood health centers employ many types of workers, from medical record personnel to speech pathologists. They provide full health services to families. Although neighborhood health facilities may be unimpressive, their services are indispensable and of high quality. In areas where there are large groups of homeless people, health centers have been established to reach out and offer health care services to these "street people."

Suicide prevention centers and crisis intervention centers operate "hot lines" where desperate, confused people can contact mental health workers. Besides providing immediate help during a crisis, health workers may refer their callers to other institutions and agencies for long-term assistance with their problems.

Hospices of the early Christian period and Middle Ages were previously discussed in this chapter. Today, the word "hospice" is used to describe an entirely different concept. "Hospice" is a program which provides care for terminally ill people and assists them and their families to cope with impending death. Home care may be provided or the person is admitted to a hospice facility. Many health workers are employed in hospices along with specially trained volunteers.

Private industry employs thousands of health workers in numerous categories. American businesses have become more aware of the value of health and wellness and, as a result, are willing to invest money in promoting the health of their employees. Today, nurses and health educators are teaching employees about proper diet, exercise, stress management, and relaxation techniques. Some companies have gyms and spas right in their buildings, and employees are encouraged to use these facilities under the supervision of an exercise **physiologist** — a person who designs a program of physical activity tailored to the needs of individual participants (**Fig. 1–4**).

Your personal physician or dentist may employ one or more assistants, perhaps a medical assistant or a dental hygienist. Emergency care centers may employ other personnel to take and process x-rays, perform laboratory tests, and to give direct care when urgently needed.

GROWTH OF HEALTH CAREERS

A single statistic will demonstrate the rapid growth of the health occupations. In 1950, the health services industry was the nation's fifth leading employer. It currently ranks as the second leading industry.

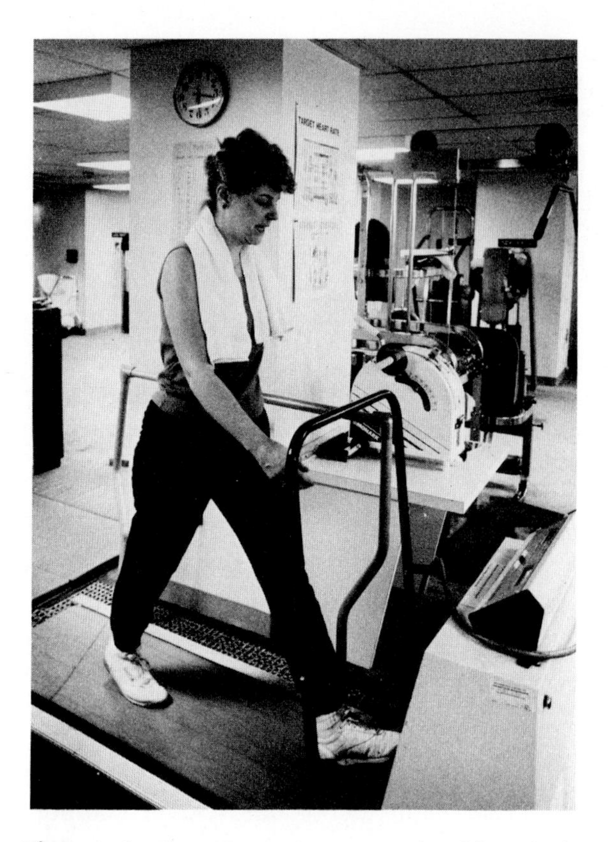

Figure 1–4. Physical activity should include aerobic exercise to promote wellness. The treadmill and other exercises such as walking, jogging, or swimming are good examples of aerobic activity. (Courtesy of Bridgeton Hospital, Bridgeton, N.J. Photo by Gary F. Cooper.)

There are many reasons why this tremendous expansion came about. Certainly, increased population, longer life span, advances in technology, public demand for quality health care, and increased awareness of the value of wellness and disease prevention all played a part. In addition, the American population is extremely mobile. Many people follow the advice, "Go west, young man." Older people, too, have gone west and south in recent years, moving into retirement communities. As populations shift, the demand for health workers also shifts. In 1986, 7.6 million workers were employed in the health industry. Projections indicate that by the year 2000 there will be 10.8 million health workers. One out of every six new jobs will be in health services (**Table 1–1**).

PROJECTED GROWTH IN THE HEALTH OCCUPATIONS 1986-2000

Jobs	1986	2000
Medical Assistants	132,000	251,000
Physical Therapists	61,000	115,000
Physical Therapy Assistants	36,000	65,000
Home Health Aides	138,000	249,000
Medical Records Personnel	40,000	70,000
Registered Nurse	1,410,000	2,020,000
Nursing Assistants	1,220,000	1,660,000

Source: United Stats Labor Department
Bureau of Labor Statistics

With further knowledge about disease and its causes, new treatments will be developed. Just as the invention of the x-ray machine led to the development of careers in radiology, so will new careers emerge to meet ongoing changes in medicine. The responsibilities of well-known careers will change and some will be transferred to other workers in newly created jobs.

In the early 1940s, nurses fluffed pillows, dusted window sills, and watered plants, but World War II changed all that. Today, nurses have responsibilities and skills that were unimaginable before. Nurses staff the Intensive Care Unit to which critically ill patients are brought for expert care. Nurses have their own private practices — nurse midwives own and operate birthing centers. In other settings, nurses operate artificial kidney machines and give highly complex care to premature infants and burn patients in specialized care centers.

Of course, some of the responsibilities formerly assigned to professional nurses have been handed over to other health workers. The licensed practical nurse is a valuable addition to the nursing team, as are the nursing assistant and the unit secretary. These workers do not water flowers and dust either — this is the work of the housekeeping department. The unit secretaries act as clerk-receptionists in patient care areas. They relieve the nursing staff of routine clerical duties, order and stock supplies, and handle a great deal of paperwork, enabling nurses to give patient care.

WHAT THIS BOOK IS ABOUT

Health Occupations — Exploration and Career Planning will explore the five major groups of health careers and the unique role that each plays in health maintenance, disease prevention, diagnosis, treatment, and rehabilitation. Although each health career has its own characteristics, each is dependent on the others. In fact, one of the satisfactions of a health career comes from working closely with other health services personnel in a cooperative effort to help people.

You will have the opportunity to try out typical tasks performed by health workers in these five categories. These activities are designed to help you develop an awareness of the types of activities and performance requirements that characterize the careers within the group of careers being studied.

The second portion of this book lays the foundation for employment in the health occupations. Communications skills, infection control, nutrition, and growth and development will be covered, as will computers in health care. Information on getting and keeping a job follows as does suggestions for further education and financing options. Career ladders and career lattices are discussed.

When you choose a health career, you will be joining a group of over 8 million workers, all of whom are playing a part in keeping our nation healthy. Each person has a unique role to play, because each has special talents and special abilities to offer. You will have the opportunity to make "the greatest use of your skills, knowledge and experience and to become a contributing member of the health care team and of your community.*

*Adapted from the Health Occupations Students of America Creed.

S·T·U·D·E·N·T A·C·T·I·V·I·T·I·E·S

1. Many charms, rituals, and superstitions are associated with illness today. What are examples of some followed by your friends and family?
2. Conduct a survey in your community to find out where health workers are employed. Include type of facility (e.g., doctor's office, daycare center, neighborhood health center), distance in miles from your home, and service offered. Bring your findings to class and discuss them.
3. Set aside a special place (file, notebook, etc.) in which to collect information concerning health careers of interest to you.
4. Research and report the contributions of one of the following people:

Lillian Wald	Elizabeth Blackwell
Mabel K. Staupers	Harry Heimlich
Julius Jacobsen	Cecily Saunders
Rachel Carson	Jonas Salk
George Cotzias	Michael DeBakey
Werner Forssmann	Denton Cooley
Christian Barnard	Joseph Lister
Robert Koch	Virginia Apgar
Francis Crick	Elisabeth Kübler-Ross
James Watson	Edwin J. Cohn
Maurice Walkins	Rosalind Franklin

5. Research and report on the development of the following inventions or discoveries:

Organ transplants	Human insulin
Lasers in medicine	Ultrasonography
Echocardiography	Tranquilizers
Microsurgery	Nuclear Magnetic Imaging (NMI)

Computerized Axial Tomography (CAT scan)

Transdermal medication delivery systems

Chapter 2

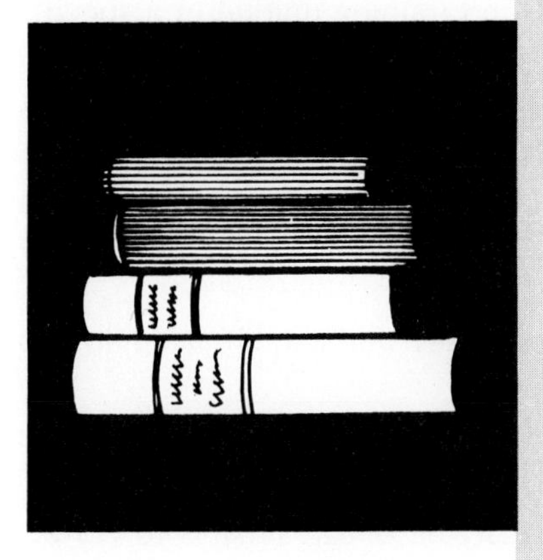

Preparing for a Health Career

Objectives

After completing this chapter, you should be able to:

- Discuss five factors to consider in choosing a career in health occupations.
- Identify by name the five groups of health occupations and two careers within each group.
- Discuss two responsibilities of each group.
- Discuss the interrelationships between three of the five groups.
- Discuss the purposes of Health Occupations Students of America (HOSA).
- Define at least 70 percent of the key terms listed for this chapter.

Key Terms

- **assistant** Performs routine procedures and tasks under the direction of the health professional, technologist, or therapist

- **career cluster** Types of jobs that are closely related because of the special responsibilities involved
- **certification** Recognition by a nongovernmental agency to an individual or institution having met certain qualifications
- **health professional** Person whose skill is based upon extensive education, knowledge, and training unique to a specific field
- **license** A document issued by a state agency which attests to the individual's competence to practice in a particular field
- **registration** A list of names of qualified practitioners in a specific health occupation which is maintained by a governmental or nongovernmental agency
- **technician** Performs procedures that require attention to technical detail
- **technologist** Applies knowledge to the practical and theoretical problems in a specific field
- **therapist** Specializes in carrying out treatments to correct or improve the function of a body part or system

DECISIONS, DECISIONS

Deciding on a career is not an easy task, especially if you want to make the decision that is best for you. Some people choose by chance — being in the right place at the right time. Others choose a career because of the influence of parents or friends. These two ways do not put you in charge of the decision-making process that will affect your life. Instead, something or someone else has taken charge.

In the past, most people made only one major career decision in their lives. Once the decision was made, it was rare that a person made a change from one career to another; the career options available simply were not as varied as they are today. There are over 20,000 different occupations in the United States, of which more than 300 job titles are represented by the health occupations field alone. Because of our rapidly changing technology, some occupations will become obsolete; new jobs will emerge to meet ever-growing demands; and existing jobs will change to accommodate new information and new skills. With this in mind, you, in the course of your health career, will probably change occupations several times as you progress in this "high-tech" area.

Choosing Your First Career

Your first choice does not "lock you into" a lifetime in a single career. Nevertheless, making a major switch from your first career choice to a totally unrelated field is unlikely. For example, it is not probable that, after your first employment as an occupational therapist, you would choose to switch to a career in the field of automobile mechanics. It is feasible, though, for you to change to a career in a related area — hospital administration, for example. In this way, the knowledge and experience you acquire in your first job is likely to be a building block to the next one.

However, your first career choice is an important one. It involves matching your interests and abilities to a specific occupation that you hope to pursue. Here are some guidelines to help you in the process of making your career decision.

First, take a good look at yourself. What do you like to do? What are your dislikes? Your own honest answers to these questions will help to put you in a better position to make a choice. If you enjoy being with people, a career that involves you directly with patients and their families may be the one most suited to you. On the other hand, you may prefer working with equipment rather than having frequent contact with patients. Careers in the medical laboratory will offer you a chance to operate intricate electronic equipment and thereby contribute toward the diagnosis of illness. Perhaps you enjoy music, or like to dance, or have a special gift for painting. These talents also have a place in health careers. Music, dance, and recreational therapists work directly with patients by conducting classes in music and recreational activities.

In order to perform effectively, a person should be in good health. But, a physical handicap is not necessarily a deterrent to a health career, provided the person is otherwise in good health. For example, a deaf or hearing impaired person may be employed in the cytology department of a medical laboratory where cells are examined microscopically to detect abnormalities in color, size, and shape. The findings are communicated in written reports so that the hearing loss does not interfere with the person's ability to carry out the job successfully.

A person confined to a wheelchair may find a rewarding career as a medical transcriber, medical secretary, or, in fact, any health career that does not require a high degree of mobility. Of course, the facility must be equipped with entrance/exit ramps and lavatories to accommodate the needs of the physically handicapped according to the Rehabilitation Act of 1973.

Next, consider your career options. One of the major reasons for a poor choice of career is the lack of factual information about the occupation — not knowing what it's all about. From a list of more than 300 health occupations titles, the average person could probably name only a small number. But just knowing the name doesn't offer many clues to what the job entails.

Using the Career Interest Chart below, check those statements which apply to your interests. Place this chart in your notebook. As you learn about each career in the five major health career groups, compare your interest statements with the information you have received about each career. A Career Interest Chart will be provided for each of the five career groups. When your career interest statement matches with the information about the specific career, you score one point.

For example, suppose you want a career which allows you to work with instruments and high-tech equipment. The career of medical laboratory technologist requires operating electron microscopes and sophisticated laboratory instruments. Therefore, your interest and the career requirements agree with each other in this one instance.

The higher the score, the more likely the career matches with your interests. The maximum score is 20 points. This is not a test but will assist you in comparing each career to your individual career requirements. Perhaps your career requirements will change as you learn more about the various health occupations. This is what career exploration is all about (**Fig. 2–1**).

MISCONCEPTIONS AND REALITIES ABOUT HEALTH CAREERS

The public sometimes gets a distorted view about just what health workers really do. Television programs frequently show the trials and

CAREER INTEREST CHART

I WANT A CAREER WHICH ALLOWS ME TO:

1. Care for people—patients or clients.	
2. Work with instruments and high tech equipment.	
3. Function as part of a team.	
4. Work independently.	
5. Be part of a large health care organization.	
6. Work flexible hours.	
7. Learn new techniques of my chosen career.	
8. Work in a "clean" environment.	
9. Operate my own business.	
10. Have a set routine of work.	
11. Be a part of a small group of health professionals.	
12. Work with infants. children. adults. older adults.	
13. Work in an area where strict adherence to procedures is required.	
14. Use my creative talents and abilities (art, music, dance, etc.).	
15. Work with well people.	
16. Work with sick people.	
17. Work with handicapped people.	
18. Wear a uniform.	
19. Wear street clothes.	
20. Earn a steady income.	

SCORE ___________

tribulations of the health worker. The doctor and the nurse are portrayed in very dramatic and exciting situations. The glamour of the life-and-death drama within a busy medical center entertains the television-viewing public, but this kind of portrayal of hospital life and health careers is misleading.

Actually, health workers are people who work with a purpose, and they generally do not resemble the glamorous actors of television shows. They perform their duties and carry out their responsibilities without public recognition and fanfare. We all have moments when we feel blue, discouraged, frustrated, and disappointed. Health workers are no different from anyone else. Every occupation, including a health career, involves some routine and unexciting tasks and long, tiring days. Rarely does a person in a health career become a millionaire, but, then, few of us do! What counts is that health careers provide adequate incomes and personal satisfaction (**Fig. 2–2**).

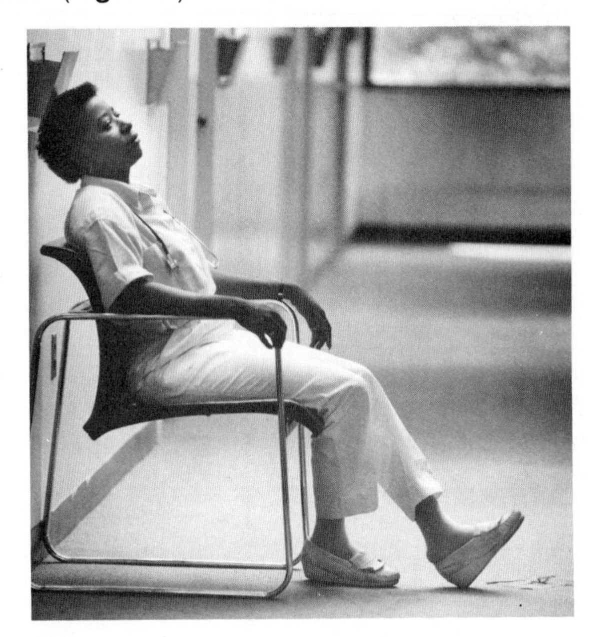

Figure 2–2. The end of a long day for a busy nurse. (Courtesy of Henry J. Austin Health Center, Trenton, N.J. Photo by Michael Mancuso.)

Incomes vary. Those who are employed by private **practitioners** may not have as many fringe benefits (health insurance, paid sick leave, etc.) as those who work in institutions; however, their work is scheduled during "preferred" times, which means they have no weekend or holiday duty and usually work daytime hours. Employment in a health care institution may require rotation among day, evening, and night shifts during the week, on weekends, and even on holidays, since the institution is open 365 days a year, 24 hours a day. Of course, employees receive added compensation for working evenings, nights, and holidays. Even so, some people consider shift work as a definite disadvantage of a health career. On the positive side, working evenings or nights allows for greater flexibility in working hours and off-duty time. Many people prefer being free during times when most people are working — stores are less crowded and recreational facilities are more accessible.

Not many occupations have the flexibility that a health career offers — not only in time but in obtaining employment anywhere in the country or world, for that matter!

REWARDS TO BE GAINED IN A HEALTH CAREER

Aside from salary, the health worker brings home a feeling of inner satisfaction. This comes both from being a part of a team working to help others and from making a personal commitment to set aside self in order to serve others. Satisfactions to be gained from a health career are numerous.

For instance, the physical therapist derives great satisfaction from assisting a patient, who has been seriously injured in an automobile accident and confined to a wheelchair, to walk with crutches. The therapist is actively involved in the needed teamwork, while providing tremendous assistance to the patient.

Those who do not work directly with patients derive their satisfactions in other ways. The dental laboratory technician who has used special talents and skills to construct a full set of dentures knows that a contribution has been made to the general well-being of another person. Those properly fitting dentures will enable that person to smile with pride, to eat most foods with ease, and to be more pleased with their general appearance.

Most of all, there are great personal rewards in knowing that your special talents are being used in significant ways. A health career is much more than a job — it's a lifetime of dedication to others. Each person in the health services has a special opportunity to improve the lives of other people.

SOME GUIDELINES YOU CAN FOLLOW

Dr. Robert Hoppock, former editorial consultant for *Career World*, a magazine for students, is a well-known guidance counselor. He gives excellent advice in "A Dozen Suggestions for Choosing a Career" (**Fig. 2–3**).

1. Choose an occupation because you like the work, not solely because of the rewards in money or prestige.
2. Choose an occupation that will use the abilities you possess.
3. Choose an occupation in which there is likely to be an active demand for workers when you are ready to go to work.
4. Do not choose an occupation because you admire someone else who chose it.
5. Avoid occupations that require abilities you do not possess.
6. Do not confuse interest and ability.
7. Before making a final choice of an occupation, find out which are **all** the things you might have to do in it. Find out which of these will take most of your time.
8. Do not expect to find a job in which you will never have to do anything that you dislike.
9. Do not stay permanently in a job in which you dislike most of the things you have to do.
10. Beware of recruiters and biased information from other sources.
11. If where you live is important to you, choose an occupation that will let you live there.
12. Take all the advice that is offered, then act on your own judgment.

Figure 2–3. A dozen suggestions for choosing a career. (By permission from Robert Hoppock, 1988.)

Remember Robert Louis Stevenson's counsel: "To know what you prefer, instead of humbly saying 'Amen' to what the world tells you you ought to prefer, is to have kept your soul alive."

GAINING YOUR FIRST EXPERIENCE

Volunteer Your Services

Consider working as a volunteer in a local hospital, nursing home, or another institution that employs health workers in the field of your interest. Such experience affords an overall picture of the facility and helps you to gain insight about the occupation in question. You learn about the general functioning of the facility and about the specific departments that perform special roles. You will have opportunities to talk with patients and their families. Also, you will observe the activities of many types of health workers: where they work, what they do, and how they function with others on the health care team. Volunteering also brings opportunities to talk with employees and learn first hand about the various jobs.

To obtain further information about volunteer activities, contact the Director of Volunteer Services at your local hospital, who will match your special interests and abilities with an appropriate volunteer service (**Fig. 2–4**).

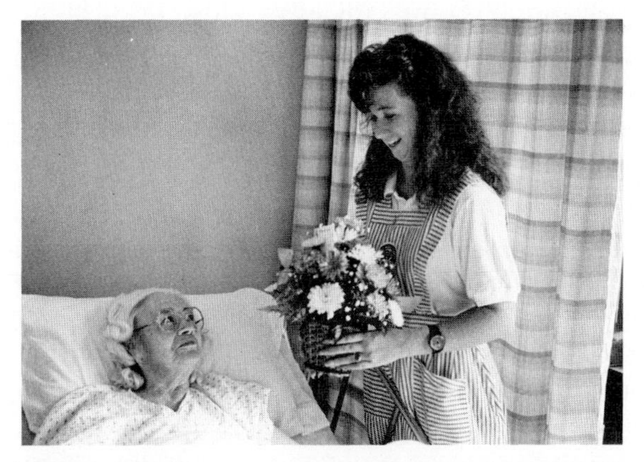

Figure 2–4. As a hospital volunteer, such as the candy striper, you get to observe different health careers and obtain experience. (Courtesy of St. Mary Hospital, Langhorne, Pa.)

Health Careers Clubs

Many schools sponsor clubs that provide members with an opportunity to gain further knowledge and experience after school hours in an area of special interest. Some examples are Computer Clubs, Math Clubs, Photography Clubs, and Drama Clubs. Also, schools offer students the opportunity to join clubs which focus on specific careers such as future lawyers, engineers, or physicians. Others offer less specific career area clubs, such as careers in computers or health careers. Through health careers clubs, students have the opportunity to investigate many health occupations. Members plan, organize, and carry out projects that involve them in community life and help them to learn more about specific health careers. Such projects include assisting voluntary health agencies in health maintenance activites, such as vision testing and blood pressure screening; planning and assisting in health fairs; planning and carrying out educational projects to acquaint elementary school students with careers in health. For example, club members may plan and carry out a program for third grade students in which the importance of brushing teeth properly is explained, the proper method of brushing is demonstrated, and the duties of the dental health team are described. To do this, club members make arrangements to visit the third grade class, then plan the educational program with the assistance of their club advisor.

Trips to visit health care facilities and programs conducted by health professionals, who speak about their careers at club meetings, are other activities which help members to learn about the wide variety of careers. Contact your guidance counselor or school nurse for information about joining a health careers club in your school or about starting one.

National Vocational Student Organizations

One of the advantages of exploring or pursuing a health career while in high school is the chance to belong to a national vocational student organization. Unlike the health careers clubs previously mentioned, students who are members of a vocational student organization conduct their activities as a part of their instructional program rather than after school.

Health Occupations Students of America (HOSA)

Health Occupations Students of America (HOSA) was founded to meet the specific needs of secondary and postsecondary students enrolled in vocational health occupations education programs and those enrolled in approved prevocational education programs. Under the guidance of the health occupations education instructor, who also serves as the HOSA chapter advisor, students form a HOSA chapter and affiliate with the state and national HOSA organizations. The purposes of HOSA are to meet the needs of health occupations education students through activities which encourage personal growth and help to develop leadership potential, explore opportunities in the health fields, and promote involvement in community service and current health care issues (**Fig. 2–5**).

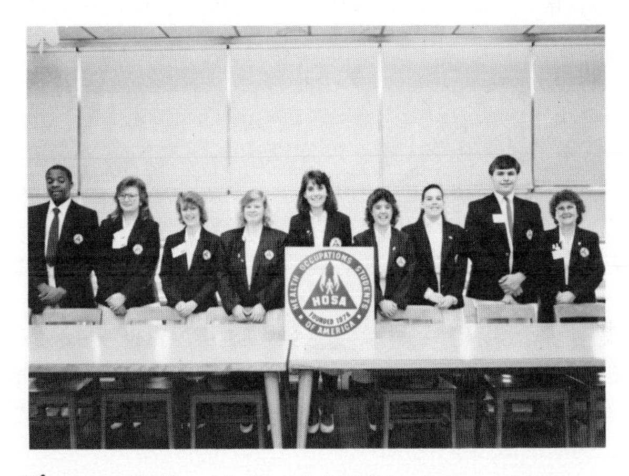

Figure 2–5. A local HOSA chapter helps to develop leadership skills through parliamentary procedures. (Courtesy of Bridgeton High School, Bridgeton, N.J.)

Through HOSA and its activities, members learn valuable skills and gain knowledge that give them a competitive edge toward employment in health occupations. More information can be obtained from:

State Supervisor, Health Occupations Education
State Department of Education
State Capital

Vocational Industrial Clubs of America (VICA)

This national vocational student organization serves students enrolled in trade, industrial, technical, and health occupations programs. VICA activities emphasize respect for the dignity of work, high standards in trade ethics, workmanship, scholarship, and safety. More information may be obtained by writing:

State Supervisor, Trade and Industrial Education
State Department of Education
State Capital

Part-time Employment

Another way to become acquainted with health careers is through part-time employment. If you are 18 years of age or older, there may be part-time employment opportunities in local health care institutions during holidays and vacations. Consult your guidance counselor for advice about securing suitable employment, as well as about the advantages and disadvantages of such work. Part-time employment should always take second place to assigned school subjects.

When you talk with a potential employer, find out if your position will include on-the-job training. If this is the case, ask who will give the training, how long it will take, and whether the employer will pay you while you learn.

When you apply for admission to a health occupations education program, be sure to mention your activities as a volunteer, part-time worker, and a health careers club or HOSA member. These activities show that your interest is based upon realistic knowledge. They also demonstrate your initiative and commitment to the field of health care.

THE FIVE MAJOR CATEGORIES OF HEALTH CAREERS

We have discussed health careers in general terms, and have suggested guidelines that might be followed in making your first career decision. The next five chapters describe the major health career categories in general and then in detail. The careers included in each group were selected because they are broadly interrelated. Each category is further divided into clusters — types of jobs that are closely associated because of the particular responsibilities involved. For example, the Dental Cluster consists of the dentist, dental hygienist, dental assistant, and dental receptionist, all of whom work together. The Dental Cluster is one component of the first category, Direct Care Careers.

Each category of health careers is special, and calls for special talents and abilities, yet each acknowledges its dependency upon the others. No single group can do the job alone and do it successfully. It takes a team approach to achieve a common goal. Listed below are the five categories of health careers and a brief introduction to acquaint you with each area.

Category 1 — Direct Care Careers

The Direct Care group is perhaps the best known of the five groups. It includes those careers that were the first to be identified as distinct entities: medicine, dentistry, and nursing — the backbone of careers in health. The function of this group is to help people maintain an optimal state of health and recover from illness and to prevent sickness. They have direct personal contact with the patient and family. Their duties center on meeting the patient's physical and emotional needs. There are five clusters of related occupations: dental, medical, nursing, social service, and mental health.

These workers may be involved in the physical care of patients (bathing, feeding, examining, prescribing, or giving treatment and medication). They may also assist the patient and family in coping emotionally and socially with difficult events, such as the serious illness or death of a family member, or a prolonged illness that saps financial resources. Because they give direct care, they are often intimately acquainted with both the physical status and the emotional makeup of their patients. In the course of their education, these workers learn how to assist people whose illnesses cause them to be afraid, irritable, or hostile. They are also in a unique position to share in a family's joy at the birth of a child or following the recovery of a seriously ill family member. They are witnesses to all levels of human emotion.

Category 2 — Diagnostic Careers

Five clusters of related occupations comprise the Diagnostic Careers category: radiologic, medical laboratory, optical, audiologic, and diagnostic equipment. The goal of this group of workers is different from that of the Direct Care category. Professional workers in Diagnostic Careers search for "cause and cure." Their work involves examining and testing body fluids, tissues, organs, and waste products in addition to photographing, by radiologic and fluoroscopic methods, body parts and their function. Their chief duty is to provide the technological backup needed for accurate diagnosis of illness. Depending on the occupation, they may have limited patient contact. Without the aid of the Diagnostic group, the Direct Care group would lack reliable, detailed information on which to base their findings, and valuable time would be lost. Thus, to a great extent, these groups are interdependent.

Category 3 — Therapeutic/Restorative Careers

Restorative therapy is the concern of workers in the Therapeutic/Restorative category. At one time, the Direct Care group encompassed the responsibilities related to restorative treatment. However, with the rapid expansion of health care technology, the need arose for personnel adequately prepared in all aspects of rehabilitation and restoration. The clusters in this group are: physical therapy, occupational therapy, respiratory therapy, rehabilitation services, dietetics, pharmacy, and reconstruction and replacement.

Category 4 — Community Health Careers

The larger community — be it a city, a village, or a small town — is the focus of personnel in Community Health Careers. The emphasis of their work is on health maintenance and on the prevention of illness that could spread throughout a community. Maintaining the purity of the public water supply, minimizing the effects of chemical and oil spills into lakes and rivers, and regulating the public health aspects of local industry are typical examples of their responsibilities. They also have an important role in community health education. Clusters within Community Health include: community services, animal care services, health education and communications, environmental health, and home health services.

Category 5 — Institutional Careers

The category of Institutional Careers is described last because these occupations serve as the underpinning, or support system, for all the other groups — Direct Care, Diagnostic, Therapeutic/Restorative, and Community Health.

The majority of all health occupations workers are employed by institutions such as hospitals, nursing homes, rehabilitation centers, etc., which serve as temporary or permanent homes for many members of society. Personnel are needed to handle finances; keep records; purchase food, furnishings, and equipment; prepare meals; keep rooms clean; and maintain a safe, healthful environment. Without the support of people in Institutional Careers, it would be virtually impossible for personnel of the other career groups to perform their jobs.

There are two main clusters in Institutional Careers: *administrative* — careers concerned with the efficient operation of a health care facility (such as nursing home administrator or medical record administrator) and *supportive* — careers concerned with the efficient maintenance of essential services (such as hospital kitchen and laundry). Supervisory personnel oversee all these activities.

IMPORTANT DEFINITIONS

Sorting out the more than 300 job titles that describe the duties of the five categories of health workers can be confusing unless some ground rules are given. Some of the terms you will meet as you explore these categories are defined to help clarify various job titles. An example for each definition is presented after a discussion of each new term.

Note that there are some exceptions to these definitions. For example, the title "electrocardiograph technician" does not precisely fit the definition of "technician," since the education required and the duties performed are not typical of a technician's work. When these exceptions do occur, an appropriate footnote will appear.

Health Professional

The professional is an individual whose skill is based upon extensive education, knowledge, and training unique to a specific field. The professional performs the most complex tasks requiring the highest degree of competence and assumes the broadest responsibility on the health care team. The educational preparation of health professionals takes place in a college or university and requires four or more years. Health professionals direct all other team members. The term "professional" also applies to the therapist and the technologist.

Example. Pathologists are medical doctors who have had the most advanced training in medical laboratory work. They supervise the work of entire staffs of clinical laboratories (laboratory aides, assistants, technicians, and technologists). Using the knowledge and skills acquired in a rigorous educational program (four years of undergraduate college studies, four years of medical school to become a doctor, and four or five years of training in a specialty), pathologists order and interpret laboratory tests. Their findings are critical to the diagnosis of disease.

Therapist

The word "therapy" means treatment, so therapists are those who specialize in carrying out treatments to correct or improve the function of a body part or system. They may be physical therapists, speech therapists or occupational therapists, to name a few.

Example. Therapists are usually educated in a four-year (or more) college program. The physical therapist has an excellent background in anatomy, physiology, and physics so that the patient's capacity for exercise as well as physical limitations can be determined. In the course of working with the patient, the therapist may plan an exercise program to strengthen the leg muscles. Hydrotherapy (hydro = water) may be used to increase blood circulation to the leg. Instructing the patient in the use of crutches, a cane, or a walker is also a physical therapist's responsibility.

Technologist

The word comes from "technology," the study of practical arts. These health workers apply their knowledge to the practical and theoretical problems in their special fields. They may develop new procedures to deal with problems encountered in their work. A four-year college program is required.

Example. The medical laboratory technologist may determine the standardized procedures to be followed by other medical laboratory personnel. They direct the activities of staff and are responsible for quality control and safety in the medical laboratory.

Technician

This term is derived from the word "technique." Health technicians are responsible for performing those procedures that require attention to technical detail. They carry out all tasks on the basis of established standards of practice. The educational program usually includes one or two years of post-high school preparation. Special attention is given to acquiring the necessary skills as well as to studying general education and science courses. The technician always works under the direction of the health professional.

Example. The environmental technician collects samples of water from oceans, bays, and rivers, as well as seaweed and floating debris. In the laboratory, these samples are tested for the presence of oxygen, nitrogen, bacteria, fungi, etc. The technician follows standardized procedures in performing these tests and submits the test results to the technologist. Should organisms or other agents be present which pose a health hazard to human, plant, or animal life, the environmental technologist has the responsibility of initiating corrective measures.

Assistant

This worker performs routine procedures and tasks under the direction of the health professional, technologist, or therapist. Preparation for this career can be completed in a one- or two-year high school or post-high school program. The educational program includes theory and practical application.

Example. In the medical laboratory, the laboratory assistant performs such routine procedures as testing urine for evidence of abnormalities including sugar, protein, and pus. The results of these findings are verified by the medical laboratory technologist or the pathologist.

Aide

The aide helps the staff in a specific area or department by performing nontechnical duties that are essential to proper functioning of the department. Preparation for this career may take place in high school, vocational/technical school, or on the job.

Example. Aides assigned to the medical laboratory see that the medical laboratory assistants, technicians, and technologists have sufficient equipment and supplies. They transport specimens from the patient care unit to the laboratory and clean and maintain laboratory equipment.

Licensure

A license to practice is mandatory in certain health occupations, of which medicine, dentistry, and nursing are the most widely known. The purpose of licensure is to assure the public that the licensee has obtained the necessary competence. Each state has its own licensing regulations, covering the occupations to be licensed, requirements to be met, and procedures for licensing. An agency of state government has the responsibility for issuing licenses.

The applicant, a graduate of an approved educational program, must take a written examination. Upon passing the examination, a license is issued to practice in that state for a given period of time (one or more years). This license confers the right to practice in a particular field and to use a specific title, e.g., licensed practical/vocational nurse. According to law, the individual must request renewal of the license.

Health care institutions such as hospitals, nursing homes, and rehabilitation centers also are licensed by an agency of state government. Rules and regulations concerning licensure are established and overseen by this agency.

Certification

A nongovernmental agency or a professional association may grant recognition to an individual who has met certain qualifications. The health worker seeking certification must be a graduate of a program recognized by the association and must have certain qualifications, such as experience in the field and membership in the appropriate professional association. Usually, a comprehensive examination is given to test knowledge and competence. When the applicant meets all the requirements and passes the examination, permission is given for the person to use the title "certified," e.g., certified dental assistant (CDA). There are also requirements for recertification.

Registration

A governmental or nongovernmental agency maintains a register of qualified practitioners in a given health occupation. Standards for placement on this list are established by the state or professional association. Those who meet these standards are entitled to use the word "registered" before their occupational title, e.g., registered physical therapist.

WHERE TO GO FOR MORE INFORMATION

It has been said that the mark of intelligent people is not that they know all the answers but that they know where to get the answers. In the five chapters to follow, lists of professional associations and organizations are provided which will give you more information about specific careers. Also, your health occupations instructor and guidance counselor may identify other resources in your community, county, and state. If you are not attending school, you will find counseling services available at public employment service offices and at reputable private counseling agencies. Remember, there are many roads to employment in the health field.

S·T·U·D·E·N·T A·C·T·I·V·I·T·I·E·S

1. Watch a television program dealing with health care personnel. How does the story compare to the real-life situation? Arrange with your instructor to discuss your observations with a panel of hospital workers.
2. What jobs in health occupations are available in your community for those who have not completed a high school education?
3. What opportunities are there for part-time employment or volunteer work in nearby health care facilities?
4. Prepare a list of personal experiences you have had with members of the five health occupations groups. Rate your experiences as excellent, very good, so-so, or poor. Discuss your experiences and ratings in class.
5. If you are not in a Health Occupations Education course in school, try to arrange a visit to a health care facility in your community. As you tour various areas, try to identify one worker from each of the health occupations groups discussed in this chapter. In your file, list the title of the worker and those activities you observed the worker performing. How many health workers did you meet who were licensed, registered, or certified?
6. Prepare a list of questions to be used when interviewing a health worker of your choice. Include such items as: Why was this career chosen? Is the work satisfying? What are the job likes and dislikes? What personality traits are needed for success in the occupation? Keep a copy in your file for future use.

Chapter 3

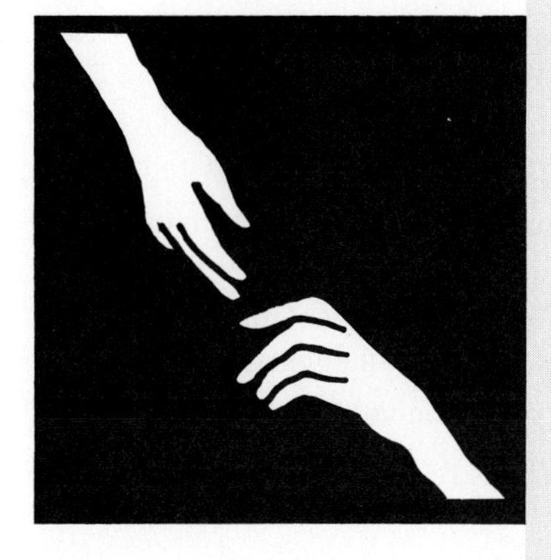

Direct Care Careers

Objectives

After completing this chapter, you should be able to:

- Name the five clusters in the Direct Care Careers group, and list three careers found in each cluster.
- Select three careers, and discuss three responsibilities of each worker in these careers.
- Identify one cluster, and discuss its relationship to two other clusters in the Direct Care Careers group.
- Define at least 70 percent of the key terms listed for this chapter.
- Perform, under supervision, three of the six suggested hands-on exploratory activities for the Direct Care Careers group. Discuss your feelings about performing them.
- Compare the advantages and disadvantages of pursuing a career in the Direct Care Careers group.

Key Terms

- **acute** Having rapid onset with severe symptoms and a short course
- **advocate** A person who supports, upholds, and defends the beliefs of another
- **auxiliary** A person who assists health professionals to accomplish given tasks, i.e., helpers or assistants
- **calculus** Hardened plaque on the surface of the teeth
- **certificate of proficiency** Recognition given for knowledge and skills acquired in a given area
- **client** A person who receives services; a customer
- **criteria** Standards of judgment; principles used in testing
- **curricula** Courses of study in a school
- **dental prophylaxis** Care necessary to assist in prevention of dental disease
- **empathy** The ability to understand and accept the situation a client or patient is experiencing without becoming emotionally involved
- **plaque** Deposits of food debris and bacteria on the surface of the teeth
- **prejudice** A preconceived opinion without knowledge, thought, or reason
- **prerequisites** Academic credits required prior to enrolling in a more advanced course
- **psychoanalysis** Method of obtaining detailed information about a person's mental and emotional experiences in order to treat the psychiatric condition
- **sympathy** The ability to react emotionally to the problems others are experiencing
- **vertebra(e)** One (or more) of the bony segments of the spinal column
- **vital signs** Temperature, pulse, and respiration

DIRECT CARE CAREER CLUSTERS

By far, the largest number of health workers are members of the Direct Care Careers. Their work goes on in schools, health maintenance organizations (HMOs), hospitals, nursing homes, and rehabilitation centers. Private offices, clinics, community emergency centers, and patients' private homes are other places where members of the Direct Care Careers also work. In addition to providing direct care to sick people, they play an active role in health maintenance and disease prevention. For example, they conduct regularly scheduled screening programs, including physical examinations, dental prophylaxis (cleaning and preventive treatment), immunization, and blood pressure reading.

There are five clusters in this group: dental, nursing, medical, mental health, and social service. Dentistry, nursing, and medicine are probably very familiar to you. Other careers include: physician assistant, emergency medical technician (EMT), surgical technologist, and geriatric aide. All of these careers will be described in this chapter.

Members of the Direct Care Careers group do not function independently but, rather, work together as a team. Traditionally, the physician heads the patient care team, but others may assume this responsibility according to the specific setting — the dentist in the dental office, the social worker in the social service department. The visiting nurse may also act as the team leader by coordinating the work of the home health aide, physical therapist, and occupational therapist. The makeup of the team changes to meet the specific needs of patients, and, frequently, those in the Restorative/Therapeutic and Diagnostic Career groups are represented.

For example, the physician and nurse consult with the hospital dietitian about a patient's nutritional requirements. If the physician has ordered a therapeutic diet, the dietitian will meet with the patient and/or his/her parents or guardian to discuss food preferences so that meals can be planned to accommodate the patient's likes and dislikes, as well as to meet nutritional needs. Throughout the patient's hospitalization, the dietitian may continue to be an active member of the team.

Frequently, the physical therapist will come to the patient's bedside to administer prescribed therapy and will report on patient progress during a team conference. Respiratory therapists, recreation therapists, and occupational therapists may all be involved in planning and evaluating patient care, treatment, and progress.

Health Care Workers on the Job

Betty Wister delivered her first baby, a girl, in the ambulance speeding to Riverview Hospital. Two EMTs from the local ambulance corps accompanied her. One EMT attended Mrs. Wister, recording her pulse and blood pressure and checking the condition of her uterus. The other EMT attended the infant. As he was about to remove mucus from the baby's mouth, he noted that the child had a right-sided cleft lip — an opening between the two parts of the upper lip, sometimes called harelip. Mrs. Wister, exhausted following the delivery, was sleeping and so was not aware of the baby's cleft lip.

When the ambulance arrived at the hospital emergency room, both Mrs. Wister and her infant were examined to detect any acute problems. Since there were none, Mrs. Wister was admitted to the maternity department where the nurses bathed her, changed her gown, and observed her for complications. After a short time, Mr. Wister arrived; both parents asked to see the baby.

Meanwhile, in the nursery, Baby Wister was visited by the pediatric resident, Dr. Elizabeth Carroll. She and the nursery nurse met with the Wisters to discuss and explain the baby's condition. After this, the infant was brought to her parents, who were extremely upset. Mrs. Wister cried uncontrollably, saying, "It was all my fault because I looked at a rabbit when I was pregnant."

Dr. Carroll explained that looking at rabbits did not cause a cleft lip and described the need for surgery to close the cleft so the baby could suck properly. The Wisters agreed to have a consultation with a plastic surgeon and to permit corrective surgery at a later date. In the meantime, the nurses taught Mrs. Wister to feed baby Lucy with an eyedropper.

Mrs. Wister was discharged from the hospital, and Lucy was transferred to the pediatric nursery in preparation for surgery. Mrs. Wister came to the hospital to feed Lucy during the day and in the evening.

The plastic surgeon and other members of the Direct Care team met and established the following goals:

1. Repair the cleft lip leaving as little residual scar tissue as possible.
2. Promote good nutrition for growth, development, and healing.
3. Prevent postoperative complications.
4. Assist Mrs. Wister in overcoming her feelings of guilt.
5. Encourage Mrs. Wister to continue to feed Lucy and to assume increasing responsibility for Lucy's care as her recovery progressed.

Each team member developed a care plan to reach these goals.

1. Nursing staff restrained Lucy to prevent her from touching the operative area. They cleansed the suture area regularly to keep it free of any drainage and to discourage the development of scar tissue. Pulling on the sutures was prevented, and measures were taken to keep Lucy from crying. The nurses fed Lucy, bathed her, and gave her "tender loving care." Of course, Mrs. Wister was the primary provider of love and mothering, and the nursing staff taught her to bathe, change, dress, and provide care for Lucy.
2. The dentist ordered an x-ray examination of Lucy's mouth to determine the presence of teeth in the gums. A dental examination was scheduled for Lucy at the age of six months to check the eruption of the baby teeth and to observe the state of her dentition.
3. The psychologist met with Mrs. Wister several times to help her understand her feelings of guilt.
4. The social worker initiated a referral to the Visiting Nurse Association (VNA). The public health nurse visited Mrs. Wister at home and helped her to prepare for Lucy's homecoming. Home health care and supervision for Lucy would be provided by the nurse.

Lucy left the hospital when she was three weeks old, and her parents were very happy to have her at home. The suture line was red and still quite visible; however, Lucy's appearance was much improved, and the Wisters were very pleased with the results of the surgery. Lucy was now being bottlefed and was gaining weight at a normal rate. Her medical and dental follow-up would continue for many years and would include speech evaluation, at the proper time, and therapy, if needed. The outlook for Lucy's normal growth and development was excellent.

CHARACTERISTICS OF WORKERS IN DIRECT CARE CAREERS

Since Direct Care workers spend most of their time with coworkers and patients, a definite asset is the ability to get along with other people, especially those who are sick, physically and emotionally dependent, demanding, or irritable. The capacity to respect each person as a unique individual and to care for all patients without manifesting prejudice of a personal nature is needed. A mature outlook is also essential: One must understand and accept the feelings of others (empathy) without becoming emotionally involved (sympathy).

Self-control is important when working with others in medical emergencies and in periods of severe stress, because the patient and family are coping with many problems. A health worker who becomes upset and loses self-control may join the ranks of those who require care! This doesn't mean that the worker should be devoid of all feeling — no one wants a robot. However, in a **critical** situation, complete self-control is required in order that lifesaving measures can be carried out quickly and efficiently.

For instance, the medical assistant has to work quickly and skillfully when a very sick patient is brought to the physician's office. There is no time for an emotional outburst. The patient must be prepared for a physical examination and examined by the physician immediately. The medical assistant needs to keep calm and to reassure the patient and family. In addition, a tactful explanation will help to reduce tension in the waiting room, since patients must now wait longer to see the physician. A sense of humor also helps to restore harmony in the office.

DENTAL CLUSTER

Sound teeth and gums are essential for proper nutrition, clear speech, desirable appearance, and overall health. Members of the dental cluster are concerned with maintenance of oral health through prevention and treatment of diseases of the mouth and through instruction of patients in oral hygiene. The dentist is the head of the dental team, which includes the dental hygienist, dental assistant, dental laboratory technician (discussed in Chapter 5), and the dental receptionist.

Dentist (DDS or DMD)

Most people are familiar with the dentist's role in repairing or treating injured and diseased teeth. Yet, a large part of dental practice is devoted to preventive care, which includes dental examination, teeth cleaning, and application of decay-preventing agents.

In the past, dental care could be obtained only in the private dental office, which was maintained by one dentist who saw one patient at a time. With population growth, this method of service became both costly and inefficient, and many people were deprived of dental care. Furthermore, a more sophisticated public began to consider good dental care a basic necessity. As a result, group practice of dentistry developed as a way of serving large numbers of people promptly and efficiently. With increasing numbers of employers offering dental care insurance as one of the fringe benefits, the demand for dental care has risen dramatically.

Many dentists work together in group practices and employ dental auxiliaries to further extend their services. Dental care is also available through public school programs, health maintenance organizations, free clinics, and at neighborhood health centers (**Fig. 3–1**).

Dental schools accept students who have completed two years of college but prefer to admit those who hold bachelor's degrees. The program is four years in length, and graduates earn either the DDS degree (Doctor of Dental Surgery) or the DMD degree (Doctor of Dental Medicine). Dental students study basic biomedical and dental sciences, diagnostic and treatment procedures, business management and ethics, dental ethics, the functions and uses of dental auxiliaries, and community health. To be qualified to practice, the prospective dentist must meet individual state requirements and pass a licensing examination.

Competition for entrance into dental school is keen, and applicants are selected with care. Dental schools seek students with better-than-average scholastic ability and artistic skill, because dentists sculpt and shape teeth replacements and reconstructions. This sculpting ability is so important that some dental schools require prospective students to take a special examination to determine their level of skill in sculpting. This test is usually taken during the second year of predental studies.

Since dental schools have specific entrance requirements, you should learn what the prerequisites are well in advance so that you will have taken the proper undergraduate courses when you apply for admission. Dental education is costly, as is establishing a private practice after

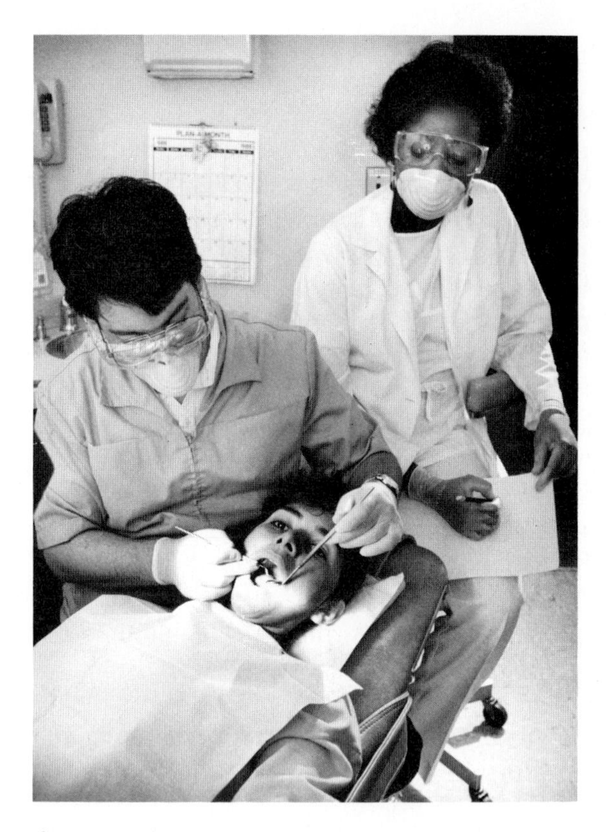

Figure 3–1. The dental team used precautionary measures to protect both client and health worker. (Courtesy of Henry J. Austin Health Center, Trenton, N.J. Photo by Michael Mancuso.)

graduation. The American Association of Dental Schools will provide specific information about admission requirements and the estimated costs of a dental education. With further education, a dentist may specialize in childhood and adolescent dentistry, tooth replacement, tooth straightening, and other specialties.

Traditionally, dentistry has been considered a career for men only. This concept is reinforced by the fact that there are few female dentists. However, the number of women enrolled in dental schools has increased significantly as women are actively recruited into the profession. Women who choose dental careers have the advantage of being able to work part-time if they want to bear children, then resume full-time practice later.

Additional information may be obtained from:

American Dental Association
211 East Chicago Avenue
Chicago, Illinois 60611

Dental Hygienist

Dental hygienists are specialists in oral health, disease prevention, and dental health education. They work mainly in private dental practice. Their responsibilities include: observing and recording the presence of disease or abnormalities of the oral cavity; exposing and developing x-rays; removing plaque, calculus, and stain from teeth above and below the gum line; cleaning and polishing teeth; making dental impressions; and applying fluorides to teeth. They also educate patients in proper oral hygiene. For example, they teach the patient how to select a toothbrush and **dentifrice**; how to brush and clean teeth to control plaque; and how diet and nutrition affect dental health. The dental hygienist may see patients twice a year and administer preventive therapy according to the dentist's prescription. If any oral diseases or abnormalities are observed, the patient is then scheduled for an appointment with the dentist.

There are two types of dental hygiene programs. Two-year associate degree programs, offered in community colleges or technical institutes, prepare graduates to work in private dental offices. Four-year baccalaureate degree programs in colleges or universities prepare graduates to work in private practice, school systems, or public health agencies, in the capacity of dental health educators and consultants.

All dental hygiene programs include courses in basic sciences, first aid, psychology, communications, dental science and techniques, health education, and clinical practice. Further education is necessary to qualify for advanced positions in teaching, administration, and public health. Dental hygienists are licensed by individual states.

For more information, write to:

American Dental Hygienists' Association
444 N. Michigan Avenue, Suite 3400
Chicago, Illinois 60611

Dental Assistant

The extra "pair of hands" in the dental office very often belongs to the dental assistant who works with the dentist at the chairside. Other patient-related duties of the assistant include: preparing fillings and cement; making plaster models from dental impressions; assisting in exposure and development of x-ray films; and cleaning and sterilizing instruments. The dental assistant also instructs patients in postoperative care, oral hygiene, and the importance of preventive dentistry (**Fig. 3–2**).

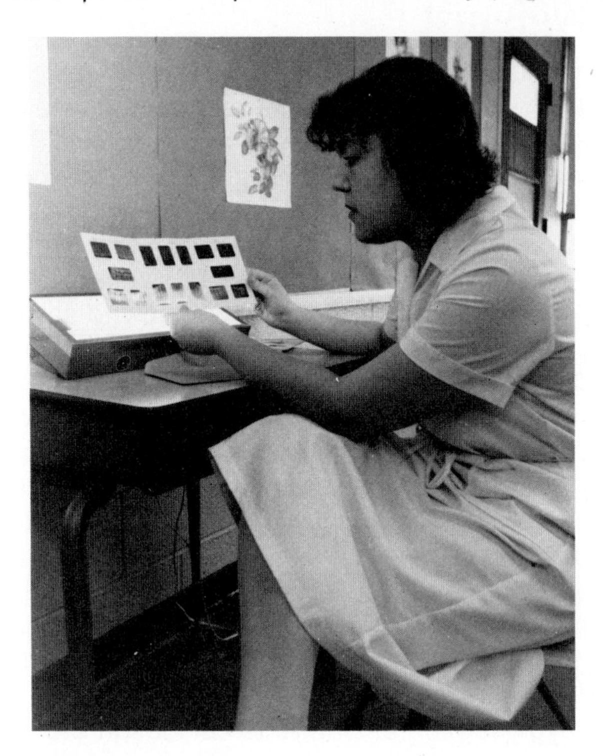

Figure 3–2. The dental assistant student examines dental radiographs. (Courtesy of Bridgeton High School, Bridgeton, N.J.)

Dental assistants who work in small offices may also assume the responsibilities of the dental receptionist, such as answering the telephone, scheduling appointments, keeping records, billing, ordering supplies, and handling other business transactions.

A few dentists hire high school graduates who have no occupational skills and train them on the job to become dental assistants. However, most dentists prefer to hire assistants who have completed a program in dental assisting in a vocational/technical school or community college.

Programs that are one year in length award a certificate of proficiency, while the two-year programs confer an associate degree. Dental assistants can be certified by meeting the requirements established by the American Dental Assistants Association.

Expanded Duties for the Dental Auxiliary

More than half the states have amended their Dental Practice Acts to permit dental auxiliary personnel (dental assistants and dental hygienists) to perform expanded duties. The American Dental Association defines "expanded role" as "anything except the cutting of soft or hard tissue." The auxiliaries carry out many intraoral (inside the mouth) procedures formerly done by the dentist. Dental auxiliaries may do the following: place, carve, and shape fillings after the dentist has prepared the cavity; remove sutures and packing; and take and develop x-rays. The definition of expanded duties varies from state to state, but this role is being incorporated into the curricula of individual dental auxiliary education programs.

More information may be obtained from:

American Dental Assistants Association
666 N. Lake Shore Drive, Suite 1130
Chicago, Illinois 60611

Dental Receptionist

The smooth running of the dental office, particularly in a group practice, is the responsibility of the dental receptionist. This staff member handles the business details of a large dental practice by scheduling appointments, sending out monthly billing statements, maintaining patient records, answering correspondence, and performing other clerical duties.

Dental receptionists are usually high school graduates who have completed business education courses and work experience programs. They may be prepared on the job by the dentist or in an educational program offered by a vocational/technical school or a private vocational school. More information about a career as a dental receptionist can be obtained from your health occupations instructor, guidance counselor, dentist, or business education teacher.

NURSING CLUSTER

The largest number of people working in health careers is found in the nursing cluster. Four occupations are represented: registered professional nurse (RN), licensed practical/vocational nurse (LPN or LVN), nursing assistant, and surgical technologist (surgical technician or operating room technician).

The registered professional nurse is the team leader who supervises the other nursing personnel. The extent and type of nursing care, and consequently the nursing personnel assigned to each patient, depend on the condition of the patient. The critically ill require the special skills and knowledge of the RN. For those whose condition is stabilized (not subject to abrupt change), the LPN may be assigned. Nursing assistants work with the professional and practical nursing staff, performing the less complex tasks in patient care. These three groups work together to provide direct care. Those in the fourth group, surgical technologists, work in the operating room with surgeons, nurses, and anesthesiologists before, during, and following surgical procedures. Opportunities for careers in the nursing cluster are available to men and women of all ages.

Professional Nurse (Registered Nurse, RN)

Professional nursing is a service, a science, and an art. RNs use the principles of biology, anatomy, physiology, microbiology, sociology, psychology, chemistry, and pharmacology in providing patient care.

Nursing is an art that calls for creativity. No two nursing situations are alike, and no two patients are alike. Registered nurses must be able to adjust to the needs of each patient and to develop individual approaches to patient care. A nursing care plan is developed for each patient on the unit. It takes into account the patient's physical, emotional, and spiritual needs. The professional nurse relies on the observations of all nursing personnel (other nurses and assistants) in formulating the plan, and all members of the nursing care staff cooperate to carry it out (**Fig. 3–3**). The duties of a professional nurse range from the relatively simple — bathing a patient — to the more complex — health counseling and patient education. Nurses may specialize in the care of children, mothers and newborn infants, the acutely ill, the mentally ill, older adults, etc. (**Fig. 3–4**). Com-

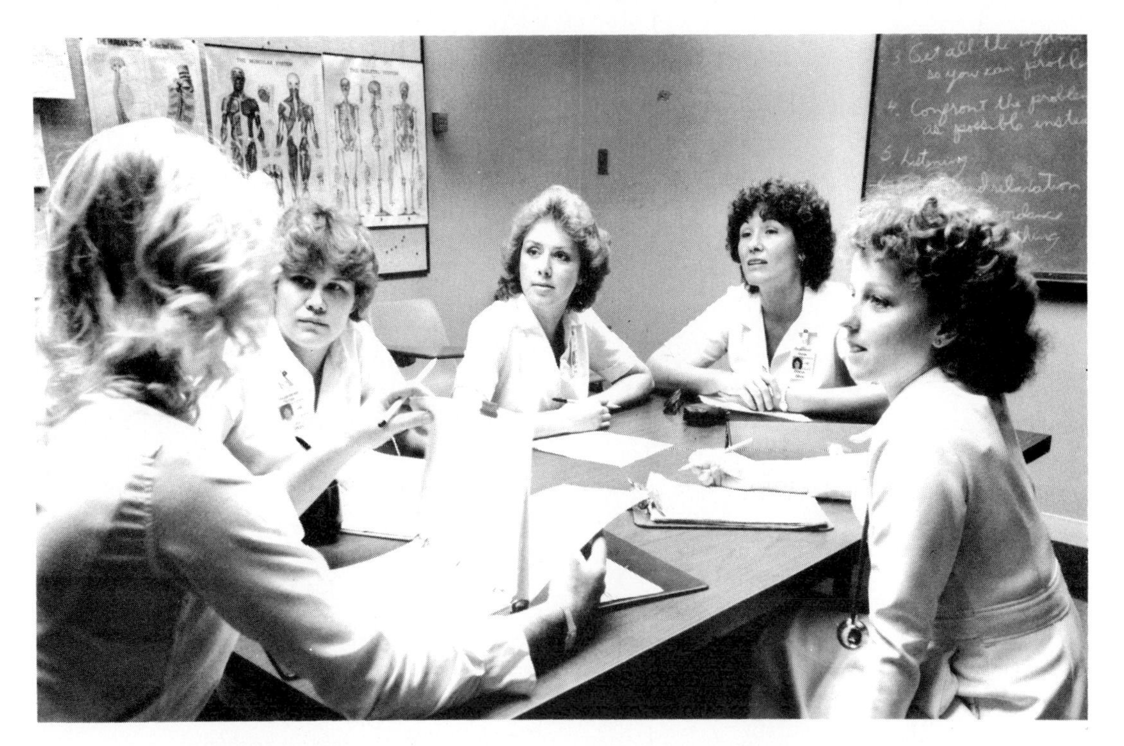

Figure 3–3. Members of the nursing team meet at the change of shift for a report on each client's progress and specific health care needs. (From Potter and Perry, *Fundamentals of Nursing,* St. Louis, The C.V. Mosby Co., 1985.)

munity health (public health) nursing is discussed in Chapter 6. Registered nurses work in many locations: hospitals, medical centers, nursing homes, schools, physicians' offices, community health facilities, industrial plants, and aboard ships.

There are three types of educational programs that prepare professional nurses to take the same state licensing examination: (1) The baccalaureate degree program (four years of college) permits further study and nursing specialization at the master's and doctoral degree levels. Only college programs can confer the degree of Bachelor of Science in Nursing (BSN). These programs prepare qualified public health nurses. (2) The associate degree program is usually offered by a community college and lasts two academic years. The degree of Associate in Applied Science in Nursing is conferred. (3) The Diploma program is based in a hospital school of nursing and requires two to three years to complete. Graduates earn a diploma in nursing. Many of these schools of nursing

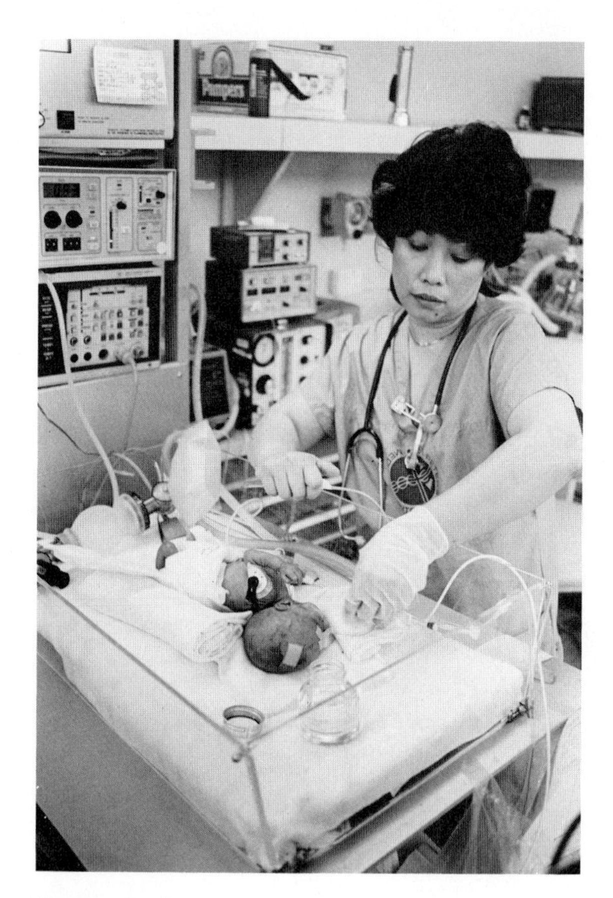

Figure 3–4. The professional nurse uses technology, skill, and tender loving care to assist this tiny patient. (Courtesy of the New Jersey Hospital Association; St. Peters Medical Center.)

have arrangements with local community colleges whereby their students take courses at the college and receive Associate in Applied Science degrees along with the diploma in nursing.

Both the diploma and the associate degree programs emphasize care of the institutionalized patient. Graduates of these programs are qualified to give bedside nursing in a hospital or nursing home, but they are not qualified for supervisory or administrative positions in nursing without further education. Graduates who wish to go on to a baccalaureate degree program after earning a diploma or an associate degree may do so but should not necessarily expect to receive full transfer credit for their previous education. Each college and university has its own policy on advanced standing.

Nurses are licensed to practice by individual states. The graduate of the nursing program usually takes the examination in the state in which the nursing program is located. The license permits the individual to practice as a registered nurse within that state only. In order to practice in another state, the nurse must apply to the appropriate state agency and meet its requirements before a license is issued.

Nurse Practitioner

One of many nursing specialties is that of nurse practitioner. As with all specialties in nursing, medicine, and dentistry, the basic requirements for beginning practice must be met — that is, the nurse must be licensed before entering an educational program to prepare for a career as a nurse practitioner. Programs vary in length from continuing education programs of nine to eighteen months to full-time graduate programs leading to a master's degree in nursing.

This specialty emerged to meet primary health care needs of people living far away from the nearest physician. Primary health care refers to meeting daily personal health needs — care given to prevent serious illness. Nurse practitioners may perform such duties as: immunizing children against certain childhood diseases; examining pregnant women and providing necessary prenatal care in uncomplicated cases; and counseling patients and their families about nutrition and the use of therapeutic diets. Nurse practitioners may work in group practices with physicians or in private practice alone or with other nurse practitioners. They are prepared to make independent judgments and assume responsibility for the primary care needs of patients.

Nurse practitioners may specialize in many areas, but the most common are pediatric care and family practice. More information about this growing field may be obtained by writing:

National League for Nursing
10 Columbus Circle
New York, New York 10019

American Nurses Association
2420 Pershing Road
Kansas City, Missouri 64108

American Academy of Nurse Practitioners
179 Princeton Boulevard
Lowell, Massachusetts 01851

Practical Nurse (LPN, LVN)

Licensed practical nurses (LPNs) or licensed vocational nurses (LVNs) in California and Texas perform many of the same duties as registered nurses. These include giving direct patient care; observing, recording, and reporting; administering treatments and medications; and assisting in rehabilitation procedures.

LPNs care for patients whose conditions do not require complex nursing care but who are relatively stable and free of complications. They also assist RNs in giving care to critically ill patients. LPNs always work under the direction of an RN or a licensed physician.

Practical nursing programs are offered in public vocational/technical schools, hospitals, and community colleges. The average length of the course is one calendar year; nursing theory and practice and selected content in the behavioral and biological sciences are included. Practical nurses are licensed to practice by individual states.

Practical nursing is considered a full-time, lifelong career in itself. However, sometimes LPNs wish to transfer into a program of professional nursing. Advanced standing, in recognition of previous practical nursing education and experience, may or may not be given by the receiving institution.

Note. THERE ARE NO CORRESPONDENCE PROGRAMS THAT WILL QUALIFY A PERSON TO TAKE THE STATE LICENSING EXAMINATION IN PRACTICAL NURSING.

Information about practical nursing may be obtained from:

National League for Nursing
10 Columbus Circle
New York, New York 10019

National Association for Practical
Nurse Education and Service, Inc.
254 West 31st Street
New York, New York 10001

National Federation of Licensed
Practical Nurses, Inc.
P.O. Box 11038
Durham, North Carolina 27703

Nursing Assistant

Nursing assistants are men and women who assist RNs and LPNs by performing uncomplicated tasks related to patient care in hospitals, nursing homes, and clinics. Their responsibilities may include: bathing and feeding patients; making beds; answering call lights; escorting patients to various departments; taking and reporting temperature, pulse, and respiration; serving meals; distributing linens; and stocking supply areas (**Fig. 3–5**).

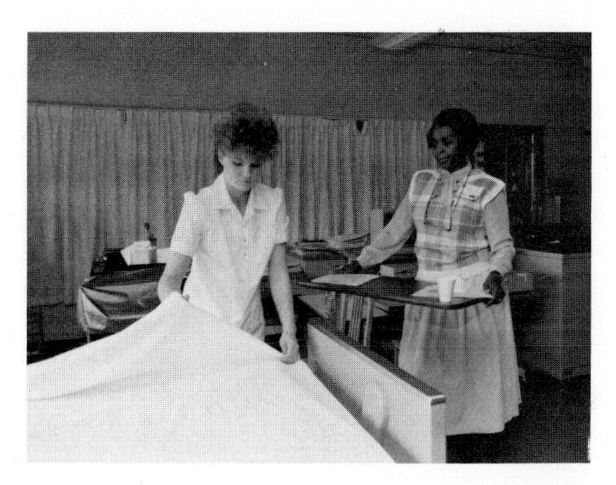

Figure 3–5. A nursing assistant student demonstrates bedmaking skills at a HOSA competition. (Courtesy of Bridgeton High School, Bridgeton, N.J.)

These health care workers may be prepared on the job or in vocational/technical schools.

Geriatric Aide

Because of the increasing number of older adults and the need to provide for their care in nursing homes and other long-term care facilities, the position of geriatric aide has developed. Geriatric aides perform tasks similar to those working in acute care hospitals. They have additional training in understanding the needs of older adults and know how to modify care procedures to meet these needs. They also learn techniques which contribute to the physical, social, and emotional well-being of the residents of these facilities.

Several states require that geriatric aides be certified prior to employment in nursing homes or other long-term care facilities. The requirements for certification vary. For further information, contact your local vocational/technical school or long-term care facility.

Surgical Technologist (Surgical Technician, Operating Room Technician)*

The surgical technologist is an important member of the operating room team, which is under the direction of the chief surgeon. Another team member is the anesthesiologist, a physician who specializes in anesthesia. This health professional administers anesthetics and keeps a constant watch on the patient's vital signs and overall condition during the operation. In each operating room, a professional nurse called the circulating nurse sees that the surgeon has the necessary equipment and supplies needed during the surgery and anticipates the needs of the scrub nurse.

Scrub nurses are professional nurses who directly assist the surgeon in complicated surgical cases by passing instruments, sutures, and sponges. In less complex surgical procedures, the surgical technologist takes the place of the scrub nurse and is assigned responsibility for preparing supplies and equipment for use in surgery; setting up and maintaining the sterile operative area; and passing the surgical instruments, sutures, and other necessary materials to the surgeon. Careful attention to sterile technique protects the patient from infection (**Fig. 3–6**).

Surgical technologists may be prepared on the job or in vocational/technical schools or community colleges. Programs range from nine months to two years in length and incorporate a study of basic surgical procedures, anatomy, physiology, microbiology, and **pathological** processes. Surgical technologists always work under the direct supervision of a registered nurse.

* Exception (see page 31).

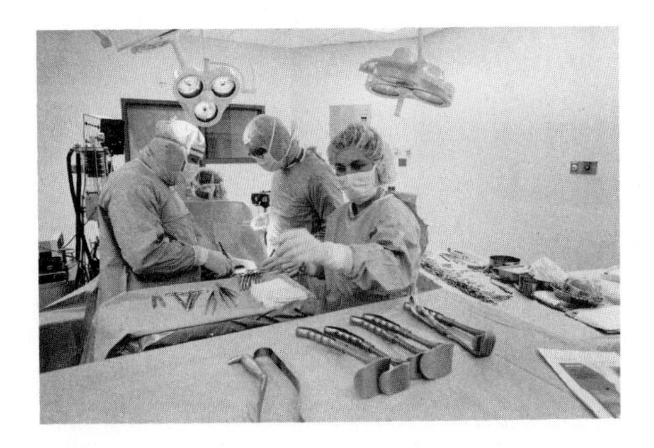

Figure 3–6. The surgical technologist functions as an important part of the operating team to assure the patient's well-being. (Courtesy of the New Jersey Hospital Association; Robert Wood Johnson Medical Center. Photo by Cliff Moore.)

Certification is granted when a technologist meets the criteria established by the Association of Surgical Technologists, Inc. This organization can provide more information. Write to:

Association of Surgical Technologists, Inc.
8307 Shaffer Parkway
Littleton, Colorado 80127

MEDICAL CLUSTER

Careers in the medical cluster are: doctor of medicine (MD), doctor of osteopathy (DO), doctor of podiatric medicine, (DMP), doctor of chiropractic (DC), physician assistant, medical assistant, and emergency medical technician (EMT). The physician — the leader of the medical team — diagnoses, prescribes treatment, and supervises care. Like other health professionals, physicians direct their efforts, in large part, toward preventing disease through regular programs of health maintenance, including regular checkups, routine immunizations, and standard screening procedures.

The other members of this cluster extend health care services by performing the technical and routine duties that allow the physician to concentrate on the patient and the specific medical problem.

Doctor of Medicine (Physician, MD)

No member of the health services is as well known or as highly respected as the doctor of medicine, and it's no wonder since we literally place our lives in the MD's hands. As leader of the medical team, the physician directs other health professionals in a plan of patient care.

Physicians must study for many years before they can be licensed to practice, and those who choose to enter a specialized medical field need additional years of education. It is difficult to be accepted into medical school because there are so many more applicants than vacancies. Only the best students are accepted; some applicants must wait as long as two years before being admitted. While most applicants have bachelor's degrees, the majority of medical schools require at least three years of college.

Students planning to enter medical school should enroll in college courses which provide them with a broad educational background in addition to the sciences. Because each medical school has specific requirements for entrance, it is important for students to obtain this information early so that they can complete the necessary prerequisites. About one to one and one-half years prior to applying to medical school, applicants are encouraged to take the Medical College Admission Test (MCAT) which measures their potential for success in medical school.

In medical school, the student spends four years in classroom and laboratory studies of medical and clinical science which include: **microbiology, anatomy, physiology, biochemistry, pathology,** and **pharmacology**. During this time, students also obtain clinical experience in hospitals and clinics. (Some medical schools now offer programs that require less time.) In most cases, a one-year internship follows graduation; if the doctor wishes to specialize, additional education, called a residency, is required. Physicians are licensed by the state in which they practice.

Acquiring a medical education and establishing a practice are extremely expensive undertakings. However, financial aid is available from many sources and is usually awarded on the basis of need.

More than 150 years ago, the first woman physician began to practice medicine in the United States, and since that time, the number of women physicians has gradually increased. Modern medicine offers many opportunities for women, as reflected in the rising number of female medical students. (About 35 percent of medical school students are women.)

For more information on careers in medicine, contact:

American Medical Association
535 N. Dearborn Street
Chicago, Illinois 60610

American Medical Women's Association
464 Grand Street
New York, New York 10002

Doctor of Osteopathy (Osteopath, DO)

In the United States, there are two approaches to medical practice. They are similar in that they utilize modern scientific methods of diagnosis and treatment, including drugs and surgery. However, osteopathic medicine emphasizes the importance of body movements to overall health. Doctors of osteopathy have had special training that enables them to recognize and correct structural problems through **manipulative therapy**, in conjunction with other methods of treatment — medication, surgery, physical therapy, etc.

There are only a few colleges of osteopathic medicine in the United States, and they require prospective students to have completed at least three, and preferably four, years of undergraduate premedical education. The four years of osteopathic medical college cover basic sciences and clinical studies, plus training in manipulative therapy. Graduates intern for one year at an approved osteopathic hospital. The number of applicants to schools of osteopathic medicine far exceeds the available openings, and only the top applicants are accepted.

Osteopathic physicians are licensed to practice medicine by individual states and, under federal law, have the same professional rights and responsibilities as medical doctors.

For further information write to:

American Osteopathic Association
212 East Ohio Street
Chicago, Illinois 60611

Doctor of Podiatric Medicine (Podiatrist, DPM)

"Oh, my aching feet!" is a familiar remark and a frequent cause for visiting a podiatrist. Very often, the foot shows the first signs of generalized disease and, if this is the case, the podiatrist will refer the patient to a physician for treatment. Gout, a type of arthritis, frequently begins with swelling, inflammation, and pain in the big toe. Yet this disease cannot be treated merely by relieving the foot discomfort, since ultimately it affects all body systems. The patient may be referred to a rheumatologist (a physician who specializes in treating arthritic conditions). Podiatrists treat ordinary foot problems with drugs, corrective devices, special shoes, and surgery (**Fig. 3–7**).

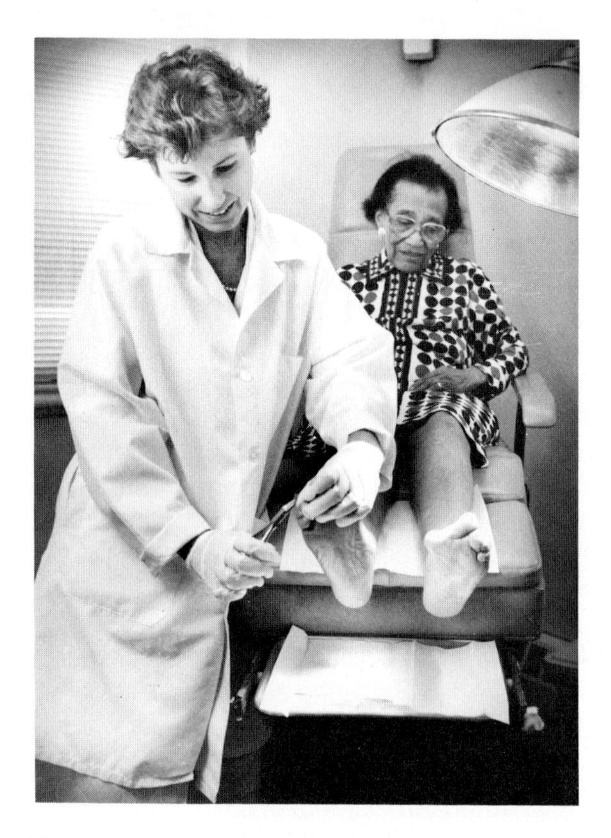

Figure 3–7. Foot deformities need the special attention of a podiatrist. (Courtesy of Henry J. Austin Health Center, Trenton, N.J. Photo by Michael Mancuso.)

Applicants for admission to colleges of podiatric medicine must complete two years of college, although most candidates have a bachelor's degree. The podiatric program is four years in duration, of which the first two years are spent in classroom and laboratory study of anatomy, bacteriology, chemistry, pathology, and physiology. The last two years are devoted to clinical training and practice. Individual states license podiatrists to practice; some states require, in addition, an internship prior to licensure. There are only six colleges of podiatric medicine in the United States, and, consequently, there is an increasing need for both additional schools and podiatrists.

Because of this shortage, the career of podiatric assistant has developed. The assistant performs some of the routine duties of foot care, such as: preparing the feet for examination; assisting the podiatrist with minor surgery in the office; and applying dressings. Some clerical and receptionist duties are also part of the job. In these ways the podiatric assistant extends the podiatrist's services.

Further information on podiatric careers may be obtained from:

American Podiatric Medical Association, Inc.
9312 Old Georgetown Road
Bethesda, Maryland 20814-1621

Doctor of Chiropractic (Chiropractor, DC)

Doctors of Chiropractic use their knowledge and skills in the treatment and prevention of disease. They concentrate on the structure and interaction of the spinal column and the effects upon the nervous system. The word **chiropractic** is a composite of two Greek words, "cheir" and "praktikox," meaning "done by hand."

Before treating the patient, the chiropractor uses standard diagnostic tests and instruments, takes and records the patient's and family's history, and performs a physical examination. This examination includes observing the patient's spine and posture, taking x-rays of the spine, and performing or ordering laboratory tests. Once the diagnosis is made, chiropractic adjustments may be performed. These include the careful application of pressure to a vertebra in order for it to function properly. Chiropractors believe that, through such adjustments, nerves and muscles related to the vertebrae will return to normal functioning. Instructing the patient about proper use of their muscles when lifting and moving as well as ordering exercises and other treatments, such as heat and massage, to help repair injured muscles and joints, are additional responsibilities of chiropractors. Their treatment, however, does not include prescribing medications or performing surgery.

Most chiropractors are in general practice and treat a variety of conditions in diverse age groups. There are 12 schools of chiropractic which are fully accredited by the Council on Chiropractic Education. Candidates for admission must have at least two years of college, including courses in biology, chemistry, and physics.

Once admitted to a school of chiropractic, the student continues the study of basic science subjects including anatomy and physiology, biochemistry, bacteriology, and pathology. This four-year program includes academic course work followed by working with patients in applying chiropractic principles.

All states require chiropractors to be licensed.

For further information about this career, write:

American Chiropractic Association
1916 Wilson Boulevard
Arlington, Virginia 22201

Physician Assistant (PA)

A developing health career is that of the physician assistant. Programs are offered by colleges and universities with schools of medicine and allied health. The average length of the program is two years which includes courses in anatomy, physiology, medical terminology, pharmacology, medical ethics, history of medicine, clinical laboratory procedures, signs and symptoms of disease, and clinical experience.

Physician assistants always work under the supervision of physicians. In the medical office, the assistant may take a patient's medical history, perform a physical examination, draw blood, and conduct routine blood and urine analyses. In the hospital, they may remove sutures and casts, treat minor injuries, and evaluate the patient's medical progress. The physician assistant never substitutes for the physician or acts as the team leader.

In some states, the physician assistant must be certified by the National Commission on Certification of Physician's Assistants. Most states require that the physician assistant register with the state agency which regulates medical practice. Many veterans who were medics are attracted to this career because it gives them a chance to use similar skills in civilian life.

For more information, write to:

Association of Physician Assistant Programs
1117 North 19th Street
Arlington, Virginia 22209

Medical Assistant

A doctor's office practice involves much more than the treatment of patients. Record keeping, correspondence, insurance claims, billing, and telephone communications are some of the routine activities that go on. Formerly, the physician could see patients and conduct office business alone or with the help of one person. Today, several people often are employed to manage the office efficiently.

The medical assistant is one of the most versatile members of the health care team, capable of handling many duties. The scope of these responsibilities includes: receiving patients and scheduling appointments, preparing and draping the patient for examination and assisting in the physical examination, performing selected diagnostic tests, arranging for hospital admission and scheduling x-ray or laboratory procedures, and keeping a variety of medical records.

The medical assistant always works under the supervision of a physician. One- or two-year programs in medical assisting are conducted in vocational/technical schools, community colleges, and private schools. Medical assistants need to be business oriented as well as people oriented. Because they are involved in many aspects of office management, the educational program includes courses in bookkeeping, insurance, and secretarial and clerical practice, including instruction in operating a computer (**Fig. 3–8**). Science-related courses include: anatomy and physiology, medical terminology, medical ethics, and clinical experience in a medical office. The program prepares students to perform administrative and patient-related duties in a physician's office.

Voluntary certification, with pediatric, administrative, or clinical specialization, is available to qualified medical assistants. Certification in more than one specialty is also possible.

For more information, contact:

American Association of Medical Assistants
20 N. Wacker Drive, Suite 1575
Chicago, Illinois 60606

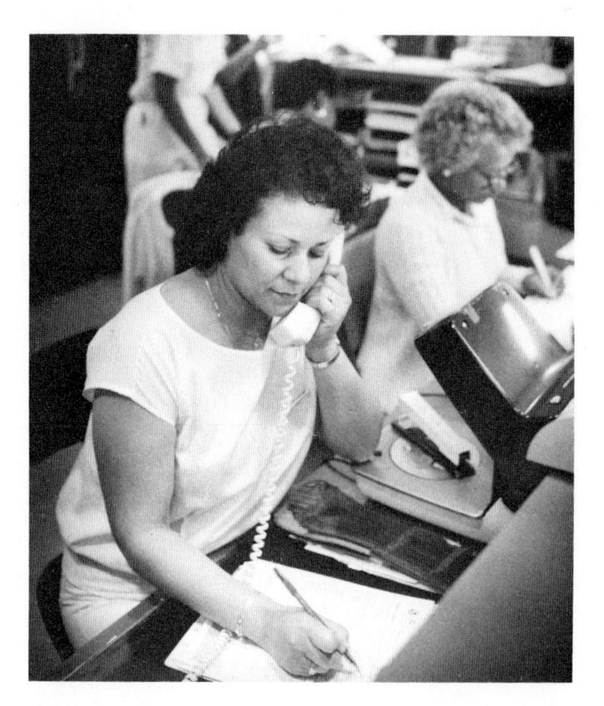

Figure 3–8. The medical assistant is vital to the smooth operation of the community health center. (Courtesy of Henry J. Austin Health Center, Trenton, N.J. Photo by Michael Mancuso.)

Emergency Medical Technician (EMT)

Medical emergencies — accident, heart attack, stroke, etc. — happen any time, any place. Usually, an ambulance is called, and the accompanying personnel are expected to give skilled first aid and to transfer the victim to a hospital quickly and safely. Men and women who are trained to provide such care are called emergency medical technicians (EMTs).

Their training qualifies them to: apply temporary splints, bandage and dress wounds, treat shock and hemorrhage, and administer artificial respiration and cardiopulmonary resuscitation. EMTs also drive ambulances, maintain emergency equipment, and operate communication equipment that relays information about the patient (e.g., blood pressure, pulse, electrocardiogram) to a hospital physician. EMTs work in fire and police departments and in ambulance rescue squads (**Fig. 3–9**).

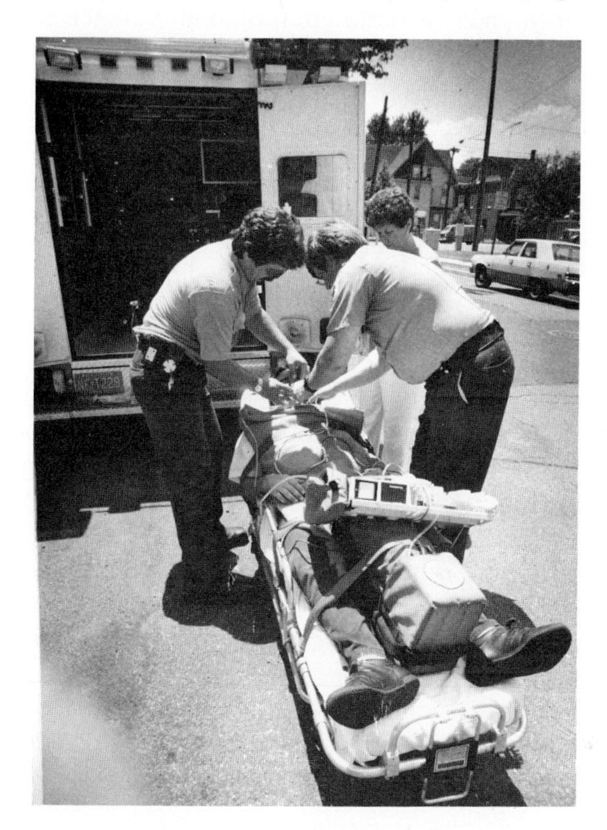

Figure 3–9. EMTs and paramedics use high-tech equipment in a life-threatening illness. (Courtesy of Rusling Hose Ambulance Corps. and Rescue Squad, Hamilton Township Div. of Health, N.J. Photo by Michael Mancuso.)

It is important to note that EMTs work under the supervision of a physician, although a physician is not usually physically present in the ambulance.

Some EMTs are salaried; others are unpaid volunteers. The length and location of their training varies in each state. Training programs may be conducted in vocational/technical schools, community colleges, police or fire academies, hospitals, or medical colleges. Standards for educational programs, certification, responsibilities, and care limitations are under the jurisdiction of each state.

For more information, write to your local ambulance or rescue squad, local police or fire department, the state Department of Health or:

National Association of Emergency Medical Technicians
9140 Ward Park
Kansas City, Missouri 64114

MENTAL HEALTH CLUSTER

Mental health personnel treat those who are emotionally disturbed or mentally retarded. This treatment may occur in psychiatric hospitals, daycare centers for the emotionally disturbed, alcoholism and drug treatment centers, private offices, special schools, or acute care hospitals.

Mental health workers are concerned about preventing mental illness and promoting mental health. Crisis "hot lines" and walk-in mental health centers provide services to people who are experiencing emotional crises. This convenient and inexpensive counseling, available in the community, offers early assistance in order to prevent a more critical situation from occurring. Staff personnel may provide treatment services or may refer clients to other agencies. The members of this cluster are psychiatrist, psychologist, mental health technician, and psychiatric aide. Others who may specialize in mental health work include professional and practical nurses, occupational therapists, and recreation, dance, and music therapists.

Psychiatrist (MD, DO)

The psychiatrist is a physician, either an MD or DO. Following graduation from medical school and an internship, the prospective psychiatrist completes a three-year residency in psychiatry to diagnose and treat mental disorders. This educational program includes formal courses, laboratory work, and supervised clinical experience. The resident physician may also undergo psychoanalysis in order to gain better self-understanding.

As leader of the mental health team, the psychiatrist identifies the patient's problems, prescribes or administers treatment, and directs overall patient care. There are many forms of treatment, including psychotherapy (specialized counseling to help patients gain self-understanding and better handle their emotional problems) and medication.

The field of psychiatry encompasses mental retardation, substance abuse, child abuse, student health, rehabilitation, research, community health, child and adolescent psychiatry, family psychiatry, etc. The psychiatrist may be employed in a private practice or in a mental health facility, such as a hospital, a school, a correctional institution, or in private industry.

For more information, write to:

American Psychiatric Association
1400 K Street, N.W.
Washington, D.C. 20005

Clinical Psychologist (Ph.D.)

Psychology is the science of the mind and behavior. A psychologist is a person who specializes in this science. Basically, psychologists attempt to understand people — their behaviors, abilities, and characteristics — and to assist clients to define their needs. Psychology is such a broad area of learning that psychologists usually concentrate on one special area such as clinical psychology. This specialty is concerned with the treatment of people who have emotional problems or illness. Therefore, it is considered to be one of the health professions. The clinical psychologist evaluates and treats emotional disorders by helping people to identify and understand their problems so that everyday living may be less stressful and more rewarding.

Eight years of study beyond high school is required to become a clinical psychologist. An undergraduate degree is mandatory for entrance into the graduate program. Because the program is so demanding, only superior students are admitted. A doctorate (Ph.D. — Doctor of Philosophy) in clinical psychology is one of the requirements for recognition by the American Board of Professional Psychology. Upon successful completion of the program, the graduate has earned the right to be called "doctor." Remember, however, that psychologists are NOT medical doctors and have received no medical training. They do not admit patients to hospitals nor do they prescribe or administer any type of medical treatment. Should any of these be necessary, the patient is referred to a psychiatrist.

Clinical psychologists use psychotherapy to treat patients individually or in a group setting. Treatment takes place in hospitals, schools, prisons, clinics, private offices, or other community settings. Specialties include family therapy, marriage counseling, substance abuse, rehabilitation, etc.

In the rehabilitation setting, the clinical psychologist helps amputees and paralyzed persons to accept and adjust to the body changes that will result in lifestyle changes. A couple experiencing marital problems may seek help from a clinical psychologist with a specialty in marriage counseling. The psychologist also instructs doctors, dentists, nurses, and hospital administrators in human behavior and how it is affected by illness.

Most states require clinical psychologists to be licensed or certified before they can practice.

More information may be obtained from:

American Psychological Association
P.O. Box 2710
Hyattsville, Maryland 20784

Mental Health Technician (Psychiatric Technician, Mental Health Technician)

A major health problem in the United States is mental illness, which requires hospitalization of millions every year. In mental institutions psychiatric technicians work in almost every patient care area — admission and discharge units, acute and chronic illness units, children's services, and geriatric units. They are also employed in transitional programs, such as community mental health centers, day-care centers, and halfway houses, where discharged clients are helped to return to life in the community. The technician is involved in the day-to-day activities of mentally retarded and emotionally ill people.

In psychiatric hospitals, technicians have a direct relationship with patients, assisting them with activities of daily living — eating, dressing, and personal hygiene. They help to promote responsibility for self-care as the patient's condition permits. For example, the technician may help a withdrawn patient to establish relationships with others. Initially, the approach may be through nonverbal means, such playing cards or checkers. Gradually, communication — either verbal or nonverbal — may be extended to other staff members and patients. In any case, the approach to patients is part of a treatment plan developed by the psychiatrist and the mental health team members.

The technician's responsibilities include: patient interviews, resocialization, and activity therapy. Technicians usually work under the supervision of a registered nurse, and they can perform basic nursing tasks, such as taking temperature, pulse, respiration, and blood pressure.

Their educational program includes courses in human growth and development, personality formation, and the nature of mental illness. They also study community mental health, specific disease conditions, disease treatment and prevention, anatomy, physiology, and basic nursing procedures. Programs for mental health technicians are usually found in two-year community colleges, and the graduate earns an Associate of Arts degree. In some states, the mental health technician must be licensed to practice.

For more information, contact:

National Association of Human Services Technologies
1127 Eleventh Street
Sacramento, California 95814

State Mental Health Services Agency, state capital

Personnel Director of your local psychiatric hospital

Psychiatric Aide

Psychiatric aides are employed in mental hospitals and in facilities for the mentally retarded, where they work closely with patients. They assist patients with routine daily activities — bedmaking, bathing, personal grooming, eating, exercise, recreation, and socializing. The aides are the "eyes and ears" of the professional staff, since they spend most of their time with patients. All of the aide's observations, reports, and comments about patient activities and behaviors are important indicators of the effectiveness of treatment. The professional staff uses this information to alter the treatment program, as indicated. Psychiatric aides are usually prepared on the job or in a short course given at a vocational school.

More information may be obtained from:

National Association of Human Services Technologies
1127 Eleventh Street
Sacramento, California 95814

Personnel Director of your local psychiatric hospital

Note. Excellent information on mental health careers is available from The National Association for Mental Health, 1800 North Kent Street, Rosslyn, Virginia 22209.

MEDICAL SOCIAL WORK CLUSTER

Basic human and social needs are intensified by illness. Patients and their families are troubled by problems related to money, housing, employment, recovery, rehabilitation, etc. Members of the social work cluster help clients arrive at solutions to these problems.

Social service personnel work with sick and well groups and individuals. They also work in a variety of settings: hospitals, guidance centers, juvenile and family courts, welfare departments, and community mental health centers. In this cluster are found the professional social worker, social health advocate, social work technician, and social work assistant.

Professional Social Worker (Social Work Practitioner)

The professional social worker is the leader of the social service team, which provides direct service to patients and families.

In the acute care hospitals, professional social workers may be responsible for discharge planning. They arrange for patients to be returned to the community with as few problems as possible. If the patient needs financial assistance, the social worker will explore possible sources of income, such as disability payment, Social Security, and welfare assistance. When the patient requires home health care, the social worker arranges for the services of a visiting nurse or homemaker/home health aide. Patients not able to return home may be transferred to nursing homes or to rehabilitation centers. In such a case, it is the social worker, acting in conjunction with the medical team and the patient's family, who makes the necessary arrangements.

A bachelor's degree from an accredited college is required for admission to a graduate school of social work. The two-year program combines class work and field experience. Half of the program is devoted to the actual experience of working with clients in the community. A few states license or certify social workers, and voluntary certification is conducted by the National Association of Social Workers.

Supportive Social Work Personnel

There are three groups of supportive personnel working under the direct supervision of the professional social worker: social health advocate, social work technician, and social work assistant. They are employed only in large health care facilities or community health departments in large urban communities. Their function is to help people meet their basic health needs, according to the specific situation. For example, they arrange transportation for medical appointments, check on broken appointments, instruct parents about the need for childhood immunizations, and cut through the "red tape" of government and health care agencies. With further education, it is possible to move up the career ladder.

Social health advocates, also known as community health aides or family aides, receive on-the-job preparation where they are employed. The program varies in length and may include some course work in a college or university. The social work technician holds an associate degree in the social sciences from a two-year community college. In some areas, graduates of a four-year college, who hold degrees in social work or social science, are employed to provide basic patient services. These workers are known as social work assistants, and they participate in staff development activities or receive on-the-job education to upgrade their skills.

For more information on careers in medical social work, contact:

National Association of Social Workers
7981 Eastern Avenue
Silver Spring, Maryland 20910

Council on Social Work Education
1744 R Street, N.W.
Washington, D.C. 20009

STUDENT ACTIVITIES

1. Select one of the health career clusters described in this chapter for further research. Which schools in your area offer educational programs in these careers? Describe the program: entrance requirements, length, tuition, fees, and scholarships available. Record this information in your file.
2. Interview a health worker from the cluster you have selected. Obtain the following information about the specific career: job description, educational preparation, beginning salary, licensure requirements, and job opportunities in the community. List the advantages and disadvantages of this career. Record in your file.
3. Perform three of the following activities that are responsibilities of workers in the Direct Care Careers (as directed by your instructor). If you are not in a Health Occupations Education Course, try to arrange to observe the performance of some of these activities:
   a. Feeding a meal to a handicapped patient
   b. Observing sterile technique
   c. Measuring and recording temperature, pulse, and respiration
   d. Observing a classmate's oral cavity and recording dental history
   e. Recording family medical history
   f. Verbal or nonverbal communication in a mental hospital.

   In your file, record the procedures completed. Briefly describe your feelings as you performed or observed these procedures.
4. Identify those who may perform the following activities:
   a. Take and record blood pressure
   b. Feed patients
   c. Perform surgery
   d. Give emergency treatment at the scene of an accident
   e. Assist a surgeon during an operation
   f. Take patient histories
   g. Find a place for a discharged patient to live

h. Treat diseased teeth
i. Help the dentist at chairside
j. Apply fluoride solution to teeth
k. Observe patients after surgery
l. Bathe patients
m. Design special shoes
n. Perform spinal adjustments.

5. Select one career discussed in this chapter. Write a letter to one organization listed in the chapter to obtain information about this career. File the information received in your special notebook.
6. Complete the Career Interest Chart for the Direct Care Careers. Obtain the chart from your instructor.

Chapter 4

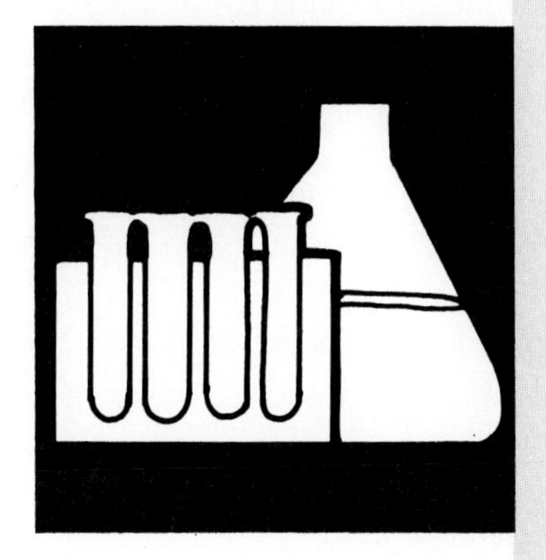

Diagnostic Careers

Objectives

After completing this chapter, you should be able to:

- Identify by name five clusters of occupations in the Diagnostic Careers and list three careers found in each cluster.
- Identify four careers and discuss three responsibilities of workers in each career.
- Compare and contrast the relationship between the Diagnostic Careers and the Direct Care Careers.
- Identify by name 10 pieces of equipment/supplies used by workers in the Diagnostic Careers.
- Discuss your feelings about performing three of the suggested "hands-on" activities in class.
- Compare the advantages and disadvantages of pursuing a career in this group.
- Define at least 70 percent of the key terms listed for this chapter.

Key Terms

• **antibody** A protein substance produced by the body in response to the presence of foreign antigens

• **antigen** A substance (poison, virus, pollen, dust) foreign to the body which stimulates the production of antibodies

• **agar** A culture media for growing bacteria

• **antitoxin** An antibody that neutralizes a specific toxin

• **benign** Not recurrent or malignant; not cancer

• **biopsy** Surgical removal of a small piece of tissue for microscopic examination

• **cataract** Clouding or opaqueness of the lens of the eye that causes decreased vision

• **CAT scan** A special type of x-ray that shows detailed internal structures in a specific layer of the body

• **diagnosis** The use of scientific and skilled methods to discover the cause and nature of a person's disease

• **electroencephalogram** A tracing of the electrical activity of the brain

• **electrodes** Small devices applied to the surface of the patient's body to measure the electrical activity of certain organs (heart and brain)

• **forensic** Pertaining to law; legal; medicine in relation to the law

• **malignant** Progressive and life threatening

• **nuclear medicine** That branch of medicine concerned with diagnostic, therapeutic, and investigative use of radioactive materials

• **ophthalmologist** A physician who specializes in the treatment of eye diseases

• **ophthalmoscope** Instrument for examining the interior of the eye

• **pathology** The study of the nature and cause of disease that involves changes in structure and function

• **peripheral vision** Side vision

- **quality control** To regulate or maintain specific standards of quality
- **radiograph** A record produced on a photographic plate, film, or paper by the action of roentgen rays or radium; specifically an x-ray photograph
- **radiogram** X-ray picture
- **serology** The scientific study of blood serum
- **sputum** Substance coughed up from the lungs and expelled through the mouth
- **Snellen chart** Chart imprinted with black letters and used for testing visual acuity
- **toxin** A poisonous substance of plant or animal origin
- **ultrasonography** Use of ultrasound to produce an image or photograph of an organ or tissue. Ultrasonic echoes are recorded as they strike tissues of different densities
- **ultrasound** Inaudible sound in the frequency range of about 20,000 to 10,000,000,000 cycles/second
- **vaccine** A suspension of infectious agents, or some part of them, given for the purpose of establishing resistance to an infectious disease

THE DIAGNOSTIC CAREER CLUSTERS

To diagnose means to identify or recognize a disease. The Diagnostic Careers group performs the tests and procedures ordered by the physician. These diagnostic studies make it possible to arrive at a determination about the presence or absence of a disease as well as its characteristics.

The tools of diagnosis range from the uncomplicated, such as the rubber hammer used to test the "knee-jerk" reflex, to highly complex precision instruments such as the electron microscope that permits magnification of up to 1 million times or more. The electrocardiograph, the x-ray machine, the stethoscope, and the sphygmomanometer (blood pressure gauge) are among the frequently used tools of diagnosis.

Computers have taken an important place in the diagnostic process. Medical laboratories have computerized automatic analyzers that can perform many diagnostic tests on a single sample of blood. Measured blood specimens are placed in test tubes in a rack and appropriate chemicals are added. The tubes are heated, agitated, or chilled as called for and then the analyzer "reads" the results, which are recorded on a computer printout. This equipment is often referred to as SMA (sequential multiple analyzer).

Computerized tomography or computerized axial tomography (CT, CAT) is a radiologic technique in which machines known as CAT or CT scanners take x-rays at multiple angles around a specific section of the body. The computer compiles all the information and produces a single composite picture of a specific "slice" of the body — e.g., abdomen, lungs, skull — on a screen.

The following belong in the Diagnostic Careers group: the radiology cluster, the medical laboratory cluster, the diagnostic equipment personnel cluster, the optical cluster, and the audiology/speech pathology cluster.

Some diagnostic personnel spend a large portion of their time operating equipment (microscopes, electrocardiographs, x-rays machines, etc.) rather than working with patients. This is particularly true in the medical laboratory where much time is devoted to preparing and examining specimens (urine, blood, tissues).

Other diagnostic personnel rely on the patient's cooperation and assistance during diagnostic procedures and have an active relationship with patients. For example, the speech pathologist tests hearing ability with the audiometer. In this test, the patient uses a predetermined signal to indicate the ability to hear various sound frequencies through earphones. Clearly, the patient must understand and cooperate with the speech pathologist in order for the test results to be accurate.

Diagnostic personnel sometimes are called upon to help police in their murder investigations. In the laboratory, samples of vital tissues would be removed and examined to determine the cause of death. The victim's body would be examined to determine the entry route of a bullet, and laboratory tests would be performed to determine whether the bullet wound was the primary cause of death. The results of the medical examination would be presented in court as sworn testimony given by the medical examiner. This branch of medicine is called forensic medicine.

Diagnostic occupations personnel are employed in hospitals, public health departments, health maintenance organizations, physicians' and dentists' offices, private medical laboratories, pharmaceutical industries, schools, and correctional facilities. Like other kinds of health care work, medical detection goes on all day and all night and does not stop during weekends and holidays.

Diagnostic careers offer employment opportunities and responsibilities in a broad range of areas. Advances in technology have created many new methods of diagnosis. Ultrasonography, computerized scanning techniques, and magnetic resonance imaging are some examples. With these technological advances, new health careers are continually emerging.

Health Care Workers on the Job

Centerton High School always played the last football game of the year on Thanksgiving morning against its arch rival, River Valley High School. Since both teams were undefeated during the season, the contest promised to be exciting.

Stan Waltkowski, Centerton's star pass receiver, wanted to win today because this was his last game before graduation. Barbara Cline wanted to do a good job today because this was her last chance to take football pictures for the River Valley High School newspaper.

The score remained tied at 7–7 until the last five minutes of the game when the Centerton offense began to press for the winning touchdown. Barbara knelt by the five-yard line and focused her camera on the goal posts. A great picture was in the making. The ball came flying through the air, and Stan caught the pass just as a River Valley player tackled him. They both fell out of bounds on the five-yard line and landed on top of Barbara!

The fans were screaming with excitement. But Barbara was unconscious; Stan sat on the grass holding his painful right ankle; and the River Valley tackle, John Daninas, was bleeding from a **laceration** near his right eye.

The injured trio was taken by ambulance to the medical center emergency department for treatment. The job of the diagnostic staff was to determine the extent of the injuries so that treatment could be started as quickly as possible.

The x-ray film of Stan's ankle was read by the radiologist and revealed no fracture. Stan was fitted with a pair of crutches and instructed to apply ice to the swelling. He went home with his parents. The next day he was to see his own physician for further treatment.

John's eye was examined by the ophthalmologist. A careful inspection with the ophthalmoscope showed no injury to the structures of the eye, and the laceration was sutured and bandaged. The doctor patched the injured area to protect John's eye and prescribed ice applications to the swollen area. The following day, the ophthalmologist would conduct a re-examination in her office.

Barbara regained consciousness and was admitted to a nursing unit for close observation. Her symptoms suggested that she might have a concussion, and the doctor wanted to rule out any brain injury. Routine blood tests and urinalysis were ordered to evaluate her general health. Special diagnostic tests, including an electroencephalogram, skull x-rays, and a CAT scan were performed to determine any nervous system problem. No abnormalities were detected, and Barbara was discharged a few days later when her symptoms subsided.

Through the efforts of the members of the diagnostic group, diagnosis and treatment were prompt and efficient.

By the way, Centerton High School won the game.

RADIOLOGY CLUSTER

A diagnostic tool familiar to most people is the x-ray machine, which makes it possible to visualize the internal structures of the body. As the x-rays pass through the body, a photograph (technically known as a radiogram) is produced on a special kind of sensitized film. Images of tissues, organs, bones, and vessels may also be recorded on film or displayed on a video monitor (**Fig. 4–1**). Sometimes, motion picture film or videotape is used. These images are studied or "read" by the radiologist who determines the diagnosis. Many treatments are based upon an accurate diagnosis using radiologic studies.

Some soft organs of the body (stomach, gallbladder, and kidneys) are not clearly visible on a standard x-ray picture, so special dyes, air, or minute quantities of radioactive material must be injected to outline or illuminate these organs so they can be examined.

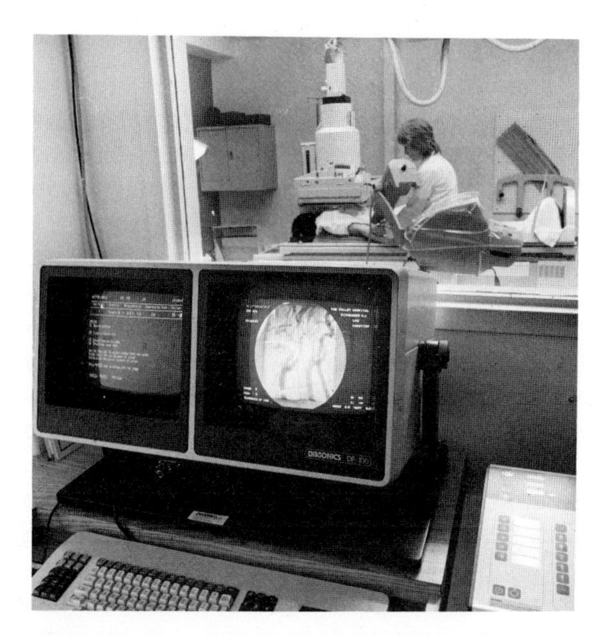

Figure 4–1. This monitor used digital subtraction angiography to provide a precise view of the arteries of the neck. (Courtesy of the New Jersey Hospital Association; Valley Hospital, Ridgewood, N.J.)

When diagnostic films of internal organs are ordered, the patient must undergo special preparation. If the bowel is to be examined, an enema is necessary. When the stomach is to be x-rayed, the patient must fast from midnight until the test is completed. The radiology department relies on the Direct Care staff to prepare patients for diagnostic radiograms. Most often, these studies are done on an outpatient basis. The physician, nurse, or medical assistant is responsible for thoroughly instructing the patients on how to prepare themselves for the test. Without the assistance of the Direct Care staff, the radiology department would be unable to perform its diagnostic work.

Radiology is one of the fastest growing fields in modern medicine and is responsible for a large part of medical diagnostic work. It has benefited from the technological growth in recent years, especially from advances in atomic physics, computers, cancer research, and specialized diagnostic equipment.

The radiology cluster includes the radiologist; the radiographer; radiation therapy technologist; nuclear medicine technologist; and sonographer.

Radiologist

A radiologist is a physician who has completed a residency in radiology. Radiologists use x-rays, radioactive substances, magnetic fields, and ultrasound waves to diagnose and treat disease. Since radiology is such a complex field, radiologists can specialize in several areas: diagnosis, treatment, and nuclear medicine. The importance of their work lies in the fact that, in many instances, treatment is based on their findings.

Often, the treatment may involve *radiotherapy*, a major weapon used in the treatment of cancer. This is an extremely potent and dangerous type of therapy — an overdose can be as deadly as the cancer for which it has been prescribed. The radiologist must select the proper radioactive material for treatment and prescribe the precise dosage (including manner of administration and the area to be treated) with accuracy and extreme caution.

Radiologists work in hospitals, private practice, industry, and community health agencies.

More information may be obtained from:

American Medical Association
535 N. Dearborn Street
Chicago, Illinois 60610

Radiographer

Radiographers comprise the largest group of workers in this cluster. Under the radiologist's supervision they take the radiograms, following a precise step-by-step procedure to ensure a quality diagnostic image (**Fig. 4–2**).

Most patients go to a hospital radiology department to have x-ray pictures taken. However, when a patient cannot be moved, a portable x-ray machine is wheeled to the bedside. Here, the radiographer accurately positions the patient's body and uses only the amount of radiation necessary to provide the desired image. The radiograms may be taken from several angles: front, back, and/or side. The films are processed in the Radiology Department by automated processing machines.

Radiograms are also taken during orthopedic (skeletal) surgery in the operating room. The radiographer wheels the x-ray machine to the op-

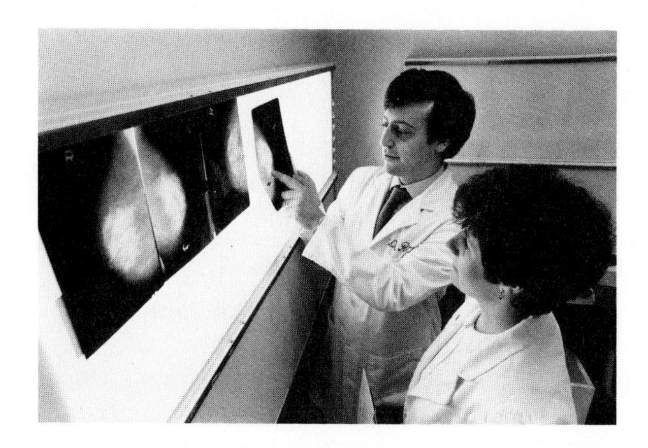

Figure 4–2. The radiologist and radiographer discuss the results of a mammogram. (Courtesy of Bridgeton Hospital, Bridgeton, N.J.)

erating room and stands by until needed. After the surgeon has inserted a metal nail, screw, or plate to hold broken parts of a bone together, the radiographer exposes films to record the placement of the device and to verify that the bone ends are aligned.

Hospital radiology departments employ clerical workers to assist in the office, but in a small, private radiology practice, the radiographer may do this work. These clerical functions may include sorting and filing films, scheduling appointments, preparing and forwarding reports, billing, and bookkeeping.

Educational programs that prepare radiographers are conducted in two-year, hospital-based certificate programs, two-year associate degree programs, and four-year baccalaureate programs. The educational program combines classroom, laboratory, and clinical experiences. Courses include: medical law and ethics, anatomy and physiology, medical terminology, radiation protection, radiation physics, principles and techniques of diagnostic imaging, radiation processing, radiographic procedures, radiographic pathology, radiobiology, introduction to computer science, and introduction to quality assurance.

It is wise to select a program that is accredited by the Committee on Allied Health Education and Accreditation of the American Medical Association. Upon completion of an accredited program, the graduate is eligible for certificaiton by the American Registry of Radiologic Technologists. Some states require that radiographers be licensed to practice.

For additional information, contact:

American Society of Radiologic Technologists
Educational Foundation, Inc.
15000 Central Avenue, S.E.
Albuquerque, New Mexico 87123

For a list of accredited programs, contact:

The American Medical Association
535 N. Dearborn Street
Chicago, Illinois 60610

Radiation Therapy Technologist

Radiation therapy involves the use of radiation to treat diseases, especially cancer. The major responsibilities of the technologist are daily patient treatments, patient support, and treatment planning (**Fig. 4–3**).

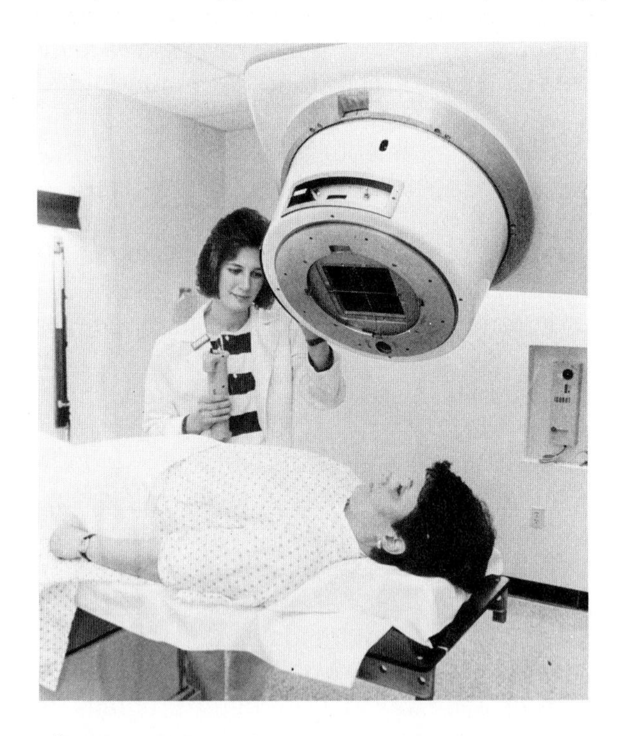

Figure 4–3. The radiation therapy technologist implements a treatment program. (Courtesy of Bridgeton Hospital, Bridgeton, N.J. Photo by Gary Cooper.)

Highly complex machines are used to deliver the radiation therapy, and the technologist must be able to operate these safely and effectively. In addition, the technologist must keep accurate records and carefully document patient treatments.

There is a great deal of interaction with cancer patients and their families because many not only fear the disease but are frightened by the treatment and equipment. The technologist is a team member working closely with physicians, nurses, and social workers to provide emotional support to the patient.

There are four types of programs available to prepare radiation therapy technologists: one-year hospital-based certificate programs, two-year hospital-based certificate programs, two-year associate degree programs, and four-year baccalaureate programs.

Admission requirements vary greatly: admission to the one-year program is restricted to radiographers who have graduated from programs accredited by the Committee on Allied Education and Accreditation (as described above). Other professionals with appropriate education and competencies may also be admitted to these one-year programs. A high school education is required for admission to the remaining programs.

Information can be obtained from both the American Medical Association, Department of Allied Health Education and Accreditation and the American Society of Radiologic Technologists (see page 82).

Nuclear Medicine Technologist

Radioactive materials are used to diagnose and treat diseases of the organs, including the thyroid, brain, lung, and liver. These structures are studied after the patient has inhaled, ingested, or been injected with a small quantity of radioactive material which is then measured with a radiation detection instrument.

The responsibilities of the nuclear medicine technologist include:

- Patient care — instructing the patient before and during nuclear procedures
- Occupational skills — preparing and administering the appropriate radioactive materials in a safe manner and then performing the desired imaging procedures
- Administrative functions — documenting the receipt, use, and disposition of radioactive materials.

Educational programs vary in length. To enter the one-year certificate program, you must be a graduate of an accredited two-year, clinically related allied health education program. Other programs are: two-year certificate program; two-year associate degree program, and four-year baccalaureate program.

Graduates are eligible for examination for registration by the American Registry of Radiologic Technologists (ARRT) or the Nuclear Medicine Technology Certification Board (NMTCB).

Information can be obtained from the American Medical Association, Department of Allied Health Education and Accreditation, and from the American Society of Radiologic Technologists (see page 82).

Sonographer

Ultrasound is one of the newest specialties in diagnosis. It is a noninvasive diagnostic technique in which reflected echos from body tissues are displayed as images on a video monitor. These images are then transferred to a film or videotape and interpreted by a physician who has specialized in ultrasound.

Programs which prepare sonographers, are: one-year certificate programs (for graduates of a two-year allied health program), two-year associate degree programs, and four-year baccalaureate programs.

A list of accredited programs in sonography can be obtained from the American Medical Association, Department of Allied Health Education and Accreditation (see page 82). Certification is available from the American Registry of Diagnostic Medical Sonographers.

MEDICAL LABORATORY CLUSTER

Medical diagnosis would not be possible without the teamwork of the medical laboratory personnel. Often, it is possible to exclude a suspected disease or to confirm the presence of a suspected disease on the basis of laboratory studies.

In the laboratory, specimens — body cells, tissues, and fluids — are examined by means of microscopes, slides, dyes, stains, and precision instruments. Medical laboratory work requires the ability to distinguish fine shadings of color, since certain test results are indicated by a change in the color of the specimen (**Fig. 4–4**).

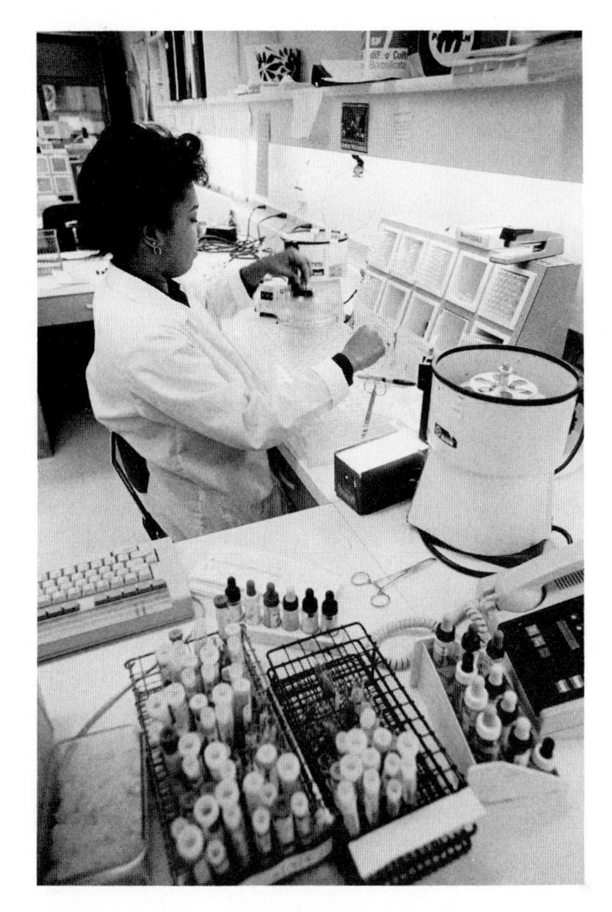

Figure 4–4. Medical laboratory personnel are a vital part of the diagnostic process. (Courtesy of the New Jersey Hospital Association, Robert Wood Johnson Medical Center. Photo by Cliff Moore.)

Most specimens required for examination are collected by Direct Care personnel in patient care areas, e.g., nursing personnel collect urine, sputum, sweat, and stool specimens; dentists and surgeons obtain tissue samples for laboratory examination. Thus, cooperation between the laboratory workers and the Direct Care personnel is essential to proper diagnosis.

Because this work does not require much physical strength, it offers excellent opportunities for physically handicapped persons, provided they are able to manipulate the equipment.

The careers in the medical laboratory cluster all offer opportunities for specialization. These careers are: pathologist, medical laboratory technologist, medical laboratory technician, cytotechnologist, and histologic technician.

Pathologist

Pathology means the scientific study of the changes caused by disease. The head of the medical laboratory is the pathologist, often called the "doctor's doctor," because the pathologist's findings often provide the basis for the physician's diagnosis, as the following examples will illustrate.

Does the physician suspect that a lump on the patient's neck might be cancerous? A biopsy (sample of tissue from the suspected site) would be obtained for examination under the microscope by the pathologist who determines whether the tissue is malignant or benign. Is the cause of a person's death in doubt? If so, the pathologist would perform an autopsy (examination of a body after death) to determine the cause.

The pathologist supervises all other personnel in the clinical laboratory and may also teach in programs for medical laboratory personnel, nurses, and physician assistants.

The pathologist is a licensed physician who has completed a four- or five-year residency, leading to certification by the American Board of Pathology.

For more information about careers in pathology, contact: the American Medical Association (see page 80) and

American Society of Clinical Pathologists
2100 W. Harrison Street
Chicago, Illinois 60612

Medical Technologist (MT [ASCP])

Medical technologists are qualified by education and experience to perform clinical laboratory tests that require the exercise of independent judgment and discretion. They have important responsibilities for patient safety in regard to blood transfusions in which certain tests are performed to determine the compatibility of blood type between donor and recipient.

Technologists are also responsible for laboratory cultures — a medium containing living microorganisms (organisms too small to be seen with the naked eye). The cultures are used to identify specific disease-producing organisms causing an infection.

Let us suppose that the physician has ordered a urine culture. The technologist would place a specimen of the patient's urine in a **culture medium** and allow it to incubate (grow) for a definite period of time to determine whether any abnormal microorganisms are present. If so, further tests would be carried out to determine which antibiotic would be an effective treatment.

Other duties of the laboratory technologist include supervision and instruction of other laboratory personnel in the performance of routine tests. Those in administrative positions handle the day-to-day operations of the laboratory, including scheduling daily assignments and evaluating staff performance. They are responsible for quality control — that is, ensuring the accuracy of test results. When questions arise about test results, the technologist is responsible for checking the equipment, chemicals, and procedures that were used and, if necessary, for performing the test again.

Some medical technologists are employed in research divisions of drug companies in the development and manufacture of new drugs. Some find employment in private clinical laboratories, health maintenance organizations, neighborhood health centers, state and local health departments, and private industry.

Medical technologists are educated in four-year colleges. Their studies include courses in chemistry, biology, and mathematics. An approved laboratory experience and specific clinical education are integral parts of the educational program. Graduates are awarded a baccalaureate degree and may take the certification examination given by the Board of Registry of the American Society of Clinical Pathologists (ASCP). The American Medical Technologists also offer a certification examination.

For more information, write to:

American Medical Technologists
710 Higgins Road
Park Ridge, Illinois 60068

American Society of Clinical Pathologists
Board of Registry
Box 12270
Chicago, Illinois 60612

Medical Laboratory Technician (MLT [ASCP])

Medical laboratory technicians are qualified by education and experience to perform clinical laboratory testing. Some of their duties include: microscopic examination of stool, identification of **antibodies** and **antitoxins,** and typing blood for transfusion (**Fig. 4–5**). The technician performs less complicated laboratory procedures than the medical technologist and does not have the supervisory or teaching responsibilities of the medical technologist.

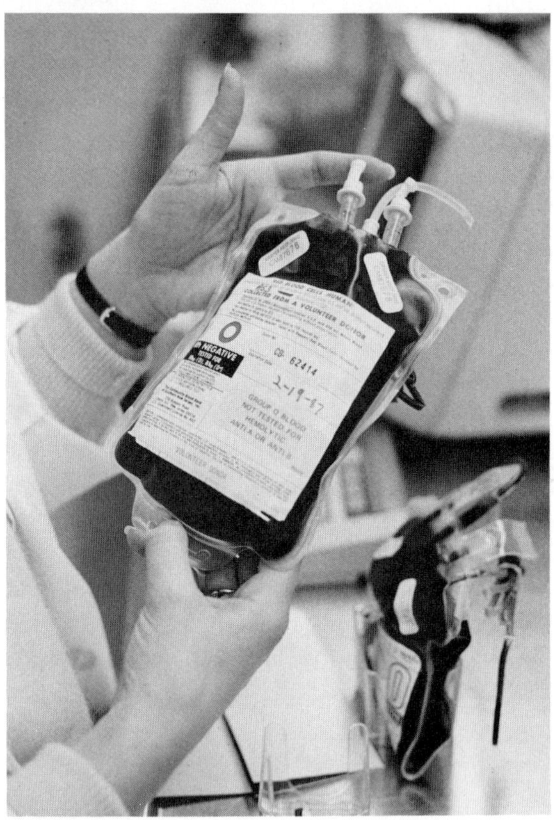

Figure 4–5. One important job of the medical laboratory technician is to check the accuracy of blood types to ensure patient safety. (Courtesy of the New Jersey Hospital Association. Photo by Cliff Moore.)

MLTs are graduates of two-year college programs. In addition to general education and science courses, the student technician receives supervised clinical experience in an approved laboratory.

Upon certification (by examination of the Board of Registry of the American Society of Clinical Pathologists), technicians may use the initials MLT (ASCP) after their names. Technicians who wish to become medical technologists may be able to transfer credits earned in their associate degree program and enroll in a university program. The American Medical Technologists also administer a certification examination and have developed a career ladder concept to allow advancement from medical laboratory technician to medical technologist.

Further information may be obtained from the American Society of Clinical Pathologists and the American Medical Technologists.

Cytotechnologist (CT [ASCP])*

Cytotechnology is the systematic study of cells. The cytotechnologist's role is to study cell samples taken from tissues in various sites of the body for evidence of cancer — a wild, disorderly growth of cells. Hopefully by the early discovery of abnormal cells, treatment can be given to destroy all such cells before they can be carried to other parts of the body.

The most common test for cancer is Papanicolaou's (Pap) smear used to detect a malignancy of the uterine cervix (the lower end of the uterus). **Saliva, spinal fluid**, sputum, and urine are among the other secretions studied.

Educational requirements for admission vary slightly from program to program, however, at least two years of college with concentration in the sciences is necessary. The educational program includes theory as well as supervised clinical study of normal human cells and abnormal cell alterations. A certificate or a degree will be awarded, depending upon the program. Certification by examination is available for cytotechnologists who have completed an accredited program or have met other requirements as established by the American Society of Clinical Pathologists, Board of Registry.

Additional information may be obtained from the American Society of Clinical Pathologists (see page 87) and from:

*Exception (see page 31).

American Society of Cytology
1015 Chestnut Street
Suite 1518
Philadelphia, Pennsylvania 19107

Histologic Technician (HT [ASCP])

Histology means the study of the microscopic structure of tissues. The histologic technician prepares portions of body tissues for microscopic examination. This is done by freezing a specimen and cutting it into paper thin slices that are mounted on slides and stained with special dyes to make the cells clearly visible under the microscope. The pathologist examines the slides and determines whether an abnormality is present. This may be done while the patient is in surgery and may determine the extent of the surgical procedure.

Histologic technicians are prepared in one- or two-year programs in a hospital laboratory or a community college. The major part of the program is spent in a clinical laboratory experience under the supervision of the pathologist and other faculty members.

Certification by examination is available through the Board of Registry of the American Society of Clinical Pathologists. Once certified, histologic technicians may use the letters HT (ASCP) after their names.

For more information, write to the American Society of Clinical Pathologists (see page 87).

DIAGNOSTIC MEDICAL EQUIPMENT PERSONNEL CLUSTER

Electrocardiograph Technician (EKG or ECG Technician)*

The means available to evaluate heart function have certainly improved since the days when the physician placed an ear on the patient's chest and listened to the heart sounds. Today, the physician listens to the patient's heart with the stethoscope but also has available the electro-

*Exception (see pages 31–32).

cardiograph (EKG or ECG) — possibly the single most important device for measuring heart function.

The technician positions both the patient and the equipment, attaches the electrodes to the patient's chest, arms, and legs, and sets the EKG dials. The machine records the electrical activity of the heart on a strip of specially coated graph paper. The strip is properly labeled with the patient's name and date and sent to the cardiologist for interpretation (**Fig. 4–6**).

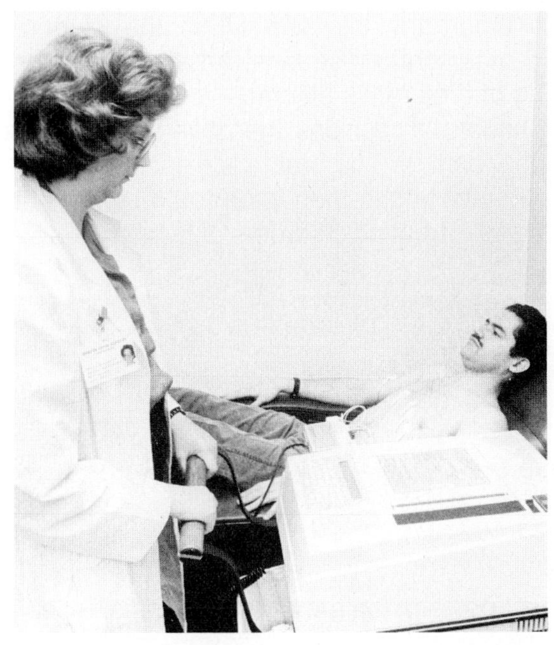

Figure 4–6. The electrocardiogram is an important device for measuring heart function. (Courtesy of Bridgeton Hospital, Bridgeton, N.J. Photo by Gary F. Cooper.

The EKG technician also maintains the equipment so that it is in proper working order. Major repairs are done by the manufacturer. Most EKG technicians are trained on the job in a hospital or by a physician.

For additional information, contact the personnel director of your local hospital or:

American Medical Association
Department of Allied Health Education and Accreditation
535 N. Dearborn Street
Chicago, Illinois 60610

Electroencephalograph Technologist (EEG Technologist or EEG Technician)*

Electroencephalography is essential in the diagnosis of epilepsy, brain tumors, and other brain diseases. An electroencephalogram (EEG) is a graphic tracing of the brain's electrical impulses.

The EEG technologist positions the patient, applies electrodes to the scalp, and sets the machine. The brain's electrical activity is then recorded on an EEG strip. The tracing is then interpreted by the neurologist, a physician who specializes in treating disorders of the nervous system (**Fig. 4–7**).

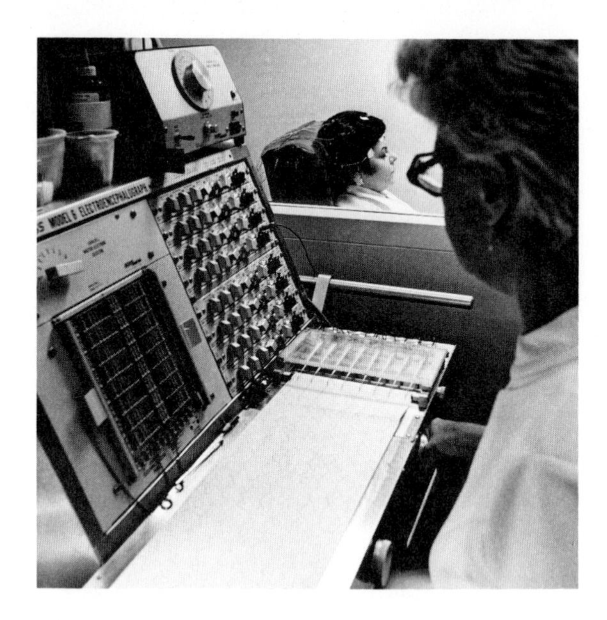

Figure 4–7. The technologist administers an EEG test to a patient. (Courtesy of the New Jersey Hospital Association; Mountainside Hospital. Photo by Irv Marks.)

*Exception (see pages 31–32).

Education may be obtained in a formal college program or in a hospital setting. The course length varies from one year to two years, and an associate degree may be awarded. Registration, by examination, is available for those technologists who meet the criteria of the American Board of Registration of EEG Technologists.

Additional information may be obtained from:

American Society of EEG Technologists
Executive Office
Sixth at Quint
Carroll, Iowa 51401

OPTICAL CLUSTER

The eye is a very delicate organ, difficult to examine because its internal structures lie behind the pupil — the window of the eye. To make it possible to examine these structures, certain medicated drops are used that dilate the pupil. With the aid of the **ophthalmoscope**, the physician can direct a light into the back of the eye and examine the interior structures. (Note that the eye is the only organ in the body where the blood vessels can be directly visualized by the examiner.) The condition of the blood vessels is a good indicator of the presence of certain **systemic diseases**, such as diabetes, arteriosclerosis, and hypertension.

Other precision instruments are used to examine the eye. Because both the eye and the examining equipment are so delicate, optical workers need steady hands and quick, skillful fingers. Since vision care specialists rely upon information from the patient to help them make a diagnosis, good communications skills and the ability to put the patient at ease are essential qualities (**Fig. 4–8**).

Two careers in this cluster carry the title of doctor — the ophthalmologist and optometrist.

Ophthalmologist (Oculist, Ophthalmic Physician)

Physicians who have graduated from medical school and have completed a residency in the treatment and prevention of eye diseases and injuries are called ophthalmologists. They use a variety of treatment

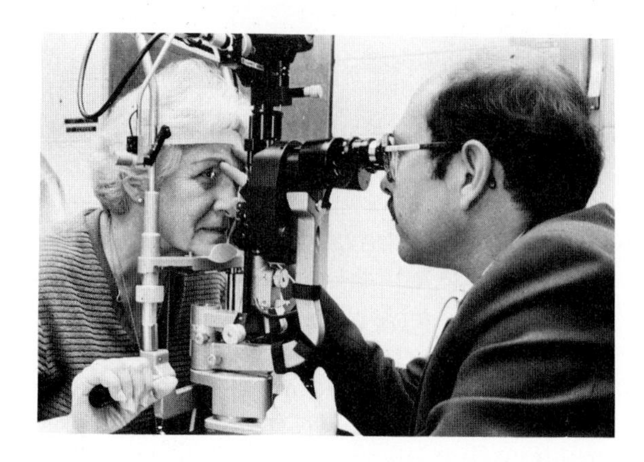

Figure 4–8. The ophthalmologist prepares the patient for treatment with the argon laser. (Courtesy of the New Jersey Hospital Association; Muhlenberg Hospital; Plainfield, N.J.)

methods, including prescription drugs, surgery, corrective exercises, contact lenses, and eyeglasses. An appreciation of the ophthalmologist's work may be gained by a brief description of the diagnosis and treatment of cataracts.

The lens of the eye is a transparent structure that lies behind the iris, colored part of eye, and the pupil. The lens focuses light rays on the retina to form an image which is then transmitted by the optic nerve to the brain. A cataract clouds the lens and makes it so opaque that the light rays cannot pass through. Patients with this condition do not see clearly, describing their vision in terms of looking out of a frosted or steamed window pane. The physician can observe the cataract with the ophthalmoscope. Cataracts can often be surgically removed with a laser beam on an outpatient (one-day) basis. A replacement lens may be implanted directly into the eye. Contact lenses and/or eyeglasses may also be prescribed to compensate for the now-missing lens.

For more information about this career, contact:

American Association of Ophthalmology
1100 17th Street, N.W.
Washington, D.C. 20036

Optometrist (Doctor of Optometry, OD)

The largest single group of vision specialists is made up of optometrists. They examine the eyes for visual deficiencies and signs of disease. If disease or injury is found, the patient is referred to an ophthalmologist for medical or surgical treatment. Optometrists prescribe eyeglasses, contact lenses, and corrective exercises to preserve or restore maximum visual efficiency. However, because they are not physicians, they do not use or prescribe medication.

A minimum of two years of college is a prerequisite to enter the four-year graduate school of optometry. This program includes courses in basic sciences; the anatomy, physiology, and pathology of the eye; optics (the use of lenses); and clinical experience. Licensure to practice optometry is required by every state. Optometrists may work in private or group practices or in interdisciplinary group practices with other health specialists. Job opportunities also exist in community health, research, teaching, and the armed forces.

For additional information, contact:

American Optometric Association
243 N. Lindberg Boulevard
St. Louis, Missouri 63141

AUDIOLOGIST/SPEECH PATHOLOGIST CLUSTER

Audiologists/speech pathologists are prepared in master's degree programs and are certified by the American Speech-Language-Hearing Association. They are employed in hospitals, schools, physicians' offices, rehabilitation centers, clinics, home health agencies, and health maintenance organizations.

The ability to speak depends upon the ability to hear. Children first learn to speak by repeating the sounds they hear. Is it any wonder that one of the first words in a toddler's vocabulary is "no"? Speech and hearing disorders may be caused by a variety of physical and emotional problems. Before the communication problem can be treated, the nature and extent of the disorder must be determined. Some of the conditions requiring speech therapy are **autism**, stroke, **cleft lip** and **cleft palate**, deafness, and impaired hearing.

Audiologists/speech pathologists use specific tests and instruments, such as the audiometer, to evaluate speech and hearing abilities. They must possess good speech and hearing themselves, since they rely upon the patient's verbal and nonverbal communication to complete the diagnostic evaluation.

More information may be obtained from:

American Speech-Language-Hearing Association
10801 Rockville Pike
Rockville, Maryland 20852

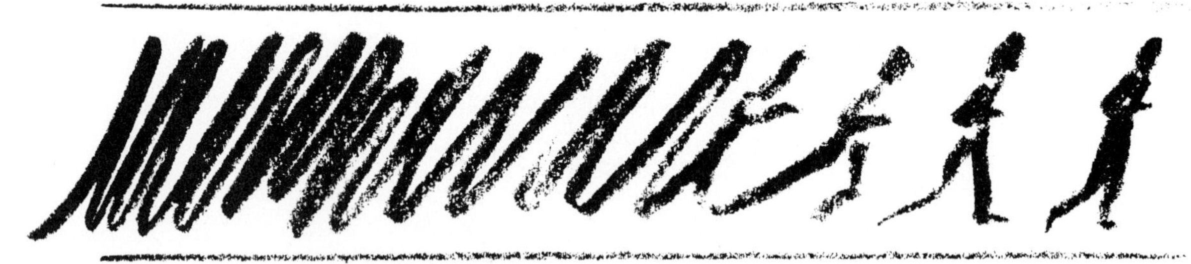

S·T·U·D·E·N·T A·C·T·I·V·I·T·I·E·S

1. Select one of the health career clusters described in this chapter for further research. Which schools in your area offer educational programs in these careers? Describe the program, including: entrance requirements, program length, tuition, fees, and available financial assistance. Record this information in your file.
2. Interview a health worker from the cluster you have selected. Gather the following information concerning the specific career: job description, educational preparation, beginning salary, licensure requirements, and job opportunities in the community. List what you feel are the advantages and disadvantages of this career.
3. List any diagnostic tests you may have had (chest x-ray, urinalysis, blood count) and note which diagnostic worker collected the specimen and/or performed the test.

4. Perform three of the following "hands-on" activities, assigned by your teacher. (Note: If you are not in a Health Occupations Education Course, try to arrange to observe the performance of some of these activities.)
   a. Perform urine analysis, including specific gravity, pH, and color and chemical reagent test sticks for glucose, albumen, and blood.
   b. Determine testing for blood type, Rh factor, hemoglobin, and sickle cell anemia.
   c. Observe a demonstration of an electrocardiograph.
   d. View developed x-ray films showing proper and improper exposures and technique.
   e. Perform the Home Eye Test for Preschoolers.

5. List the title of the diagnostic staff member who performs the following functions:
   a. Takes x-ray pictures
   b. Obtains blood samples
   c. Obtains urine specimens
   d. Examines blood samples
   e. Analyzes urine samples
   f. Takes electroencephalograms
   g. Interprets x-ray pictures
   h. Collects spinal fluid
   i. Interprets electro-encephalograms
   j. Analyzes spinal fluid
   k. Examines healthy eyes
   l. Examines and treats injured and diseased eyes
   m. Prescribes eyeglasses
   n. Takes electrocardiograms
   o. Interprets electrocardiograms
   p. Tests for hearing loss
   q. Stains small samples of tissue for microscopic examination.

Chapter 5

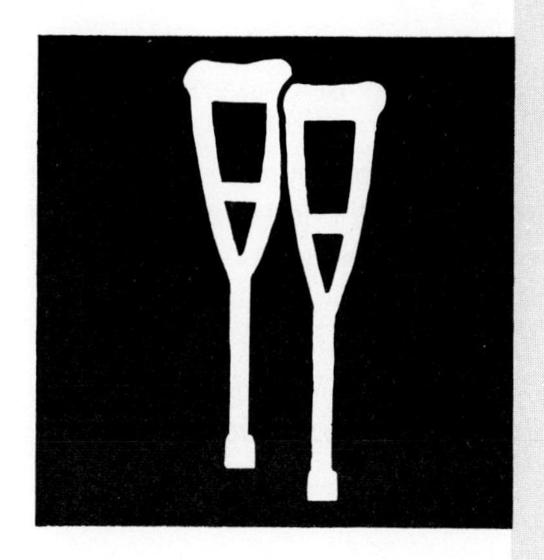

Therapeutic/ Restorative Careers

Objectives

After completing this chapter, you should be able to:

- Identify by name four of seven clusters in the Restorative/ Therapeutic group.
- Select five careers and identify three activities performed by each worker.
- Compare and contrast the relationship of the Restorative/Therapeutic Careers group to careers in Diagnostic and Direct Care.
- Identify by name 10 pieces of equipment used by workers in this group.
- Perform three of the suggested "hands-on" exploratory activities for the Restorative/Therapeutic group. Discuss your feelings about performing them.
- Compare the advantages and disadvantages of pursuing careers in this occupational group.

• Define at least 70 percent of the key terms listed in this chapter.

Key Terms

• **ADL (Activities of Daily Living)** Tasks which a person performs without conscious effort every day

• **apprenticeship** An educational program involving a minimum of 2,000 hours of on-the-job supervision and 144 hours per year of related instruction in technical subjects to supplement employment training in a skilled trade

• **controlled substance** A habit-forming drug that requires special handling and recording as per federal law

• **manual dexterity** Skill in using the hands and fingers

• **orthosis** A brace or other device applied to an existing part of the body to improve functioning

• **physiatrist** A physician who is a specialist in rehabilitation and physical medicine

• **prosthesis** An artificial substitute or replacement for a missing part

• **rehabilitation** Process whereby a person returns to maximum functioning capacity given the nature of the disability

• **restorative (tion)** Promoting a return to health

• **sensory perception** Ability to use one's senses effectively

• **therapy** Application of techniques or treatments to combat disease

THE THERAPEUTIC/RESTORATIVE CAREER CLUSTERS

In this chapter, we shall be looking at careers in the Therapeutic/Restorative group: Physical Therapy Cluster; Occupational Therapy Cluster; Respiratory Therapy Cluster; Specialized Rehabilitation Services Cluster; Reconstruction and Replacement Cluster; Dietetic Cluster; and Pharmacy Cluster. Those who do this work are specifically trained to help disabled patients return to normal life within the limitations of their handicaps. Because there are many kinds of handicaps, there is a wide range of occupations within this health care category.

During the **acute stage of an illness**, when the patient spends most of the time in bed, therapeutic and restorative care are often provided by members of the Direct Care Careers group. However, some therapeutic/restorative workers (e.g., **respiratory therapist**, **physical therapist**) come to the patient's bedside to administer special treatments. Others who may provide therapy during the acute phase of illness are the pharmacist and the **dietitian**, although they may have limited patient contact.

Following the acute stage of an illness, recovery becomes an active process involving the patient and health care personnel. Various departments of the health facility provide therapy: physical therapy, occupational therapy, speech and hearing therapy, recreation therapy, dance therapy, and music therapy. Whatever specific form it takes, the essential purpose is always the same — to help the patient, through various kinds of training, aids, and adjustments, to resume the normal activities of independent living. A course of therapy must be designed for each individual case, so therapeutic programs are always prescribed by the patient's physician.

Physical therapy helps to restore muscular strength and coordination through exercise and the use of special devices, such as braces, crutches, and artificial limbs. Many of these devices (prostheses and orthoses) are designed and manufactured by therapeutic/restorative workers.

Occupational therapists teach useful and creative skills to patients who have either physical or emotional illnesses. Therapists in various specialized fields assist those who must make difficult adjustments to physical handicaps, such as blindness or paralysis, or to chronic or prolonged illness. They design and carry out programs of skill training and adaptation and retrain patients in those skills and functions that must be relearned following an illness or disability.

Following an illness or injury, some patients may require special assistance in readjusting to home, family, the community, and employment. Social workers, vocational rehabilitation counselors, psychologists, and psychiatrists provide this help.

Since there are so many occupations in this group of careers, it is difficult to compile a list of personal characteristics that will apply to all. In most cases, manual dexterity is an essential quality. Some workers rarely see patients (e.g., the dental laboratory technician), so the ability to work with people is not essential for this career. But others, including therapists and their auxiliaries, spend almost all of their time with patients and must be able to establish good personal relationships.

Therapeutic careers offer opportunities to use a variety of talents, interests, and skills. Some jobs require a great deal of physical stamina and patience; some demand ingenuity and creative talent in the arts.

The health workers who cooperate in a plan to restore body function and independent living constitute the rehabilitation team. Most of the careers discussed in this chapter will be represented on this team, which is headed by a physiatrist — a physician who is a specialist in rehabilitation and physical medicine.

General information on the many careers in this group may be obtained from:

National Easter Seal Society
2023 West Ogden Avenue
Chicago, Illinois 60612

National Rehabilitation Association
1522 K Street, N.W.
Washington, D.C. 20005

HEALTH CARE WORKERS ON THE JOB

It was a hot, humid day. Kevin and his buddies climbed into his pickup truck and drove to Greenwood Lake for an afternoon swim. The water was cool and refreshing. After some roughhousing, Kevin challenged Don to a race from the end of the dock to the raft in the center of the lake. Both were members of their high school swim team, the current state champion. The other boys counted off for the race to begin, "One, two, three — go!"

Kevin and Don ran to the end of the dock and dove in. Don swam swiftly toward the raft, but Kevin did not surface! After several minutes, the boys on the dock jumped into the water and began diving for Kevin. They grabbed his body and dragged him to shore. He was not breathing but did have a faint pulse. Mouth-to-mouth resuscitation was started, and an ambulance was called.

Kevin regained consciousness before he was taken to the hospital. His legs felt dead, and he could not move them. He remembered hitting his back on a log under the water.

He was admitted to the Intensive Care Unit of Greenwood Hospital. X-ray studies revealed a compression fracture of the lumbar vertebrae, causing permanent damage to the spinal cord and lower limb paralysis. Kevin required expert care from the physicians and nurses to prevent complications and to prepare him for rehabilitation.

When Kevin's condition became stable, he was transferred to a rehabilitation center in a nearby city. This center was quite different from the hospital. Meals were served in a dining room; patients assumed responsibility for taking their own showers; and everyone was up and about, actively participating in a rehabilitation program.

Kevin met with the physiatrist and other members of the rehabilitation team (physical therapist, occupational therapist, recreation therapist, orthotist, nurse, and social worker). Together, they established the following rehabilitation goals:

1. Strengthen arm muscles for crutchwalking.
2. Fit leg braces for walking.

3. Maintain balanced nutrition for strength and energy.
4. Prevent complications, such as pneumonia, muscle weakness, and decubiti (bed sores).
5. Continue education, and try to complete senior year of high school.

Each team member developed a care plan to reach these goals:

1. The physiatrist tested Kevin's physical ability to determine the extent of injury and supervised the rehabilitation program.
2. The nursing staff helped Kevin to master in-bed and chair exercises to strengthen his arm muscles. They also took measures to prevent complications such as decubiti, pneumonia, and joint deformities.
3. The physical therapy staff taught Kevin to use a wheelchair as a preliminary means of mobility. When his braces arrived, the physical therapist taught him to use them to walk between parallel bars and, finally, to walk with crutches.
4. The occupational therapy staff planned activities that allowed Kevin to use his upper arm and trunk muscles. He learned woodworking, weaving at a large loom, and printing on the printing press.
5. The recreation therapy team got Kevin "in the swim" at the center's pool through water activities and exercises which were planned by the physical and recreation therapists.
6. The orthotist measured and fitted Kevin with braces designed to strengthen and support his legs for crutchwalking.
7. The social worker arranged for Kevin to have tutors so that he could complete his high school education.
8. The vocational rehabilitation counselor kept in touch with Kevin, his parents, and the rehabilitation team to plan for his activities after high school. Kevin had expressed an interest in a health career. Through a testing and counseling program, Kevin was able to investigate various careers and to make a realistic choice.

Kevin went home every weekend, for Thanksgiving, and for a week at Christmas. By Easter, he was back at school and graduated with his class in June.

Through the work of the Therapeutic/Restorative Careers group, Kevin was returned, as far as possible, to full functioning. He is now enrolled in a community college program where he is studying to become a medical laboratory technician.

PHYSICAL THERAPY CLUSTER

Physical Therapist (Registered Physical Therapist, RPT)

Physical therapists do not prescribe or administer medications. Instead, they use techniques of exercise, massage, and applications of heat, cold, water, electricity, and ultrasound. For example, heat applied by means of radiant heat lamps, electric heating pads, or paraffin baths reduces pain, relaxes muscles, and improves blood circulation. Ice placed on an injured area reduces swelling and pain and stops hemorrhage. When used, ultrasound eases inflamed joints and nerves.

The equipment in the physical therapy department includes parallel bars, stationary bicycles, weights and pulleys, dumbbells, whirlpools, and, often, a swimming pool. Swimming and water exercises are a major part of many treatment programs. So is posture training, because orthopedic deformities can develop in bones that are healing.

After a serious illness or injury, many patients need retraining before they can walk again or perform the routine tasks of bathing, dressing, grooming, and eating. Physical therapists use various mechanical devices and manual treatments to help patients develop and strengthen muscular coordination (**Fig. 5–1**).

Before designing a therapeutic program, the therapist evaluates the patient's muscle strength, balance, range of joint motion, motor abilities, sensory perception, and ability to understand and follow instructions. Based on these findings, the therapist determines the patient's readiness to participate in an activity program, such as walking with the help of crutches.

The goals of therapy are then determined. For example, the physiatrist and the therapist may decide that the patient should be able to walk using a cane within a certain time and should be able to perform the activities of daily living (ADL). ADL are those tasks which a healthy person performs without conscious effort every day, such as dressing, bathing, grooming, and eating. A plan of treatment is then designed to accomplish these goals. This plan may include exercises to strengthen leg muscles, walking between the parallel bars to improve coordination and build confidence, and similar activities. The patient also learns how to do other activities with the aid of a cane, such as climbing stairs, and getting into and

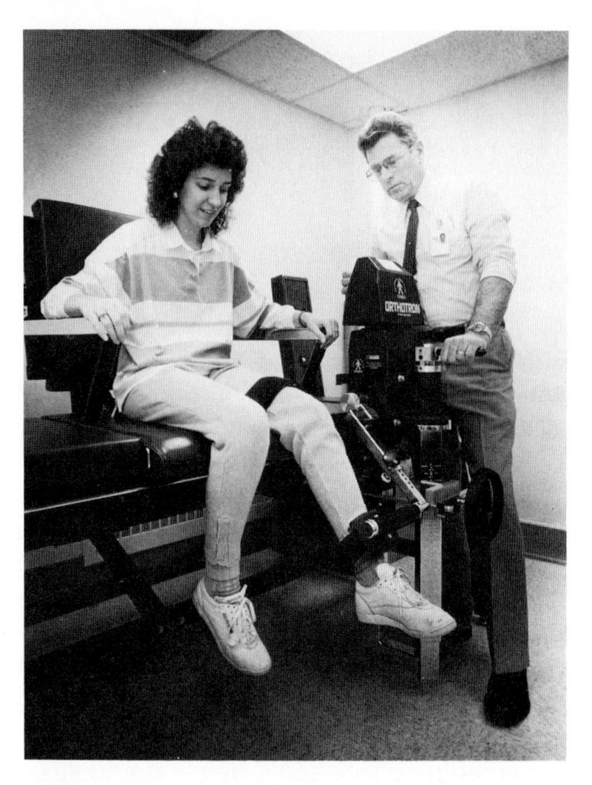

Figure 5–1. Muscle strength is evaluated by the physical therapist. (Courtesy of Bridgeton Hospital, Bridgeton, N.J. Photo by Gary Cooper.)

out of the bathtub or shower. Initially, the therapist helps the patient to perform these tasks. As the patient gains increasing independence, assistance is gradually withdrawn (**Fig. 5–2**).

Therapists try to set realistic goals for their patients. Treatment is conducted in a series of graduated steps that are always within the patient's range of capability. Sometimes walking, even with special devices, such as canes, walkers, braces, and crutches, is not possible. In that case, the patient is taught to travel by wheelchair and to perform ADL even though mobility is greatly restricted.

Those who benefit from physical therapy include handicapped children, amputees, arthritics, and those with spinal cord and brain injuries, fractures, and burns.

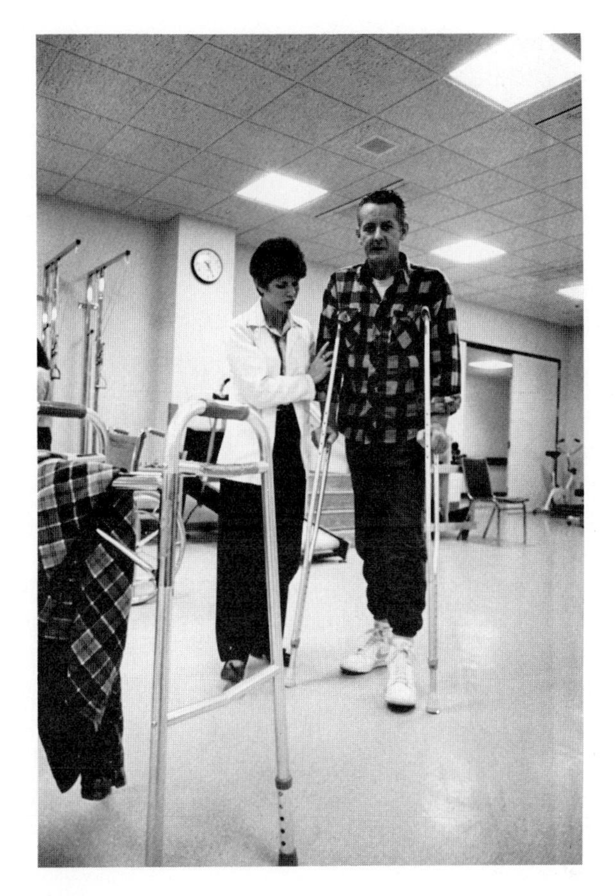

Figure 5–2. The physical therapist teaches the client to use crutches properly. (Courtesy of St. Mary Hospital, Langhorne, Pa.)

Physical therapists, employed by home health agencies, provide therapy to patients in their own homes. This is a valuable service to the many people who are homebound and cannot travel to a hospital for therapy. An additional benefit to these patients is learning to perform ADL in their own homes.

Programs in physical therapy are conducted in colleges and universities. They offer three types of educational programs: a four-year bachelor's degree to the high school graduate; a 12-month (certificate) program to those who hold a bachelor's degree in another field; and a master's degree program to those with a bachelor's degree who meet special entrance requirements. In all states, physical therapists must be licensed to practice. There never seem to be enough physical therapists to meet the demand. As a result of this shortage, two health careers, physical therapy assistant and physical therapy aide, have been developed.

Physical Therapy Assistant

Physical therapy assistants are skilled health technicians who work under the therapist's direction and assist with patient care. Their responsibilities include teaching patients to walk with canes and crutches using proper gait and instructing them to perform ADL. Assistants also perform selected treatments, supervise exercises, and maintain equipment and supplies.

Programs for physical therapy assistants are conducted in community colleges and technical institutes. These two-year programs award an associate degree in applied science. Students take courses in general education, anatomy, physiology, biology, and physical therapy assisting. They also receive clinical practice in a hospital physical therapy department. In some states, assistants are licensed to practice. Those who wish to become physical therapists may return to college to complete the preparation for this degree and then may apply for licensure as physical therapists.

Physical Therapy Aide

Physical therapy aides carry out the nontechnical duties in the physical therapy department. They prepare treatment rooms for patients receiving therapy, clean whirlpool tanks, and stock linens. Aides order supplies, such as crutches, canes, walkers, and other devices needed by therapists and assistants. A physical therapy aide is prepared on the job by the employer or completes an educational program offered by a vocational/technical school.

For further information on careers in physical therapy, write:

American Physical Therapy Association
1111 North Fairfax Street
Alexandria, Virginia 22314

Athletic Trainer

Are you an avid sports fan? Then the career of athletic trainer may be the one for you. The role of this health professional is to help athletes to perform their skills in competitive sports by using techniques to prevent injury. These techniques include devising and supervising muscle strengthening and conditioning exercises, checking equipment for possible problems, and taping joints particularly susceptible to injury prior to an athletic event. Making injury pads, installing face guards, and assisting in the purchase and fitting of new equipment are other responsibilities assumed by the athletic trainer.

They are among the first health professionals at the accident scene to treat an injured athlete. Proper emergency care is critical to preventing further injury. Following the physician's examination, trainers use a variety of treatments for sports injuries. They use applications of heat and cold by means of whirlpool baths or ice packs and apply elastic bandages to injured **extremities**. Following the initial treatment, athletic trainers carry out a rehabilitation program developed by the physician, including exercise, massage, and other therapies. Additional duties include keeping the locker room clean and stocked with necessary supplies.

Preparing for this career requires a college degree with emphasis on anatomy, physiology, and kinesiology — the study of movement of the body in relation to anatomy. Following graduation from college and obtaining certification by the American Red Cross in first aid and cardiopulmonary resuscitation (CPR) and successful completion of an emergency medical technician (EMT) program, athletic trainers may seek certification from the National Athletic Trainer Association. Once certified, they must continue to maintain and update their knowledge and skills through approved continuing education programs.

For further information about this growing field, write:

The National Athletic Trainers Association
1001 East 4th Street
Greenville, North Carolina 27834

American Athletic Trainers Association
and Certification Board
600 West Duarte Road
Arcadia, California 91006

OCCUPATIONAL THERAPY CLUSTER

Occupational Therapist (Registered Occupational Therapist, OTR)

Purposeful activity, rather than mere busywork, is a major part of the treatment plan for certain emotional and physical disorders. Occupational therapy, a plan of directed creative activity, helps patients to develop new interests and gain self-confidence. The mastery of new skills that strengthen muscles and improve fine muscle coordination and dexterity, especially of the arms, hands, and fingers, helps the patient to become independent in the activities of daily living. This provides the basis for further training that may lead to employment and total independence. The goal of independence varies for each individual. To a young man or woman, it may mean gainful employment; to a child, a return to school; to an older adult, a more active life. The occupational therapist tailors the treatment plan to match these individual goals. To do this, familiarity with each patient's background and interests as well as knowledge of the handicap are essential.

Therapists also teach people to adapt to physical handicaps. For example, when patients are unable to eat with regular utensils, they are taught how to use special self-help devices, such as a guard to keep food from slipping off the plate.

Occupational therapy helps emotionally disabled persons to progress toward psychological adjustment. Many activities are designed to allow patients to express their emotions (anger, fear, unworthiness, etc.) in a harmless, socially acceptable manner. One such activity might be sanding a length of wood — the harder a patient sands, the more anger and hostility is released! (This same activity could also be used with a physically disabled person to strengthen the wrist and arm muscles.) Patients with emotional illnesses are also encouraged to paint, sculpt, or draw as ways of expressing their fears and anxieties.

Occupational therapy is sometimes described as "curing by doing." When patients perform activities or tasks independently, they are taking an active and positive role in their own recovery process. In other words, their cure begins when they start doing the prescribed activity.

The concept of "curing by doing" is not new. It originated with the Roman physician, Galen, in A.D. 172 and has been used in therapeutic programs ever since. It became a widely used approach after World War

II, when occupational therapists were in great demand to train disabled veterans in new skills and to help them make the difficult physical and emotional adjustments to living with handicaps.

Occupational therapists rely on arts and crafts in patient therapy, weaving, knitting, painting, ceramics, leathercraft, woodwork, and macrame. Therapists test the patient's hand, finger, wrist, and arm to assess coordination, dexterity, and strength before beginning any type of skill training, such as typing or machine sewing. In addition, homemaking skills are taught to both men and women so they can assume housekeeping responsibilities when they return home (**Fig. 5–3**).

The equipment used in occupational therapy is as diverse as the needs of the patients. It might include looms, checkers, typewriter, balls

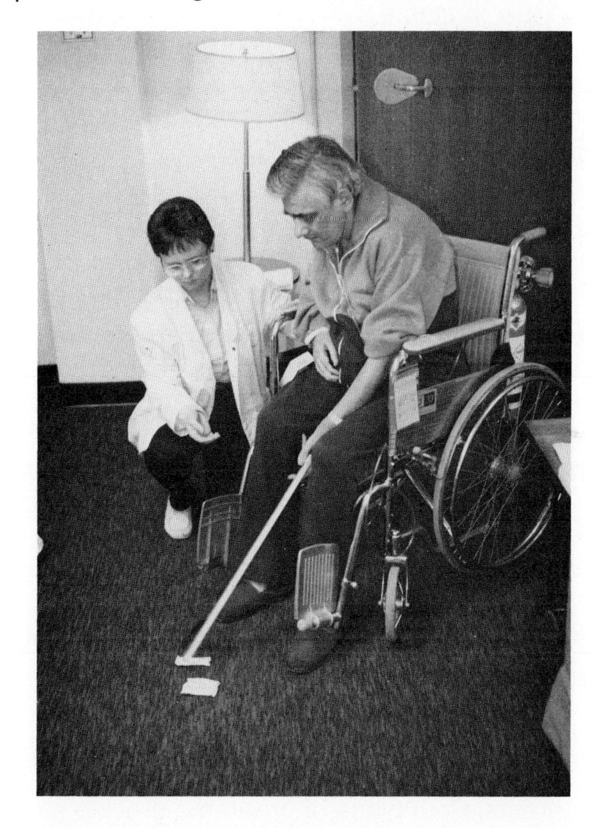

Figure 5–3. The client must often re-learn how to perform various tasks. (Courtesy of St. Lawrence Rehabilitation Center, Lawrenceville, N.J.)

and blocks, a potter's wheel, modeling clay, printing press, saws, nuts, bolts, hammers, and nails.

Occupational therapy patients are of all ages, from small children to older adults, and their disabilities are just as varied — arthritis, stroke, birth defects, cerebral palsy, psychiatric illness, heart disease, orthopedic problems, spinal cord injuries, and learning disabilities.

Programs in occupational therapy are conducted in colleges that award a bachelor's degree. Six to nine months of these four-year programs are spent in the hospital and other community health care agencies gaining clinical experience under the supervision of the college faculty. There are also postbaccalaureate certificate and master's degree programs for those who hold degrees in other fields. Graduates are eligible to take the national certification examination given by the American Occupational Therapy Association. After passing the examination, the therapist is qualified to practice as an OTR and to become a registered member of the Association. About one-third of the states require occupational therapists to be licensed.

Occupational Therapy Assistant (Certified Occupational Therapy Assistant, COTA)

Occupational therapy assistants extend the services of the therapist by assuming some of the teaching duties and by helping patients to accomplish various activities. They instruct patients in arts and crafts and assist them in working with large floor looms, printing presses, and other equipment. At the beginning of the therapy session, the assistant prepares and lays out all of the work material needed by each patient. The tools, supplies, and equipment are maintained by the assistant, who may also teach ADL.

Programs that prepare occupational therapy assistants include two-year associate degree programs in community colleges or one-year vocational school programs. Both types of programs provide supervised clinical experiences. Graduates of programs approved by the AOTA (American Occupational Therapy Association) are eligible to take the certification examination and become Association members.

Occupational Therapy Aide

Occupational therapy aides work in rehabilitation programs in hospitals and other institutions. They help therapists and assistants with routine duties, including cleaning, stocking, and ordering equipment and supplies. Aides are prepared in programs offered by vocational/technical schools or trained on the job by therapists. Aides always work under the supervision of the occupational therapist.

Additional information on occupational therapy careers may be obtained from:

American Occupational Therapy Association
1383 Piccard Drive
Rockville, Maryland 20850

RESPIRATORY THERAPY CLUSTER

Respiratory Therapist (RRT)

Breathing is an automatic function; we inhale and exhale at a regular rate, usually without any effort or strain. But when breathing is irregular, labored, or interrupted, great discomfort and irreversible damage to vital organs may occur.

If this happens, the patient requires assistance so that normal breathing and heart-lung function will be restored. Oxygen is administered by the respiratory therapist who follows the physician's orders. This gas may be given in many ways — through a face mask, ventilator, or a nasal cannula. Other medical gases such as carbon dioxide are also used in the treatment of respiratory problems. Like oxygen, these may be administered alone or in combination with medications that are dispensed as an aerosol or mist.

Respiratory function tests conducted by the therapist determine the effect of disease upon the lungs and the effectiveness of therapy. All treatments and tests are ordered by the physician.

One such test measures vital capacity — the ability to inhale enough air into the lungs to breathe efficiently. After inhaling deeply, the patient blows out all the air into an empty bag or deflated balloon attached to a measuring device. The volume of expelled air is recorded on the device to give an immediate reading of vital capacity (**Fig. 5–4**).

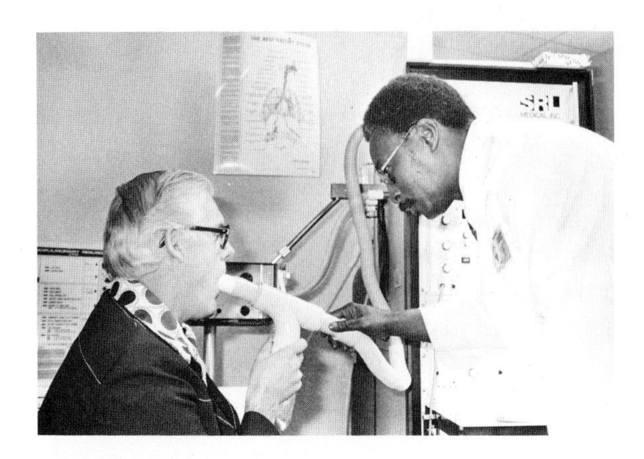

Figure 5–4. Measuring vital capacity of the lungs requires careful attention by the respiratory therapist. (Courtesy of New Jersey Hospital Association, Hamilton Hospital, Hamilton, N.J. Photo by John A. Leone.)

Besides indicating existing respiratory problems, this test gives an early warning of conditions such as emphysema so that early treatment can begin.

Therapists teach patients breathing exercises to improve respiratory function and explain the proper use of respiratory equipment at home. In addition, they teach hospital staff skills in providing respiratory care to patients. They are also responsible for the management and supervision of their department and for the in-service education of the hospital staff. Therapists may specialize in particular aspects of education, research, and patient care.

Two-year programs in respiratory therapy are offered by hospitals and community colleges. There are also four-year programs leading to a bachelor's degree. These programs are approved by the Committee on Allied Health Education and Accreditation of the American Medical Association. Registration is available from the National Board of Respiratory Care upon completion of special requirements.

Respiratory Therapy Technician (Certified Respiratory Therapy Technician, CRTT)

The training of technicians emphasizes the techniques of therapy. They administer routine respiratory therapy and care. They initiate continuous oxygen therapy and visit all patients regularly to check the equipment for proper functioning. Special treatments, such as the administration of medical gases under pressure, are given by the technician. These treatments help patients to cough and expel any material in the lungs that could interfere with breathing. Ordering supplies, maintaining equipment, billing, and keeping records are additional responsibilities.

Educational programs for respiratory technicians are usually one year in length. These are offered by vocational/technical schools, community colleges, and hospitals. Certification as a respiratory technician is available after completion of the required educational program and job experience.

Respiratory Therapy Assistant

The primary work of respiratory therapy assistants is to clean, disinfect, and sterilize equipment, though they also perform routine clerical duties. They have very limited patient contact. Assistants are educated in short-term programs in vocational schools or on the job.

Information about careers in respiratory therapy may be obtained from:

American Association for Respiratory Therapy
1720 Regal Row
Dallas, Texas 75235

SPECIALIZED REHABILITATION SERVICES CLUSTER

Physically and emotionally handicapped persons may benefit from a wide range of rehabilitation services, depending on their needs. These services include recreation, music, and dance therapy; corrective therapy; homemaking training; and speech and language therapy. This is the most diversified cluster in all the Therapeutic/Restorative Careers — perhaps in all of the health occupations groups.

Recreation Therapist

The word "recreation" suggests another word — fun. Can therapy be fun? Of course! Have you ever watched a game of wheelchair basketball?

It offers excitement, exercise, challenge, and a good time. Recreation therapy plays an important part in rehabilitation by promoting the social, emotional, and physical well-being of the handicapped person. A wide range of activities — games, sports, drama, crafts, indoor parties, beach parties and cookouts — is planned and carried out by recreation therapists. Therapy takes place in hospitals, nursing homes, senior centers, summer camps, and rehabilitation centers. People of all ages enjoy and benefit from recreation therapy — those who are permanently institutionalized as well as those who will be returning to the community (**Fig. 5–5**).

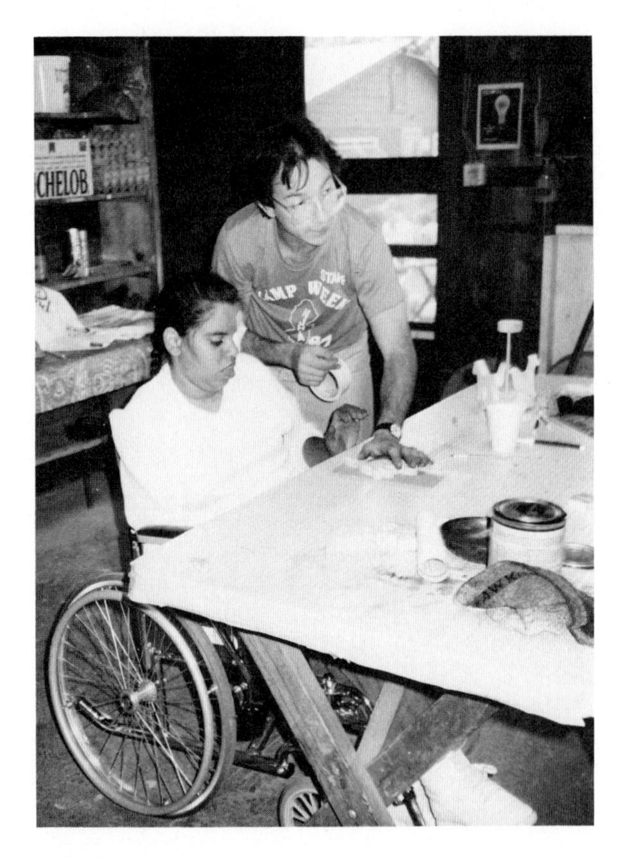

Figure 5–5. The recreation therapist is employed in a variety of settings, such as this special camp for handicapped persons. (Courtesy of St. Lawrence Rehabilitation Center, Lawrenceville, N.J.)

Recreation therapists are prepared in college programs that offer a degree in therapeutic recreation or may earn a degree in physical education supplemented by courses in art, music, and drama. Master's degree programs, with therapeutic recreation as a major, are also available. Almost all programs provide internships or on-the-job clinical experiences under the supervision of experienced recreation therapists.

Recreation Therapy Aides

Aides are employed to assist with the activities of recreation therapy. Some of their duties include: maintaining equipment and supplies; scheduling recreation activities; decorating for holiday celebrations; and ordering food and beverages for parties. Aides are trained on the job by the recreation therapist.

For further information about careers in recreation therapy, contact:

National Therapeutic Recreation Society
3101 Park Center Drive
Alexandria, Virginia 22302

Music Therapist

The influence of music toward effecting change in mood and behavior has been recognized for centuries. Physicians in classical Greece were aware that music had soothing and calming effects upon disturbed persons. In Biblical times, David played the harp and sang to cheer King Saul. As a part of everyday life, music lifts the spirits, quickens the step, eases loneliness, and adds brightness to dull routines. Music therapy means the methodical use of music as part of the treatment of persons with social, emotional, and physical handicaps. The therapist plans and directs vocal, instrumental, rhythm, and listening activities for patients. Therapists work with all age groups although handicapped children make up the largest group currently served by music therapists.

This career offers opportunities for serious musicians, because it gives them the opportunity to perform music, to improvise, and to work with other musicians. Proficiency in at least one musical instrument is required, and the ability to play a portable instrument, such as the guitar, accordion, or flute, is desirable. Programs in music therapy lead to a bachelor's degree. A six-month period of clinical experience in an approved music therapy program in a hospital or community mental health center takes place after the college course work is completed but before the degree is granted.

More information regarding careers in music therapy may be obtained from:

National Association for Music Therapy
1133 15th Street, N.W.
Washington, D.C. 20005

Dance Therapist

Dance is used to help people express feelings and emotions, while providing movement and exercise that is therapeutic and enjoyable. A person's physical coordination often is improved by moving rhythmically to music. Dancing also is a part of the resocialization process for emotionally disturbed persons.

Dance therapists are prepared in master's degree programs where they study dance therapy (including special techniques for various client populations), develop administrative and research skills, and receive a supervised clinical experience in a patient care area. To become a dance therapist, it is necessary to have a creative talent in dance. This is an exciting career and a relatively new one. Because it is new, there are only a few educational programs currently available.

A listing of schools and additional information on dance therapy careers may be obtained from:

American Dance Therapy Association
2000 Century Plaza
Columbia, Maryland 21044

Corrective Therapist

In the later stages of physical rehabilitation, some patients may benefit from special training that is not included in standard treatment plans. Corrective therapy is not the same as physical therapy, although corrective therapists do help patients to function as efficiently as possible. However, their treatment builds upon the work already completed in physical and occupational therapy programs. They teach physically handicapped people to drive specially equipped cars, guide blind persons in the initial stages of training for independent movement, and teach patients to use braces and artificial limbs.

Most therapists have a degree in physical education and have completed a period of clinical experience. This career is highly specialized, and the opportunities for employment are growing due to the increased awareness of the needs of handicapped and disabled persons. Corrective therapists work mainly in veterans hospitals, rehabilitation centers, nursing homes, and special schools and centers for the handicapped.

More information may be obtained from:

American Kinesiotherapy Association, Inc.
259-08 148th Road
Rosedale, New York 11422

Home Economists in Rehabilitation

Sometimes people need help to learn or relearn homemaking skills after an accident, injury, or illness. The person with a heart condition needs to learn work simplification techniques so that everyday activities can be carried out independently. Very often, a handicapped person may have to learn these techniques so that another family member can assume the role of breadwinner.

A college undergraduate program in home economics, with concentration in rehabilitation, is the preparation for this career.

More information may be obtained from:

American Home Economics Association
2010 Massachusetts Avenue, N.W.
Washington, D.C. 20036

Speech-Language Pathologist and Audiologist

It is estimated that in the United States one of every ten persons has a speech, language, or hearing problem. Speech-language pathologists help clients, such as children with cleft palates or cerebral palsy and stroke victims, to communicate in as nearly normal a way as possible. Audiologists test hearing-impaired clients and help them select appropriate hearing aids. They are employed in hospitals, schools, home health agencies, clinics, rehabilitation centers, and in private practice (**Fig. 5–6**).

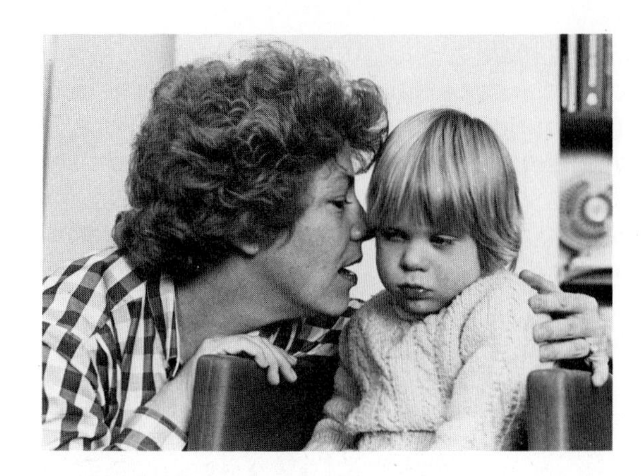

Figure 5–6. A close relationship often develops between the speech therapist and client. (Courtesy of Morristown Memorial Hospital, Morristown, N.J. Photo by Grace Moore.)

Most of these health career workers have master's degrees in this field. Many states now require speech-language pathologists and audiologists to be licensed. Certification is available from the American Speech-Language-Hearing Association, which also offers more information about career opportunities. Write:

American Speech-Language-Hearing Association
10801 Rockville Pike
Rockville, Maryland 20852

RECONSTRUCTION AND REPLACEMENT CLUSTER

The men and women working in this cluster are artisans who construct the full or additional replacement parts that are essential to successful rehabilitation. Their products include artificial limbs, braces, dentures, and eyeglasses.

Orthotist and Prosthetist

Orthotists make and fit orthopedic braces that correct physical defects, provide support, and increase functional ability. Prosthetists make and fit artificial limbs to replace those amputated due to accident, surgery, or congenital defect (**Fig. 5–7**). Orthotists and prosthetists design these appliances, which are fashioned of foam, leather, steel, or plastic, according to medical prescription. The devices are made to order for individual clients and must be fitted and refitted during the construction period. The inspection, repair, and maintenance of prostheses and orthoses are ongoing responsibilities of the orthotist and prosthetist.

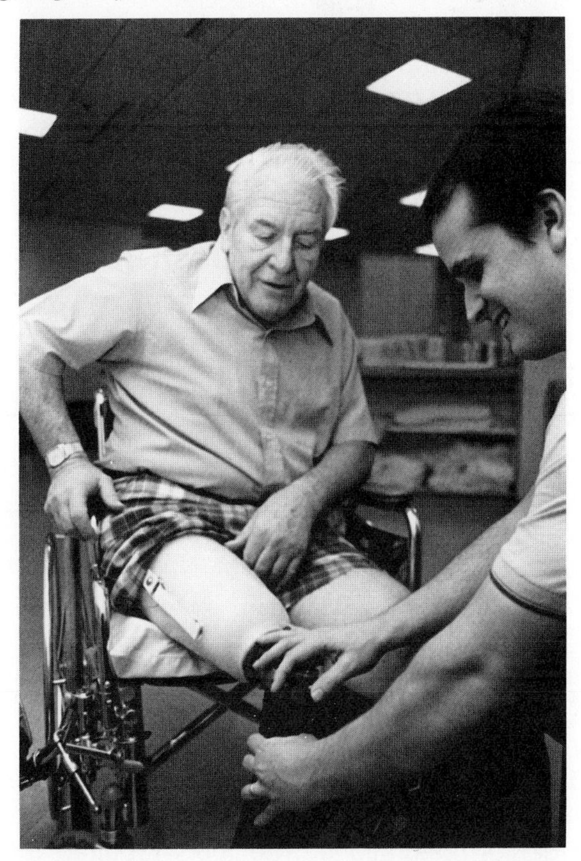

Figure 5–7. A properly fitted artificial leg is the goal of the prosthetist. (Courtesy of St. Mary Hospital, Langhorne, Pa.)

In order to meet specific patient needs, this work demands skill in handling tools as well as true creative talent.

Before 1975, orthotists and prosthetists were prepared in a four-year apprenticeship program. They took some specified college courses and were certified after passing an examination given by the American Board for Certification in Orthotics and Prosthetics. Today, educational programs, located in community colleges and universities, include classroom work and actual shop work.

Orthotic/Prosthetic Assistant

The orthotic/prosthetic assistant works under the direct supervision of the orthotist/prosthetist and shares responsibility for making and fitting appliances. A high school graduate who has completed three years of an accredited apprenticeship program is eligible to take the examination to become certified as a prosthetic assistant.

Orthotic/Prosthetic Technician

These technicians are responsible for making either parts of braces or prostheses or for the complete device. They do not fit the devices. Technicians must complete a two-year preparation program in the orthotist/prosthetist's workshop and must pass the technician certification examination.

For further information, contact:

American Orthotic and Prosthetic Association
1440 North Street, N.W.
Washington, D.C. 20005

Dental Laboratory Technician

The men and women who make and repair dentures, crowns, bridges, and inlays according to the dentist's prescription are called dental laboratory technicians. They use gold, silver, plastics, and ceramics in the preparation of dental restorations. The tools required for this work are quite delicate. Excellent color discrimination is essential because the technician must recognize fine degrees of shading when matching artificial teeth to natural ones. Patience and meticulous attention to detail are essential qualities. Since the work is not strenuous, this is a health career well suited to the physically challenged (**Fig. 5–8**).

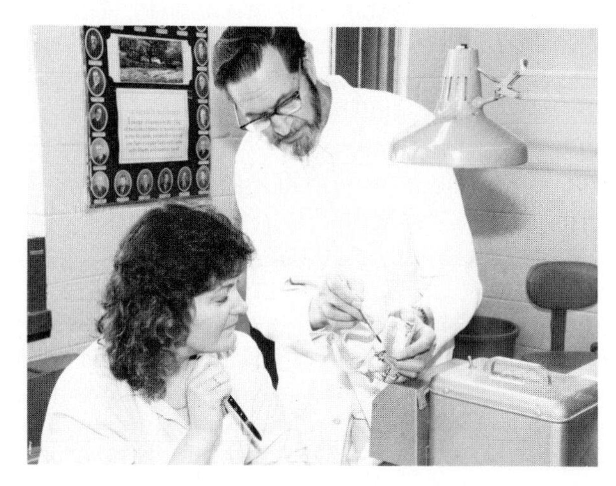

Figure 5–8. The dental laboratory technician instructor explains the details of a properly constructed set of dentures. (Courtesy of Camden County Voc/Tech School, Sicklerville, N.J.)

Dental laboratory technicians learn their skills on the job as apprentices in a dental laboratory or in formal educational programs of two years' duration. These programs are offered by vocational/technical schools and community colleges, with the first year spent on academic studies and the second on supervised training in a dental laboratory.

More information about this career may be obtained from:

National Association of Dental Laboratories
3801 Mount Vernon Avenue
Alexandria, Virginia 22305

Optician and Optical Technician

The history of eyeglasses probably began as early as the tenth century in China. In 1629, a guild of British spectacle makers was granted a charter that permitted them to establish a business for the manufacture of spectacles. Benjamin Franklin is credited with the invention of bifocal glasses, which he himself wore. Dispensing opticians fit eyeglasses and lenses exactly according to the optometrist's or ophthalmologist's prescription.

Because of the popularity of contact lenses, dispensing opticians have greater scope of responsibility. Contact lenses will fit correctly only if the shape of the cornea is accurately measured. The wearer must be taught how to insert, remove, and care for the lenses. Periodic checkups by the optician are needed to verify that the contact lenses continue to fit properly and that they are crystal clear.

Dispensing opticians are prepared in a one- or two-year program offered by a community college or vocational school. Some opticians learn on the job through an apprenticeship. In some states, opticians must be licensed to practice. Many dispensing opticians operate their own businesses.

Optical technicians follow blueprints and do the actual grinding of the lens surfaces, either in a dispensing optician's shop (benchroom) or in the benchroom of a large company that manufactures corrective lenses.

Optical technicians usually are prepared in a two-year apprenticeship program or, in some instances, a school of opticianry, a vocational/technical school, or a community college.

More information about careers in opticianry may be obtained from:

Opticians Association of America
10341 Democracy Lane
P.O. Box 10110
Fairfax, Virginia 22030

Orthoptist

Crossed eyes hinder proper vision and thereby interfere with learning. The orthoptist is a specialist in the treatment of crossed eyes. Rather than employing surgery for the condition, the orthoptist prescribes exercises that increase and strengthen coordination of both eyes so that they focus properly. The orthoptist is primarily an instructor, educating those — especially children and young adults — who have visual problems.

The basic requirements for this career are two years of college preparation and a program in orthoptics. This program is usually two years in length including clinical experience. Certification by the American Orthoptic Council is granted after the applicant passes a certifying examination. Although it is not required by state law, 95 percent of practicing orthoptists obtain certification. The orthoptist always works under the supervision of an ophthalmologist.

Since programs in orthoptic training vary, further information should be obtained from:

American Orthoptic Council
3914 Nakoma Road
Madison, Wisconsin 53711

DIETETIC CLUSTER

Millions of people in underdeveloped countries live in a state of near starvation; you probably have seen newspaper pictures or television programs depicting their misery. These poorly nourished people are easy prey to scurvy, pellagra, and anemia (all caused by vitamin deficiencies) and to other diseases associated with poor diet. Also, because they are inadequately fed, they are **vulnerable** to such diseases as pneumonia and tuberculosis.

Proper nutrition is an important part of the treatment of many health problems. Some diseases can be cured or controlled by diet alone — not necessarily a complicated diet but one that is well balanced and nutritionally sound. There is nothing mysterious about proper nutrition. It is based on providing a variety of foods from each of the food groups. By following good dietary habits, we can help ourselves stay well. However, during periods of illness, we often need to depend upon others to see to it that we are properly nourished, and this is where the dietetic personnel come in.

There is a large group of people within hospitals and other health care agencies who prepare food and plan menus and diets. Dietetics is a rapidly expanding field with a good future for those who are seeking a people-oriented career.

Dietitian

Dietitians are experts in the art of feeding. They apply management principles to planning and directing food service programs while providing people with balanced, attractive meals.

There are six specialty areas in which dietitians may perform their services.

The Clinical Dietitian. Responsible for the nutritional care (dietary treatment) of patients. This member of the medical team provides nutrition advice, counseling, and specific meal plans as part of treatment. The dietitian must be certain that patients' therapeutic diets also meet their nutritional needs. An example would be a low-calorie diet that must meet the patient's daily nutritional requirements, even though the calorie intake is drastically reduced.

The Community Dietitian. Advises clients and families on the selection of proper foods for balanced nutrition. He/she also coordinates programs for the public on nutrition awareness and disease prevention in day-care centers, public health agencies, and community health centers.

The Management Dietitian. Specializes in food systems or clinical management by planning food service programs in health care facilities, restaurants, cafeterias, and schools. Personnel management, including provision for employee training programs, are other responsibilities of this dietitian.

The Educator Dietitian. Conducts nutrition research and teaches nutrition science and food systems management in hospitals, colleges, and universities.

The Business Dietitian. Acts as a food, nutrition, and marketing specialist to corporations in food product development. Also, these dietitians represent food, nutrition, and equipment product accounts.

The Consultant Dietitian. Practices independently. Counseling patients in nursing homes; authoring nutrition books; advising food industries; providing nutritional programs for dancers, athletes, and others; and consulting with business and industry regarding fitness programs for employees are some of the possibilities.

More dietitians are employed in hospitals than in any other agency. However, their services are also in demand in universities and colleges, hotels, schools, child care centers, neighborhood health centers, and health maintenance organizations — almost any place that is concerned with the preparation and service of well-prepared and nourishing food (**Fig. 5–9**).

Dietitians are graduates of accredited colleges who have completed a program that meets the criteria of the American Dietetic Association (ADA). This association sets experience standards, which must be met before dietitians can be registered. When these requirements have been

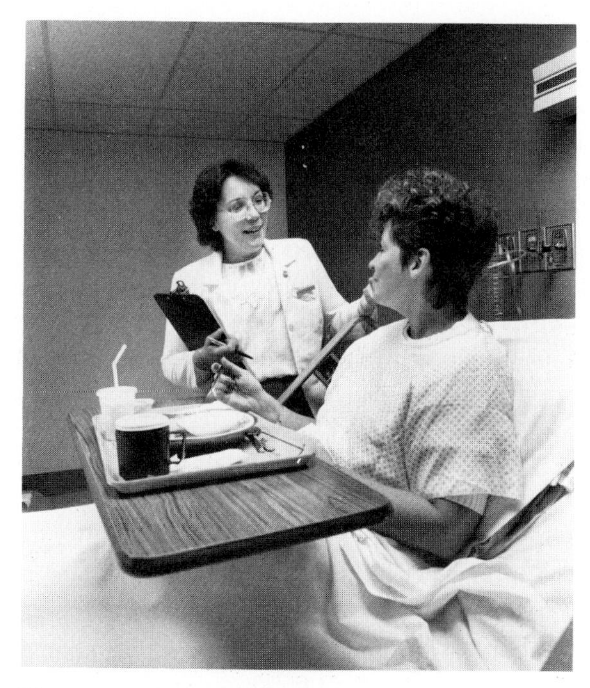

Figure 5–9. The clinical dietitian discusses with the client a special diet prescribed by the physician. (Courtesy of Bridgeton Hospital, Bridgeton, N.J.)

met, the dietitian is eligible to take a national examination. The title RD (Registered Dietitian) is used by qualified members of the Association.

Because of a shortage of professional dietitians, the American Dietetic Association has established a category of support personnel: the dietetic technician.

Dietetic Technician

The technician specializes in one of two areas, *food systems management or nutrition care.* Those who are employed in food systems management are members of the food service team. Under the supervision of the dietitian, the technician supervises the support staff, monitors cost control procedures, and sees that quality assurance procedures are implemented.

Technicians in the nutrition care area take diet histories, calculate nutritional intake, evaluate dietary problems, counsel individuals or small groups about proper nutrition, and develop nutrition care plans for clients. Dietetic technicians always work under the supervision of or in consultation with a dietitian.

The educational preparation of a dietetic technician requires an associate degree in an ADA-approved Dietetic Technician Program. The Commission on Dietetic Registration of the American Dietetic Association provides a **credentialing** examination for qualified graduates.

For more information on dietary careers, contact:

American Dietetic Association
430 North Michigan Avenue
Chicago, Illinois 60611-4085

PHARMACY CLUSTER

Pharmacist (Registered Pharmacist, RP)

Pharmacists are specialists in knowledge of drugs — their composition, properties, manufacture, uses, actions, and effects. Most pharmacists work in community pharmacies where they compound and dispense medications according to medical prescription. They maintain records of prescriptions (called "patient drug profiles") to help prevent undesirable reactions that could result from a patient's taking a combination of incompatible drugs. Most pharmacies use computers to record transactions and maintain patient records. Pharmacists employed in retail drug stores may also dispense health supplies and sickroom equipment and may advise their customers about the purchase of nonprescription drugs.

Hospital pharmacists dispense drugs according to the physician's prescription, but they rarely see any patients since most medications are sent to patient care units and are administered by nursing personnel. The pharmacist is a consultant to the physicians and nurses and conducts in-service programs in drug therapy for them. Pharmacists also consult with nursing home personnel regarding drug therapy for older adults.

The hospital pharmacy stocks large quantities of medications and sterile solutions. They must be stored at the proper temperatures, protected from contamination, and used before their expiration date. Inventory and quality control are the responsibility of the pharmacist. Pharmacists must maintain careful records of all controlled substances stocked and dispensed, and these records must be available for examination by federal officials on request. Since the hospital pharmacy never closes, a registered pharmacist must be on duty at all times (**Fig. 5–10**).

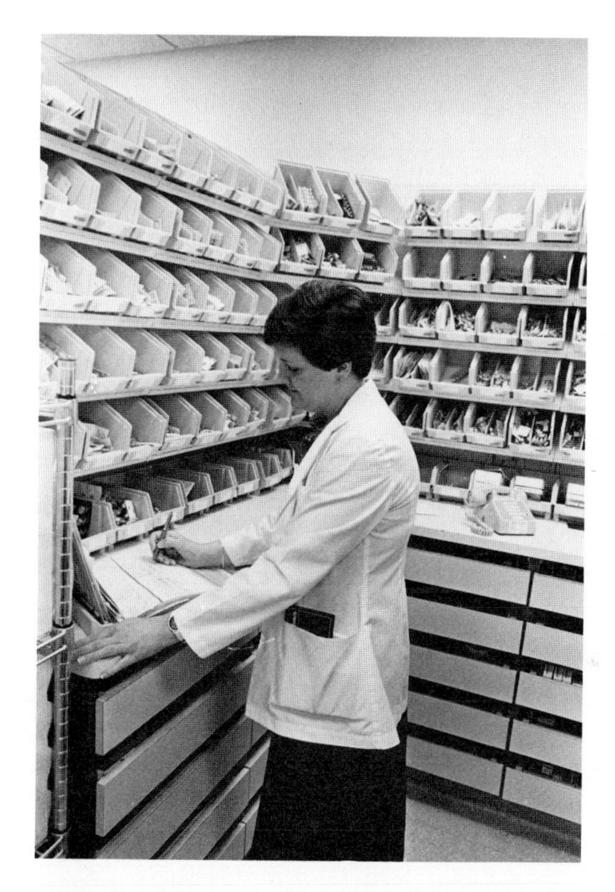

Figure 5–10. The hospital pharmacist dispenses all medications used in the hospital. (Courtesy of St. Mary Hospital, Langhorne, Pa.)

Programs in accredited schools of pharmacy are usually five years in length, although some include a required or optional sixth year. Applicants must have completed one or two years of undergraduate preparatory study. The pharmaceutical program emphasizes basic sciences, especially chemistry, physics, and biology. It also includes extensive study of drugs, a clinical pharmacy experience, and a required one-year internship. Pharmacists must pass a licensing examination given by the state Board of Pharmacy.

Pharmacy Assistant

Some hospital pharmacies and retail drug stores employ men and women to help maintain inventory control and product storage and to handle routine clerical duties. These assistants are usually prepared on the job. They work under the direct supervision of the pharmacist and never dispense or handle medications.

For more information about a career in pharmacy, contact:

American Association of Colleges of Pharmacy
Office of Student Affairs
4630 Montgomery Avenue, Suite 201
Bethesda, Maryland 20014

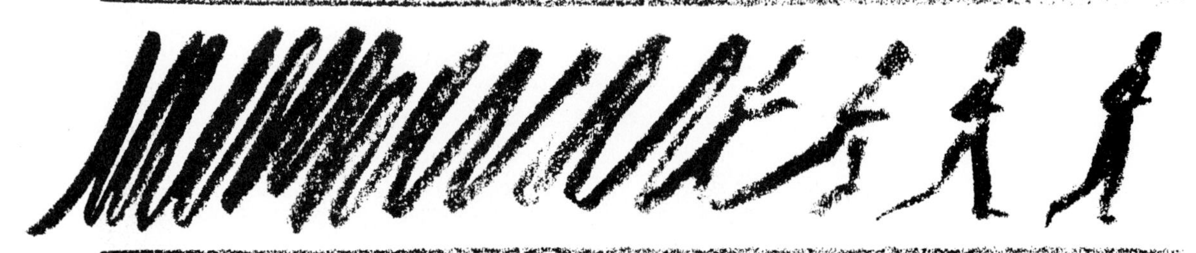

S·T·U·D·E·N·T A·C·T·I·V·I·T·I·E·S

1. Many of the health workers described in this chapter are employed in your community. Are all the therapeutic clusters represented? Every career? (Check with local health agencies, rehabilitation centers, mental health centers, and with your physician, dentist, and instructor.)

2. Select one of the health careers in the Therapeutic/Restorative group for further research. What schools in or near your community offer educational programs in these careers? Describe the program, including: entrance requirements, length of program, tuition fees, and available scholarships. Compare the advantages and disadvantages. Record information in your file.

3. Perform three of the following "hands-on" exploratory activities as assigned by your instructor. (Note: If you are not enrolled in a Health Occupations Education course, try to arrange to observe the performance of some of these activities.)
   a. Assessing effects of dance and music upon others
   b. Measuring for crutches, adjusting underarm crutches, and assisting with crutchwalking
   c. Taking family medication inventory
   d. Preparing a well-balanced menu for one day
   e. Measuring facial contours for eyeglass frames
   f. Recording speech on a tape recorder and critiquing the playback.

   Keep a record of the procedures completed or observed. Briefly describe how you felt about performing or observing each activity.

4. Identify the health worker who may perform the following activity:
   a. Constructs false teeth
   b. Fits eyeglasses
   c. Teaches crutchwalking
   d. Teaches basketweaving
   e. Teaches typing
   f. Administers oxygen
   g. Takes patients bowling
   h. Works with patients using rhythm and music
   i. Teaches the amputee how to get on and off a bus
   j. Works with blind people
   k. Assists the handicapped to return to gainful employment
   l. Builds and fits braces and prostheses
   m. Teaches patients about therapeutic diets
   n. Fills prescriptions
   o. Teaches eye exercises
   p. Evaluates hearing aids
   q. Grinds eyeglass lenses.

5. Select one career discussed in this chapter. Write a letter to one organization listed in the chapter to obtain information about this career. File the information received in your notebook.

6. Complete the Career Interest Chart for the Therapeutic/Restorative Careers. Obtain the chart from your instructor.

Chapter 6

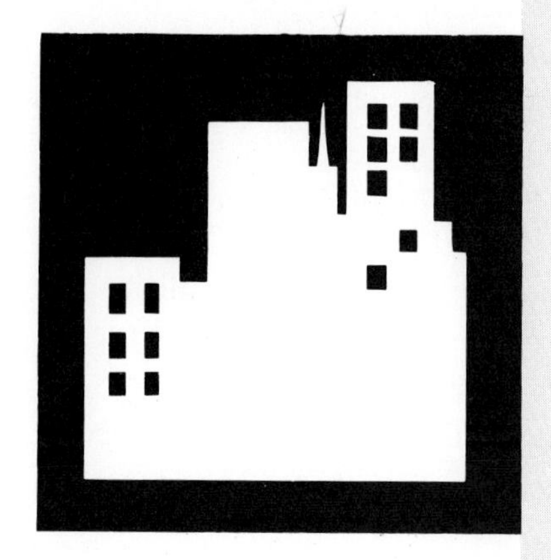

Community Health Careers

Objectives

After completing this chapter, you should be able to:

- Identify by name four clusters of occupations in the Community Health Careers and list three careers found in each.
- Identify five careers and discuss three responsibilities of each.
- Discuss the relationship between the Community Health Careers and the other three groups of careers.
- Name four agencies devoted to community health and describe three functions of each agency.
- Discuss your feelings about performing three of the suggested "hands-on" exploratory activities in class.
- Compare the advantages and disadvantages of pursuing a career in Community Health.
- Define 70 percent of the key terms listed for this chapter.

Key Terms

- **antitoxins** Substances manufactured by the body in response to the presence of toxins
- **official community health agencies** Governmental agencies which are created by public ordinance and obtain their funds from tax revenues
- **pest control** Elimination of animals and insects harmful to humans
- **pollution** To make impure; to contaminate with waste
- **potable** Suitable for drinking
- **solid waste** Refuse, such as garbage or rubbish
- **toxicology** A science that deals with toxic substances
- **toxins** Poisonous substances of plant or animal origin
- **vital statistics** A record of births, deaths, and marriages in a specific geographic area
- **voluntary community health agencies** Agencies that are privately funded and operated

THE COMMUNITY HEALTH CAREERS CLUSTERS

In parts of Asia, Africa, and South America, diseases like **typhus, typhoid fever,** and **cholera** still claim thousands of lives. Some fatal diseases, caused by bacteria that breed in contaminated food, water, and garbage, spread rapidly through towns and villages, leaving many inhabitants dead before the diseases can be controlled.

Such diseases are virtually unknown in the United States, Canada, and Western Europe today, because of strict enforcement of public health and safety laws. These laws govern building codes, industrial safety, and fire regulations, as well as measures to ensure community health.

In this chapter, we shall be looking at careers in community health. All aspects of community health work are essential to the public welfare, because it deals with anything that pertains to the community and its environment — prevention and control of communicable disease, purity of the public water supply, regulation of waste disposal, restaurant inspection, etc.

Each municipality has enacted ordinances that establish the responsibility for safeguarding the health of its citizens, and the funds to carry out this responsibility come from local taxes. Activities are grouped into several broad categories: vital statistics (which includes recording of births, deaths, and marriages); communicable disease control; maternal and child health services; health education; environmental health; and chronic disease control.

Official health agencies exist at every level of government, and their operating funds come from taxes. Local communities (townships, boroughs, counties, and cities) have their own health departments, administered by the Board of Health. States, too, maintain health departments, as does the federal government through the Department of Health and Human Services.

The World Health Organization (WHO), a part of the United Nations, is concerned with the health of the international community. Some health problems (pollution of oceans, **malnutrition, epidemic** disease, and starvation) can be prevented, solved, or controlled only through an agency that fosters international cooperation. Conferences on major worldwide health issues, such as acquired immune deficiency syndrome (AIDS), are sponsored regularly by WHO.

Voluntary health agencies, like the American Cancer Society, are privately operated and financed. Most voluntary agencies are organized to meet a specific need within the community. One example is the local Heart Association, which is concerned with the prevention of heart and vascular disease. This voluntary agency conducts free educational and screening programs to detect high blood pressure, trains people in first aid for heart attacks, carries out research projects, and teaches about proper diet to prevent heart disease and promote health.

Both public and voluntary agencies are concerned with mental health, too, and operate public education programs, as well as free or low-cost clinics.

Sometimes, diseases for which there is no known cure can be prevented by inoculation. Public health agencies organize and conduct **immunization** programs against **poliomyelitis, tetanus, influenza,** and other diseases. They regularly offer free examinations that can indicate the possible presence of **cancer, diabetes, glaucoma,** and **hypertension** (**Fig. 6–1**).

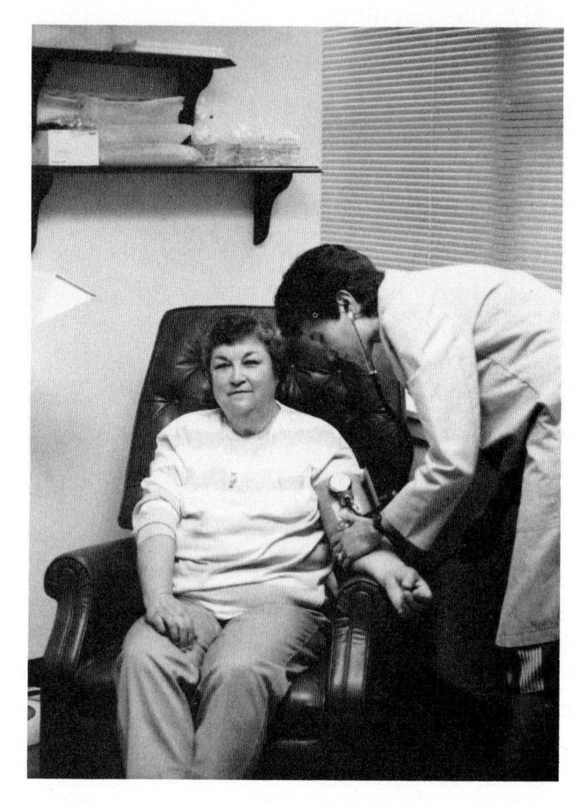

Figure 6–1. A community health care worker takes a client's blood pressure. (Courtesy of Visiting Nurse Association of Trenton, N.J.)

American citizens traveling to certain parts of the world must be immunized against **smallpox**, typhoid, and typhus, so they will not contract one of these diseases and transmit it to others when they return home. A quarantine officer of the U.S. Public Health Service inspects all incoming airplanes and ships from foreign ports to ensure that passengers, crew members, and cargo are cleared for entry into the United States.

Despite these precautions, on a rare occasion, a person may develop smallpox or typhoid fever after arriving in the United States. In that case, the person is quarantined, or isolated, from other people. Anyone who has had contact with the sick person will be located and tested for the presence of the disease.

Free clinics and multimedia information campaigns represent major public health efforts to bring serious health problems — such as AIDS, drug abuse, venereal disease, child abuse, and teenage pregnancy — under control or to prevent their development.

Members of the Community Health Careers are employed in large cities and small towns, as well as in rural districts and isolated mountain and desert regions, both in this country and abroad. An important personal characteristic is flexibility, because the community health worker needs to adjust to many changes in work situations, coworkers, and clients. The clusters in this group are: Community Services Cluster; Environmental Health Cluster; Animal Care Services Cluster; Health Education and Communications Cluster; and Home Health Care Cluster.

HEALTH CARE WORKERS ON THE JOB

The water filtration plant in Compton served 250,000 people in that community and three nearby suburbs. On Sunday of Labor Day weekend, one of the valves on a pump failed to close, and the entire plant was flooded by incoming contaminated river water. After the fire department pumped out the water, the damage was surveyed. One large pump sending pure water into the system had been completely soaked. This pump was removed and returned to the manufacturer to be dried in a large oven — an operation that would take four to five days. The increased water pressure had also caused a large crack in a **concrete conduit**. Four to five days would be required to patch the concrete and to allow it to dry.

The Compton reservoir held enough water for only one to two days. Clearly, the community would soon be without safe drinking water. The mayor and city council held a meeting with public health officials. They defined the most urgent problems arising from the pump failure at the plant as follows:

1. Acute shortage of water
2. Possible contamination of water in the system due to low pressure
3. Inadequate water pressure for firefighting
4. Shortage of water supply to schools, hospitals, and nursing homes
5. Shortage of water to retail food establishments (restaurants, supermarkets, delicatessens, meat markets) for adequate sanitation.

The mayors and health officers of the four communities declared a severe water emergency. Bathing, dishwashing, car washing, clothes washing, and watering of lawns were forbidden by law for the duration of the water crisis. Citizens were encouraged to use disposable plates and plastic utensils. Parents were urged to use disposable diapers for their babies.

Public health educators took advantage of all the local media to teach the citizens how to treat water to make it **potable**. (Water is made safe to drink by boiling it or adding purifying tablets to it.) Nutritionists demonstrated waterless methods of cooking, such as baking. Some retail food stores and restaurants closed, while others obtained their own water supply from private sources and remained open. Every food service business that served the public had to be inspected by sanitarians and certified as safe to operate during the crisis.

Public health planners and sanitary engineers estimated that on the third day of the crisis, Compton's water taps would be dry. They arranged to use other sources of potable water. The National Guard and nearby Army and Air Force bases sent tank trucks full of water for use by Compton residents. These were stationed at central locations, so people could fill containers with water. Environmental technicians tested samples of these water sources to be sure they were safe.

Long-range plans to ensure alternate water supplies were also being developed. The Compton water mains were to be connected to those of outlying water companies by volunteer firefighters. Water would be pumped through their hoses until permanent water mains could be installed. Men and women from all over the state volunteered to help Compton during the crisis. Rural fire companies sent their water tankers to stand by the city firehouses in case of emergency. One hospital in Compton had an emergency **artesian well**, but the others had no water at all. The health officer dispatched a tank truck, or "water buffalo," to each patient care facility.

Toilet flushing was a major problem. Some "gray water" (untreated surface water from ponds and lakes) was available at central locations. But, mainly, swimming pools were drained, and streams were tapped to provide water to dump into toilets. Business and industries rented portable toilet facilities for temporary use.

The only people who weren't worried were the school children. There was no school — and no baths! After a few days, nearby communities opened their school shower facilities so that Compton citizens could bathe.

After six days, the water plant was repaired, but it took another week before full output was restored. During that time, water purity was determined by environmental health personnel. Finally, two weeks later, the water crisis was over.

COMMUNITY SERVICES CLUSTER

Public Health Statistician

This career offers an opportunity to use mathematics in a health occupation. Vital statistics, census reports, and records of certain diseases are the basis for analyzing and evaluating existing health conditions and forecasting trends. Numerical facts about health and illness are also used to plan and evaluate programs and to allocate resources to those places where services are needed.

Statisticians design questionnaires to gather facts about health and disease. They gather and analyze the resulting data which are then sent to community agencies. This statistical research enables local agencies to anticipate health needs and services. For example, if statistical data showed a sharp increase in cases of **silicosis** in a coal mining community, public health workers would be dispatched to the area to check conditions in the mines, measure toxic emissions in the air, and help care for victims.

Statisticians design controlled experiments to determine the effectiveness of new drugs. For example, in one study, a new drug to treat arthritis was tested. A sample group of patients with specific symptoms was studied in clinical trials. Private physicians were asked to invite appropriate patients for participation in the research. The new drug was then added to the patients' usual treatment programs. Diagnostic tests such as blood studies, joint examinations, and x-ray studies were conducted at regular intervals to determine whether any changes had occurred in the patients' physical conditions. All of the information was gathered and converted by the statistician into numerical information called data. Mathematical calculations were used to interpret the findings and thereby determine the effectiveness of the drug, the incidence of side effects, and any other significant findings.

Public health statisticians are responsible for preparing clear, concise, and accurate reports of their findings. They must be well versed in the operation of computers and their functions since electronic data processing equipment is used to collect, store, analyze, and retrieve health facts and figures.

The basic education for a public health statistician is four years of college with emphasis on mathematics, statistics, and computers. Knowledge of the social, biological, and physical sciences is also required. Graduate education is essential for advancement in this career. Most statisticians are employed in official health agencies.

Statistical Clerk

Clerical duties, plus the collection and computation of basic statistical facts, are usually the responsibilities of the statistical clerk. These workers do not make statistical projections or long-range forecasts. They compile information, such as the number of births or deaths in the community in a given year. These data are then utilized by statisticians. A high school diploma, clerical and computer skills, as well as mathematical ability are needed for this work. However, there is little or no opportunity for advancement in a statistical career without a college degree.

Information on careers in health statistics may be obtained from:

American Statistical Association
806 15th Street, N.W., Suite 640
Washington, D.C. 20005

Association of Schools of Public Health
1015 15th Street, N.W., Suite 404
Washington, D.C. 20005

Health Officer

The health officer is usually the head of the public health staff and is responsible for the overall administration of local official agencies. The health needs of the community are evaluated by the health officer who develops and implements plans to meet these needs. Many specialists in the areas of environmental health, vital statistics, public health nursing, and health education work with the health officer. The final and ultimate responsibility for enforcing the community's public health laws rests with the health officer.

Some health officers are physicians or veterinarians with advanced education and experience in public health. Sometimes health officers are lay persons who have met certain standards established by the state health department. A master's degree in public health is the usual educational requirement. Many states require licensure for health officers.

For further information about this work, contact:

American Public Health Association
1015 18th Street, N.W.
Washington, D.C. 20036

ENVIRONMENTAL HEALTH CLUSTER

Sanitarian (Environmental Health Specialist)

Sanitary standards for food, water supply, sewage, garbage disposal, housing, camps, swimming pools, etc., are regulated by federal, state, and local legislation. These laws are interpreted and enforced by sanitarians who plan, develop, and administer environmental health programs. They work closely with other community health workers in disease investigation, disaster and emergency aid, community surveys to detect urgent health needs, health education, and health promotion.

Most sanitarians are employed in local health or agriculture departments. Some are experts in specialized fields, such as milk and dairy products, housing, institutional sanitation, waste disposal and control, water supply, pest control, occupational health, and air pollution. This is not desk work — most of the time is spent out of doors. This career offers rapid change and constant challenge. Just as one environmental health problem is solved, there seems to be another waiting for attention.

To become a sanitarian, a bachelor's degree in environmental health is needed. Graduate education in public health is required for advancement to management level. The American Public Health Association recommends the specific courses that are incorporated in college educational programs. Many states provide for the registration of sanitarians.

More information may be obtained from:

American Public Health Association
1015 18th Street, N.W.
Washington, D.C. 20036

National Environmental Health Association
720 S. Colorado Boulevard, Suite 970, South Tower
Denver, Colorado 80222

Sanitary Engineer

Official health agencies employ sanitary engineers who have the following responsibilities: review and approve designs for water purification and waste disposal systems, inspect and supervise water purification facilities, sewage treatment, and solid waste disposal. The sanitary engineer ensures the safety of drinking water in every city in the United States — a vital service essential to human health.

As technology progresses, hazards to a healthy environment increase. Because of this, sanitary engineering is constantly faced with new challenges. Some of its current concerns are: use of insecticides, pesticides, and herbicides; city planning; noise pollution and abatement; shellfish contamination; and protection measures.

An example of a sanitary engineer's role can be found in the northeastern United States where commercial fishing along 100 miles of river was banned when fish were found to contain toxic levels of certain chemicals. Furthermore, two electrical plants in this region were forced to stop discharging harmful chemical waste into the waterway.

Sanitary engineers must complete a four-year college program in engineering and obtain a master's degree in the sanitary and public health sciences. Engineers are registered and licensed by individual states and may be certified by the American Academy of Sanitary Engineers.

Sanitary engineers are employed by public health agencies, private consulting firms, and industries.

For more information, write to:

American Academy of Environmental Engineers
P.O. Box 1278
Rockville, Maryland 20850

American Public Health Association
1015 18th Street, N.W.
Washington, D.C. 20036

Environmental Technician and Aide

Samples of water, food, and air are collected and prepared for public health laboratory analysis by environmental technicians, who also assist in performing tests of these samples. They are members of a group of environmental specialists (sanitarians, chemists, engineers, and educators) who work in water, refuse, and sewage treatment facilities. Most technicians are employed by public health agencies, although some work in private industry (**Fig. 6–2**).

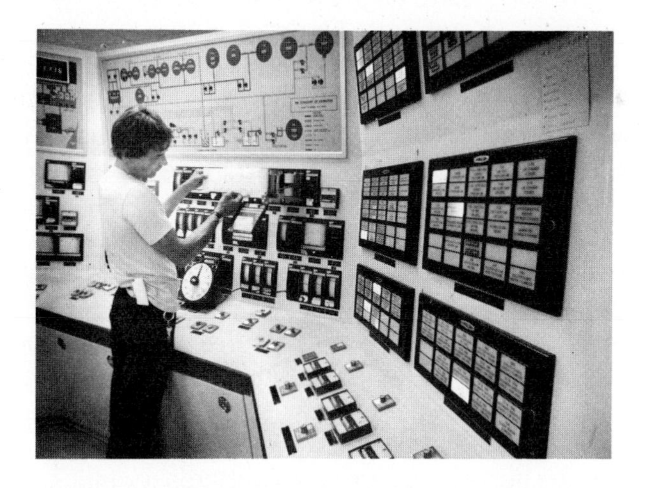

Figure 6–2. Monitoring the flow of wastewater is important to the health of a community. (Courtesy of Hamilton Township Department of Water Pollution Control, N.J.)

Technicians are prepared in two-year community college programs in environmental technology. Depending on the receiving college, some of these courses may be credited toward a bachelor's degree in environmental sciences or engineering.

Environmental aides, under the supervision of engineers and technicians, perform the routine duties of environmental health programs. Many aides are employed in water supply and treatment facilities, waste disposal and collection, community sanitation, industrial safety, and air pollution control. For example, in a neighborhood where vacant lots or abandoned structures are infested with rats, the aides may set out traps or chemicals and then dispose of the dead rats. Aides are usually trained on the job, in short-term courses in vocational schools, or in special training projects.

For information about a career as an environmental technician or environmental aide, contact:

American Public Health Association
1015 18th Street, N.W.
Washington, D.C. 20036

Environmental Management Association
1019 Highland Avenue
Key Largo, Florida 33540

The job of maintaining a safe environment is not solely the responsibility of the workers we have discussed. An army of people is involved in accomplishing this goal. The muscle behind these jobs comes from blue-collar workers who operate and maintain the machinery and equipment needed to do the job. Two examples are workers in plants who recycle water by removing industrial wastes and sewage and operators of tractors, bulldozers, and other earth-moving equipment who bury refuse. While they are not health workers in the sense we have been using the term, they, nevertheless, make a valuable contribution to community health.

Employees of government-run agriculture and labor departments have responsibilities for setting safety standards in industry in general; overseeing the safety and purity of drugs, cosmetics, and foods; and regulating the use of insecticides and pesticides. Among the job titles that apply to these occupations are: biologist, entomologist (studies insects), ecologist (studies habitat), safety engineer, chemist, and agronomist (studies farming).

If you are interested in an environmental career, you may obtain more information about each specialty from your guidance counselor. Specific information may be obtained from:

American Industrial Hygiene Association
475 Wolf Ledger Parkway
Akron, Ohio 44311

National Environmental Health Association
720 S. Colorado Boulevard, Suite 970, South Tower
Denver, Colorado 80222

ANIMAL CARE SERVICES CLUSTER

Veterinarian (Doctor of Veterinary Medicine, DVM)

Veterinary medicine goes back to ancient times. In fact, there are Egyptian records of drug prescriptions used to treat diseases of dogs and cows.

While more than half of all veterinarians maintain a private practice, others work in public health and research, and at zoos, circuses, and racetracks. They attend sick and injured animals, prevent animal disease through vaccination programs, and offer instruction to owners about animal care and nutrition (**Fig. 6–3**). A less well-known but equally important part of their work is to protect humans from diseases that can be carried by animals, e.g., tuberculosis.

Rabies, a disease that is almost always fatal, is transmitted to humans through a bite or a scratch from an infected animal — usually a dog. Infected squirrels and bats are also known to transmit rabies to humans.

Rabies can be prevented in dogs and cats by routine immunization with a rabies vaccine. In many communities, this vaccination is a prerequisite for obtaining a dog license. The Public Health Department conducts clinics where veterinarians inoculate pets at a lesser cost than a private veterinarian.

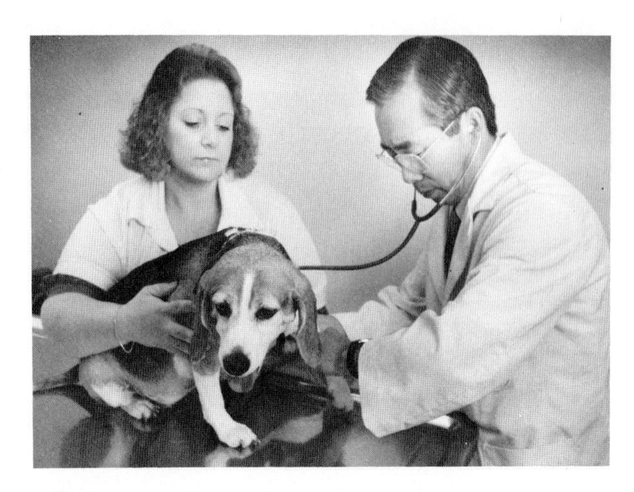

Figure 6–3. The veterinary team works together to conduct a physical exam. (Courtesy of Yardville Animal Hospital, Yardville, N.J. Photo by Michael Mancuso.)

Animals suspected of having the disease are captured by an animal warden and observed closely by the veterinarian for two weeks. If no symptoms appear, the disease is virtually ruled out. However, if disease symptoms appear, the animal is destroyed, and its brain is examined for evidence of rabies. If there is any question about the presence of rabies in the animal, the veterinarian will instruct that the bitten person be treated immediately for rabies.

Veterinary research has been instrumental in the development of vaccines, antitoxins, and artificial heart valves. New drugs and chemicals are first laboratory-tested to learn whether they cause toxic and cumulative effects in animals before they are prescribed for people. The health of the animals that are slaughtered for human consumption is constantly protected by the veterinarian who oversees livestock health.

Veterinary schools accept students who have completed a minimum of two years of college, but most are college graduates. The four-year study of veterinary medicine includes courses in animal anatomy, physiology, microbiology, biochemistry, pharmacology, and animal diseases. Clinical study and practice include all areas of veterinary work. Graduates receive the degree of Doctor of Veterinary Medicine. Veterinarians may specialize in the care of large animals or small animals (companion animals or pets). Veterinarians are licensed by individual states.

For more information about a career in veterinary medicine, contact:

American Veterinary Medical Association
930 North Meacham Road
Schaumburg, Illinois 60172

U.S. Department of Health and Human Services
HRSA–Bureau of Health Professions
5600 Fishers Lane
Rockville, Maryland 20857

Veterinary Science Technician (Animal Care Technician, Laboratory Animal Technician)

Animal technicians support and complement the work of veterinarians. Technicians work in specialty areas: care of sick animals, laboratory research, and meat inspection and regulation.

Educational programs in veterinary science technology are usually two years long and offered by community colleges. Studies include basic social and physical sciences; comparative anatomy; animal health, disease, care, and nutrition; and laboratory animal methods. Additional courses in meat inspection and regulatory veterinary medicine may be available for elective study.

More information on this career may be obtained from:

American Veterinary Medical Association
930 North Meacham Road
Schaumburg, Illinois 60172

U.S. Department of Health and Human Services
HSRA–Bureau of Health Professions
5600 Fishers Lane
Rockville, Maryland 20857

HEALTH EDUCATION AND COMMUNICATIONS CLUSTER

Health Educator

Providing the community with health care information is the responsibility of health educators. They teach the importance of regular health checkups, the need for vaccinations and immunizations, the dangers of smoking, and methods to prevent certain types of diseases.

Health educators lecture to civic associations, labor unions, service clubs, and similar organizations. They prepare and distribute leaflets, films, slides, and posters. They may also communicate through the mass media — newspaper, radio, television, and magazines. They are employed in official and voluntary public health agencies, hospitals, agricultural extension services, schools, neighborhood health centers, family planning centers, and clinics.

Educational programs to prepare health educators are found in four-year colleges. Master's degree programs are required for more advanced positions.

Further information may be obtained from:

Association for Advancement of Health Education
1900 Association Drive
Reston, Virginia 22091

Society for Public Health Education
703 Market Street, Suite 535
San Francisco, California 94103

Association of Schools of Public Health (see page 140).

Nutritionist

Nutritionists instruct people about the proper foods to include in meal planning in order to maintain good health. They also instruct those on limited budgets in buying food and in preparing economical meals for their families. Nutritionists are experts in normal nutrition. They serve as consultants to the members of the community health team. They are usually employed in a health department or an agricultural extension service. Educational programs for nutritionists are similar to those for dietitians.

Further information is available from the American Dietetic Association (see Dietitian, Chapter 5, page 128).

Medical Illustrator and Medical Photographer

The medical illustrator combines scientific training with artistic skill to record medical events, such as surgical procedures, and to graphically display body structures. Sketches, photographs, models, slides, and vidoetapes are prepared by the medical artist for use in professional and community education.

Candidates seeking admission to an educational program in medical illustration must submit a portfolio of their art work for evaluation by the school's admission committee. Academic ability is also taken into consideration. Programs are available at both the bachelor's and master's degree levels, and both provide extensive training in art and the biological sciences. This is a highly specialized and competitive field, and only a handful of students are admitted each year. Most jobs are found in large medical centers in metropolitan areas.

Other programs in the related fields of medical photography and medical communications are available in some areas of the United States, although many persons enter these careers from other health occupations.

Additional information about these careers may be obtained from:

Association of Medical Illustrators
2692 Huguenot Springs Road
Midlothian, Virginia 23113

Health Sciences Communications Association
6105 Lindell Boulevard
St. Louis, Missouri 63113

HOME HEALTH CARE CLUSTER

Public Health Nurse (Community Health Nurse, Visiting Nurse)

Community health nurses provide highly skilled care for clients at home, bridging the gap between hospitalization and health. A nursing care plan is developed to meet the needs of each client and may include: drug administration and intravenous therapy, dressing changes, client education in self-care, arranging for home health aide assistance, obtaining special medical equipment and supplies, and teaching the family how to care for the client (**Fig. 6–4**).

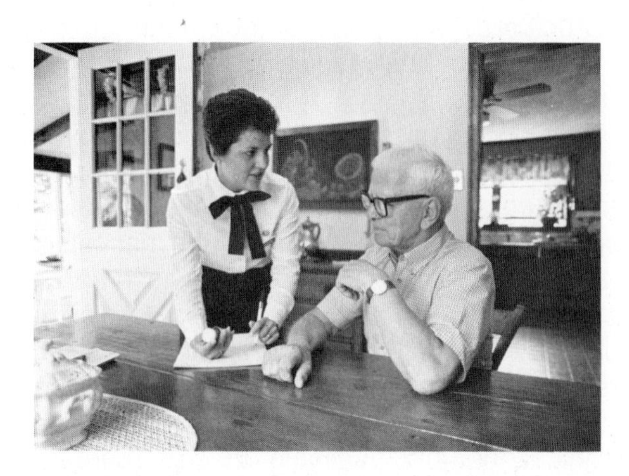

Figure 6–4. A community health nurse and client review daily medication. (Courtesy of St. Mary Hospital, Langhorne, Pa.)

Community health nurses also offer services to healthy individuals. They teach mothers to care for newborn infants especially in high-risk cases like multiple births, premature infants, and teenage mothers. In senior citizen housing centers, the nurse is a friend and counselor, advising the older person about health practices and seeking medical care. Educating individuals about proper diet and adequate nutrition is an important part of the nurse's responsibility. When necessary, the public health nurse refers clients to other members of the health team or other health agencies. The nurse coordinates the services provided by other health workers who care for the client at home (occupational, physical, speech, and respiratory therapists; social workers; nutritionists; home health aides, etc.).

Home health care is not the only setting where community health nursing is practiced. Public health nurses are employed in schools, industries, day-care centers, public health clinics, senior citizen centers, and neighborhood health centers (**Fig. 6–5**). They also work in hospitals, rehabilitation centers, and nursing homes. In these settings, they arrange for home health care for clients being discharged from the facility.

Registered nurses who are graduates of baccalaureate degree schools of nursing are prepared for beginning level positions in community health nursing. On-the-job experience is required for advancement to a first level supervisory position, and a master's degree in public health nursing is necessary for advancement to an administrative position.

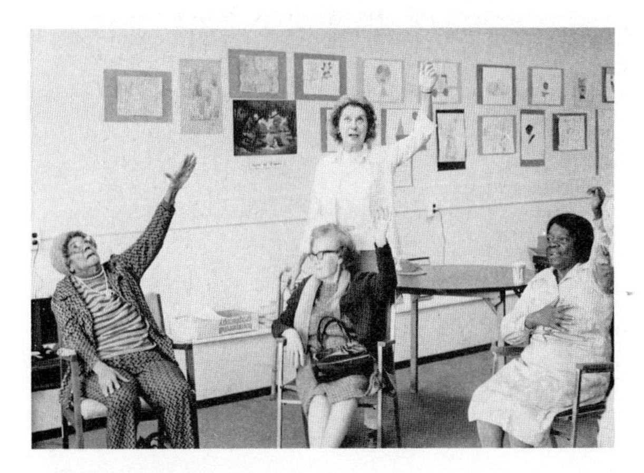

Figure 6–5. This exercise class for older adults is conducted by a community health nurse. (Courtesy of Mercer Street Friends Center, Trenton, N.J.)

The demand for nursing services in the home continues to increase, as clients have shorter hospital stays. Their return home often requires complex nursing care. Licensed practical nurses may also be employed in community health nursing. Specific information on nursing careers in community health may be obtained from:

National League for Nursing
10 Columbus Circle
New York, New York 10019

Homemaker/Home Health Aide

Home health agencies employ homemakers, home health aides, community health nurses, and therapists who give direct care to sick people at home. Persons who are homebound due to an illness or a handicap may require assistance with physical activities and homemaking.

The home health aide provides routine physical care for the patient such as bathing and exercising; preparing, serving, and feeding meals; assisting the client in taking prescribed medication; and reporting observations to the professional nurse who is the assigned case manager (**Fig. 6–6**).

Homemakers are mainly concerned with the housekeeping duties. They clean, shop, and cook for an invalid or a handicapped person.

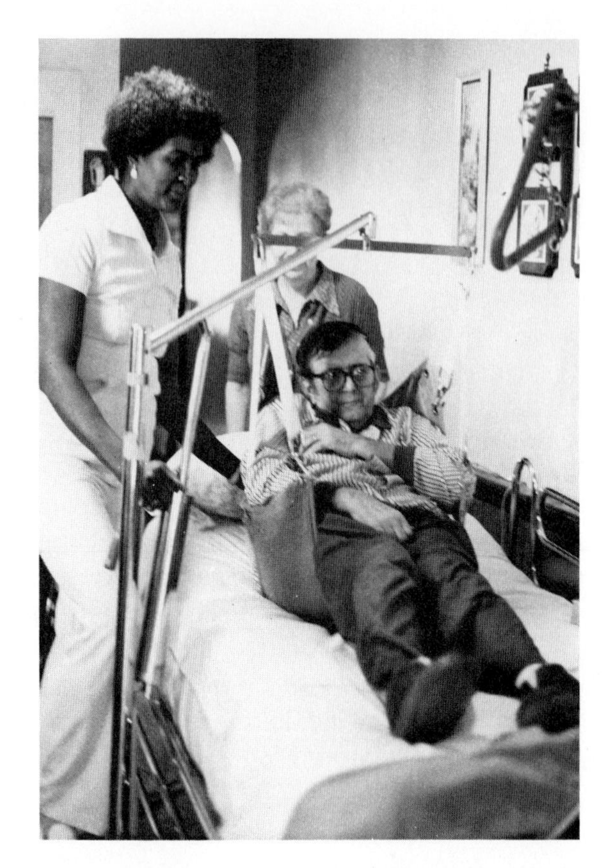

Figure 6–6. A home health aide uses a mechanical lift to return a client to bed. (Courtesy of Mercer Street Friends Center, Trenton, N.J.)

Homemakers may run the household and take care of the children when the caregiver is hospitalized or sick at home.

Homemakers and home health aides are employed by health departments, social service agencies, voluntary community health agencies, and commercial home health agencies.

Short-term educational programs to prepare homemaker-home health aides are conducted by vocational schools and health agencies. Some states require certification for home health aides.

More information may be obtained from the state Department of Health, state capital. Any local home health agency that employs homemaker-home health aides can tell you where to obtain training, or you may contact:

National HomeCaring Council
235 Park Avenue South
New York, New York 10003

OTHER HOME HEALTH SERVICES

Institutionalization often can be avoided or shortened because of the services available from a home health care agency in the community. Visiting nurse associations, health departments, home care departments of general hospitals, and other health care facilities provide many services on a part-time basis for the homebound client.

Health care personnel — physicians, community health nurses, home health aides, physical therapists, speech pathologists, audiologists, occupational therapists, social workers, and nutritionists — are employed in community health care agencies. Because hospital care is so costly, only those with acute illnesses stay for any length of time. Those with long-term illnesses are often discharged before they have fully recovered. Home health care services are in great demand and job opportunities will continue to grow. Diagnostic medical laboratory studies, dental treatment, and home-delivered meals are but a few examples of the services offered.

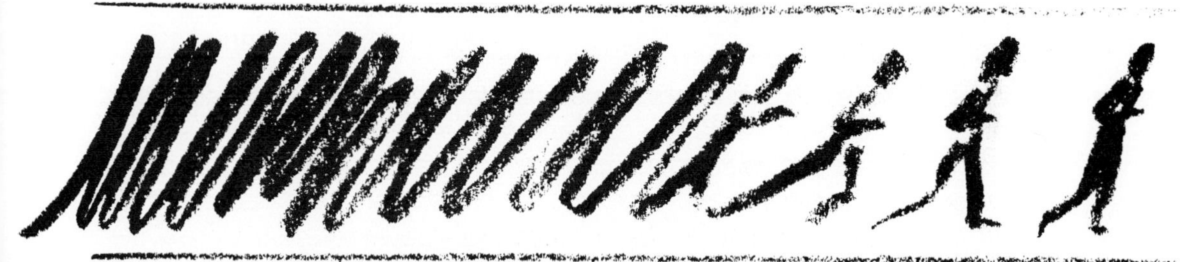

S·T·U·D·E·N·T A·C·T·I·V·I·T·I·E·S

1. What is the source of potable water in your home? Which agency or individual tests the water in your community? How often?
2. How is sewage removed from your home? Which agency or person assures the proper functioning of the system? How often?
3. Does you neighborhood restaurant, delicatessen, or supermarket have a certificate relating to sanitary conditions issued by the Health De-

partment? Ask the owner/manager what steps are involved in inspection before a certificate is issued.

4. Prepare a list of schools and colleges in your area that offer training in the occupations found in the Community Health Careers group.
5. Perform three of the six "hands-on" exploratory activities as assigned by your teacher. (Note: If you are not enrolled in a Health Occupations Education course, try to observe some of these activities below.)
   a. Surveying and inspecting school cafeteria or retail food establishment
   b. Researching a health problem in the community and developing plans for a community health education program
   c. Developing a questionnaire and conducting a statistical survey of communicable diseases contracted by classmates
   d. Determining smoke density and water pollution levels
   e. Conducting a safety survey in school
   f. Determining fat content in ground beef.
6. Identify the person who would perform the following activity:
   a. Care for sick animals
   b. Educate the public in health maintenance and disease prevention
   c. Test water for purity
   d. Obtain samples of fish, meat, and milk for laboratory examination
   e. Collect and analyze vital statistics
   f. Supervise all public health activities in a community
   g. Give skilled care to sick people in their homes
   h. Perform housekeeping duties for aged or sick persons
   i. Give basic physical care to homebound sick persons
   j. Teach economical ways to purchase and prepare foods.

Chapter 7

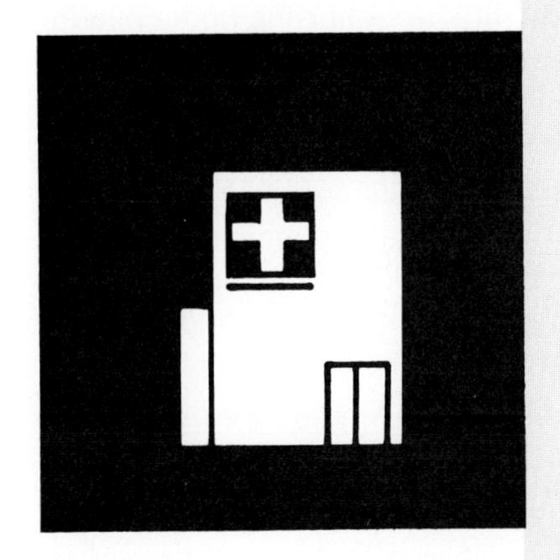

Institutional Careers

Objectives

After completing this chapter, you should be able to:

- Identify by name five occupations from each cluster in the Institutional Careers and list three careers found in each cluster.
- Select four careers and discuss three responsibilities of each worker.
- Discuss the relationship of the Institutional Careers to the other four groups of careers.
- Explain three ways in which this group is different from all the others.
- Compare the advantages and disadvantages of pursuing a career in this group.
- Define 70 percent of the key terms for this chapter.

Key Terms

- **hospital** Institution for medical and surgical treatment of the sick and injured

- **house staff** The interns and resident physicians of a hospital who work under the direction of the general staff of physicians
- **inpatient** The hospital patient who receives lodging and food as well as treatment
- **intermediate care facility** A nursing home offering personal care and help with daily living activities along with less extensive nursing care than a skilled nursing facility; a place for persons who are unable to live alone but do not require constant nursing care or supervision
- **medical center** An institution which has as its primary goal the care of the sick and injured and is also involved in promoting community health and conducting professional education and medical research
- **outpatient** A person who is not lodged or fed in a hospital but who visits it for diagnosis and treatment
- **pastoral** Pertaining to religious needs and spiritual life
- **patient** One who is sick with, or being treated for, an illness or injury
- **resident** A person who resides in a nursing home
- **skilled nursing facility** A nursing home that provides 24-hour care for chronically ill and disabled persons

THE INSTITUTIONAL CAREERS CLUSTERS

There are approximately 7,000 hospitals in the United States. There are thousands more nursing homes, including intermediate care facilities (ICF) and skilled nursing facilities (SNF), rehabilitation centers, and a variety of inpatient care facilities. Millions of people utilize the expert medical, diagnostic, treatment, and rehabilitation services located in these facilities. These services are provided by workers in the

Direct Care, Diagnostic, and Therapeutic/Restorative Careers, while the day-to-day activities necessary to keep these institutions running efficiently and to ensure a high quality of patient/resident care are performed by those employed in Institutional careers.

Conducting the "business" of the institution is the responsibility of the workers in the Administrative cluster: the health care administrator (hospital, nursing home, medical center), purchasing agent, public relations director, personnel manager, health unit coordinators, unit/ward clerks, medical record and clerical personnel. They work primarily in the office areas of the institution and have limited contact with patients/residents. Some personal qualifications needed, besides an interest in business and management, are the ability to sort, organize, and store information and materials and a liking for detailed precision work utilizing computerized data equipment.

Personnel in the Supportive Cluster provide services that meet both everyday needs and emergency situations. They are employed in the housekeeping, maintenance, laundry, dietary, and supply departments, but they perform their work in any area of the hospital. Some supportive workers have regular contact with patients, for example, those who do the housekeeping and serve the meals. Others, such as laundry workers, may never see patients. Each institution depends upon supportive personnel to provide the services vital to patient/resident care, safety, and comfort.

HEALTH CARE WORKERS ON THE JOB

At 1:30 P.M., the weather bureau released a traveler's warning of heavy, drifting snow, and the Office of Disaster Control declared a snow emergency. Schools, offices, and industrial plants closed early so that people could get home before transportation came to a halt. All moving automobiles were required to have snow tires or chains. How would Riverton Medical Center continue to meet patient needs?

At 2:00 P.M., the administrator of the Medical Center met with the staff to implement the snow emergency plan. All department managers surveyed their staff members to determine the number of employees who were able to remain at the Medical Center for extra duty on the evening or night shift. Regular evening employees began to arrive early, but those from outlying areas called to report transportation problems. The combined volunteer and regularly scheduled staff provided adequate personnel to meet patient needs. Several physicians volunteered to stay at the Medical Center to assist the house staff in the event of emergencies.

The Medical Center would be having unexpected guests (its own staff) for the night, and several departments took special steps to prepare for them. The admitting department ran a computer check to locate the available empty beds. The admitting officer tallied the number of employees staying for the night and assigned them to patient rooms from the empty bed list. Extra bed linens, gowns, robes, and towels were readied by the laundry and sent to the "guest" rooms. The purchasing agent provided toilet articles, soap, toothpaste and toothbrushes, razors, and other items from the storeroom. Extra food was prepared and the hours of the employees' dining room were extended. Coffee and sandwiches would be available all night. All department directors (nursing, radiology, laboratory, dietary) arranged an on-duty/off-duty schedule for the next two shifts. Everyone had time to eat dinner and sleep, but patient care was not neglected. A midnight meeting was scheduled to review the staffing pattern for the next day.

The administrator remained at the Medical Center to coordinate and evaluate the emergency snow plan. Other management personnel who stayed included the director of nurses, chief medical technologist, chief radiologic technologist, pharmacist, laundry manager, admitting officer, food service manager, and chief engineer.

At the midnight meeting, the administrator reported that the storm was over but that twelve inches of snow had fallen. The maintenance department was plowing the driveways, sidewalks, and parking lots. The Disaster Control Center reported that public transportation would be available for most of the incoming day-shift employees.

The snow emergency plan was working, and all departments were functioning without problems. The crisis was over.

ADMINISTRATIVE CLUSTER

Health Service Administrator (Health Services Manager, Health Care Administrator)

A medical center is a complex organization made up of many people in many departments who share the primary goal of caring for the sick and injured and helping them return to the community restored to health when possible. Their other responsibilities include medical research, professional education, and community health promotion. All departments — nursing, pharmacy, radiology, laboratory, laundry, kitchen, and others — must work together smoothly in order for the medical center to achieve its goals.

A nursing home is a facility which provides care at different levels — usually, it is for elderly people and others who can no longer live independently because of physical or mental impairment, **emotional trauma,** or **chronic** illness. Nursing homes provide dietary, **therapeutic,** social, **pastoral,** recreational, and nursing services. People who live in nursing homes are called residents rather than patients because the nursing home really is their home.

No matter what the facility is called, the administrator is the executive who coordinates the activities of the various departments and ensures that staffing and equipment needs are met. The governing body of the institution (a board of trustees or a governmental agency) hires the administrator, who acts as its representative.

By seeing that high standards of health care are enforced, the administrator seeks to gain accreditation for the institution. For the medical center, this recognition comes from the Joint Commission on the Accreditation of Hospitals (JCAH), an agency that establishes standards of quality. Nursing homes are inspected and licensed by individual states and must meet additional specific requirements to be certified to participate in Medicare and Medicaid programs.

Fund-raising, to prevent deficits or to expand facilities, is a major duty of the administrator who works with community members in an effort to raise monies for the expansion of institutional services and the expansion or renovation of buildings. The administrator enlists the aid of labor unions, large industries, and other community groups to pledge donations for new building campaigns. Construction of health care facilities is also funded through governmental grants and loans. The administrator prepares the applications and proposals to request this money and must fully describe the use of such funds. The application may be reviewed by a regional or state health planning agency. They can recommend the expansion and help the institution to fund the building. They may suggest changes in the plans.

The administrator's day may involve meetings, evaluations, budget reviews, correspondence, speeches — in other words, an executive's typical day. At any time, an ordinary, busy day may be interrupted by an emergency, such as a major disaster (fire, natural disaster, or accident) that sends many new patients to the medical center. In this case, the administrator will alert the managers of various departments to prepare them for the arrival of an unknown number of patients. Arrangements must be made for beds and for emergency treatment areas. The schedules of physicians, nurses, and other medical center staff may have to be rearranged to provide care for the injured. Ambulances must be dispatched to the disaster scene, and administrative workers must be prepared to handle the admitting and processing responsibilities.

Education for a career in health services administration is at the graduate level. The first year of the program is spent in academic studies concentrating on business management and the second year in an administrative residency, a period of in-facility preparation and experience. It is not necessary to be a doctor or a nurse before becoming a hospital administrator, although a medical background may be helpful.

Additional information on this career may be obtained from:

American College of Health Care Administrators
8120 Woodmont Avenue, Suite 200
Bethesda, Maryland 20814

American College of Health Care Executives
840 N. Lake Shore Drive
Chicago, Illinois 60611

American Health Care Association
1200 15th Street, N.W.
Washington, D.C. 20005

Association of University Programs in Health Administration
1911 N. Fort Myer Drive
Suite 503
Arlington, Virginia 22209

Director of Human Resources

Like all organizations, a health care facility is only as good as its employees. The director of human resources finds the best-qualified people to fill job openings. Advertisements are placed in newspapers and journals; applicants are interviewed and recommended for hiring. Other responsibilities of the director of human resources include: updating and revising personnel policies at regular intervals, publishing these policies and distributing them to all employees, and writing job descriptions (in cooperation with department managers) to be used in personnel recruitment.

The final decision in all hiring is the responsibility of the department manager who consults with the director of human resources in selecting from a group of qualified candidates. Most of the activities of the director of human resources involves working with the staff of the institution. There is little or no patient contact.

Directors of human resources have college degrees in personnel services or a related field. They become specialists in health care personnel through their work experience.

More information may be obtained from your guidance counselor and from:

American Hospital Association
840 N. Lake Shore Drive
Chicago, Illinois 60611

Note: Some agencies employ nurse recruiters whose responsibilities are to seek out registered professional nurses and licensed practical nurses to work in that institution. These recruiters are registered professional nurses with a bachelor's degree, who have become specialists in this field through experience and additional education.

Comptroller, Business Manager, Controller

Good business practices and careful money management are important parts of running a health care institution. The comptroller supervises the receipt and disbursement of all funds, approves expenditures, and keeps all financial records for audit.

Comptrollers have at least a bachelor's degree in accounting or business administration including extensive background using computers. In addition, several years of experience in hospital accounting and supervision are required. The comptroller may also be the manager of the institution's business department, supervising accountants, billing clerks, cashiers, admitting officers, payroll personnel, and others.

Accountant

Accountants keep records of all financial transactions and compile reports from this information. Through cost accounting, they determine the cost for institutional services. Accountants are directly responsible to the comptroller. A college education in accounting is required for this work, and a bachelor's degree is necessary for advancement. It is absolutely essential to be familiar with computerized accounting records and the various types of computer programs used in this occupation.

Admitting Officer

The first contact a patient or family has with an institution takes place in the admitting office. It is here that the patient/resident (or family member) furnishes all the information necessary to begin the institutional record known as the *chart*. The admitting officer explains the institution's rates, charges, services, and policies regarding payment of bills. The patient/resident goes to an assigned room in the appropriate area of the institution. All transfers and discharges of patients/residents are recorded by the admitting officer, who also maintains the daily census (patient/resident count). In the case of hospitals and medical centers, the admitting officer maintains a list of empty beds (beds available for emergency admissions). In large institutions, the admitting officer may supervise additional admitting personnel.

Educational requirements for this position vary. Many institutions require a college degree in social science or business administration, plus one or two years of experience in a health care institution. Often, registered nurses are employed in this position. High school graduates may be employed in other clerical positions in the admitting office, but additional education is required for advancement. Again, computer skills are essential, and a knowledge of medical terminology is required.

Other Hospital Business Careers

Opportunities exist for high school business education graduates in many areas including the credit and payroll departments.

For information on all business careers in hospitals, write to:

Healthcare Financial Management Association
1900 Spring Road
Oak Brook, Illinois 60521

Public Relations Director

The public relations director and staff keep the public informed about the role of the institution in the community and in the field of medical treatment and research. The institution's goals, programs, and services are explained through the news media, institutional publications, tours, and community events.

The public relations director selects newsworthy events to bring to the public's attention. Suppose a staff surgeon successfully performs intricate heart surgery that has never been done in the community. Suppose a resident of the nursing home celebrates a 100th birthday. The community is made aware of these outstanding accomplishments at local institutions.

Often, the public relations director takes part in fund-raising efforts, laying the groundwork for large-scale community support through publicity campaigns, fund appeals, and benefit dinners and parties. Another major responsibility is to keep the community or region informed about changes in institutional services and policies, planned expansion, or necessary cutbacks.

In addition to projecting the institution's image to the community, the public relations department also promotes the facility within its own walls. It publishes house magazines or newsletters for employees, plans award ceremonies for volunteer workers, and arranges service award recognition for employees.

Most public relations directors have college degrees in public relations or journalism. They should be familiar with computers, especially word processing and desktop publishing software. Medical photographers may also be employed in the public relations department of very large institutions.

For more information on this career, contact your guidance counselor or the public relations director of your local hospital.

Volunteers, Director of Volunteer Service

Volunteers are unpaid workers who give their time and talents to the institution, assisting the staff and patients/residents in many ways. Volunteers may feed patients/residents, read to them, or write letters for them. They deliver mail, gifts, and flowers to patients/residents, stock the library cart and take it from room to room, and so on. Volunteers work on a part-time basis and are trained by the head of the department to which they are assigned or by the director of volunteers (**Fig. 7–1**).

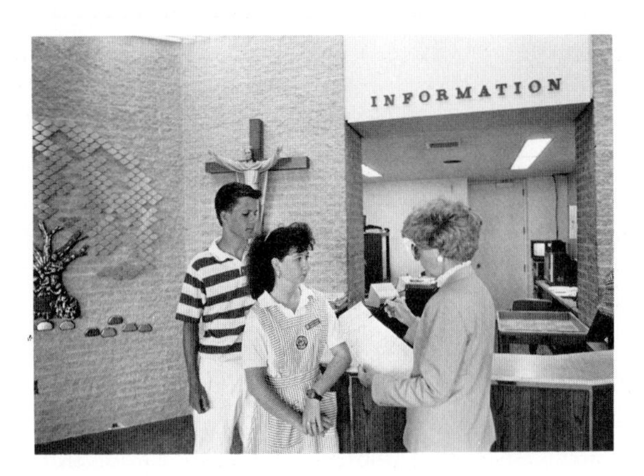

Figure 7–1. The director of volunteers assigns duties. (Courtesy of St. Mary Hospital, Langhorne, Pa.)

Not all volunteers are assigned to patient/resident care services. Some work in reception areas where they answer the telephone and give information and directions to visitors. Others may work in the gift shop or coffee shop. Experienced volunteers are often called on to help with fund-raising activities.

As institutions come to rely more on volunteer services, opportunities for directors of volunteers are expanding, especially in small- and middle-sized facilities throughout the United States. Large institutions have employed this type of worker for many years.

Further information about this career is available from your guidance counselor, local hospital, and from:

American Hospital Association
840 N. Lake Shore Drive
Chicago, Illinois 60611

Medical Record Administrator, Registered Record Administrator (RRA)

Every person who enters the health care delivery system has a permanent record containing information about one's progress during illness or after an injury. For inpatients and residents, this record is compiled from the clinical chart and includes the medical history and physical examination reports; physicians' and nurses' progress notes; reports of diagnostic tests; diet and medication records; and reports from the surgical, pathological, and restorative therapy departments.

These records are compiled, stored, and retained for retrieval in the medical record department. Records of past illnesses are furnished to physicians if a patient returns for further medical care. Documentation of the patient's/resident's medical evaluation and treatment is essential to the institution's financial reimbursement. Also, certain data are extracted from these records for preparation of statistical reports used by public health officials, medical researchers, and health care administrators. Computers and microfilm are used in the management of health information systems. These have reduced the handling of large volumes of paper to manageable size (**Fig. 7–2**).

The medical record administrator develops health information systems for: quality patient care, facility reimbursement, medical research, health planning, and health care evaluation. The statistics gathered by the medical record administrator provide valuable information about the use of hospital facilities and may be used in planning for expansion or reduction of plant and/or services.

There are two types of educational programs for medical record administrators. (1) High school graduates may enter a college undergraduate program with a major in medical record administration. (2) College

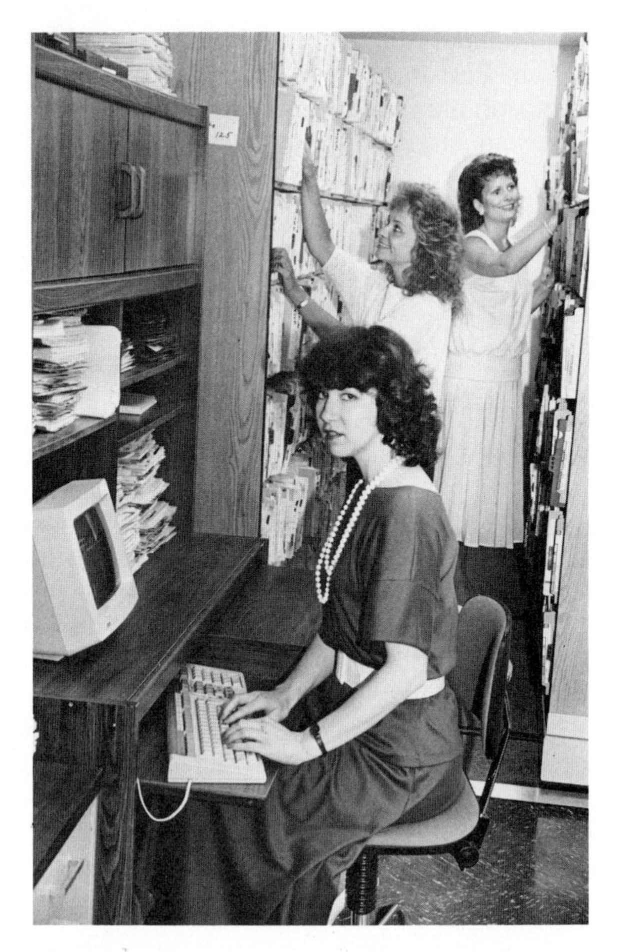

Figure 7–2. Patient records are compiled and stored by medical record personnel. (Courtesy of St. Mary Hospital, Langhorne, Pa.)

graduates, who have certain prerequisite courses, may earn a post-graduate certificate in medical record administration.

The curriculum for accredited medical record administrator programs includes anatomy and physiology, medical terminology, fundamentals of medical science, record management, health information systems, computer science, business administration, financial management, **medico-legal** aspects, quality assurance, statistics, and research methods. There is also a supervised clinical practice in the medical record department of an approved health care facility.

Registration is available through the American Medical Record Association.

Medical Record Technician, Accredited Record Technician (ART)

Medical record technicians transcribe medical reports by: inputting and retrieving computerized health data; compiling various administrative and health statistics; and coding symptoms, diseases, operations, procedures, and other therapies according to recognized classification systems. They also maintain and use a variety of health record indexes, special registries, and storage and retrieval systems. Charts are reviewed for completeness and accuracy according to established standards. Technicians control the usage and release of health information. For instance, they may take records to court as evidence or provide records for review by lawyers, insurance company representatives, or police.

Programs for medical record technicians are one or two years long. They are conducted in hospitals, community colleges, and universities. Graduates are eligible to take a national accreditation examination to become Accredited Record Technicians (ART). In small hospitals, nursing homes, and health maintenance organizations, technicians may be employed as department directors.

Medical Record Clerk

High school graduates with good typing and filing skills perform clerical duties in the medical record department.

The American Medical Record Association offers an independent study program in medical record technology. After meeting certain requirements, graduates of the independent study program can apply to take the national accrediting examination and become an ART.

For additional information, contact:

American Medical Record Association
875 N. Michigan Avenue
Suite 1850
Chicago, Illinois 60611

Medical Secretary

A knowledge of medical terminology enables the medical secretary to transcribe patients' records from dictation, to assist in preparing research reports, and to complete many types of medical forms, records, and manuscripts. Medical secretaries are employed in various places — physicians' offices, medical record departments, health agencies, medical and nursing schools, and medical book publishing companies.

Community colleges and technical schools offer programs in medical secretarial science, including word processing and other types of computer software. Some high school programs are offered jointly through a health occupations education program and the business education department.

For more information, contact your guidance counselor or local community college.

SUPPORTIVE CLUSTER

Laundry Manager and Laundry Workers

The linens required for every hospital bed include two sheets, two pillow cases, one mattress cover, one bedspread, two towels, and one washcloth. Multiply the total of these pieces by the number of hospital beds, and you will have some idea of the volume of laundry used daily in every hospital. Then come the diapers, patient gowns, and curtains. A king-size washload (**Fig. 7–3**).

Many workers, supervised by the laundry manager, are needed to handle the enormous job of washing, finishing, mending, sorting, removing stains, and maintaining inventories. Some institutions do not employ laundry workers but, instead, contract the job to an independent company.

Laundry workers are high school graduates who receive on-the-job training. They perform heavy work in a hot, humid environment and may come in contact with hazardous materials. There is little opportunity for advancement.

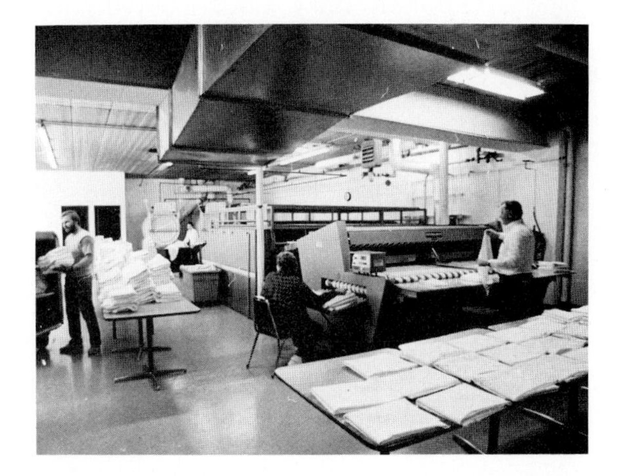

Figure 7–3. Many workers are needed to handle the laundry in a health care institution. (Courtesy of Bridgeton Hospital, Bridgeton, N.J. Photo by Gary F. Cooper.)

Executive Housekeeper, Housekeeper

Keeping the patient/resident environment clean and orderly is the job of the housekeeping department. The overall appearance of the institution is a factor in the physical comfort and well-being of patients, but of even greater importance is preventing the spread of infection.

The work of the housekeeping department is directed by the executive housekeeper who is also responsible for training new employees, planning work schedules, selecting cleaning methods, and inspecting and evaluating staff performance.

A college education in institutional management or home economics is needed to qualify for a position as an executive housekeeper. A bachelor of science degree in institutional management is a definite advantage.

When the "house" to be kept is a hospital or nursing home, the assistance of many people is necessary. There are essentially two categories of work: (1) heavy housecleaning, such as washing walls and windows; scrubbing and waxing floors; and removing and rehanging drapes, curtains, and blinds; (2) light daily housekeeping in patient/resident rooms, offices, and other areas.

Some institutions contract with "outside" companies for housekeeping services.

For more information, contact your local health care institution or:

American Health Care Association
1200 15th Street, N.W.
Washington, D.C. 20005

Environmental Management Association
1019 Highland Avenue
Largo, Florida 33540

American Hospital Association
840 N. Lake Shore Drive
Chicago, Illinois 60611

Dietary Service

Dietary and food services careers and related information are found on page 127 in Chapter 5.

Purchasing Agent, Storekeeper, Stock Clerk

All the shopping for the institution is done by the purchasing agent who buys equipment, supplies, and outside services. Samples of new products are tested by the staff of the institution; they report their findings to the purchasing department. For example, the nursing department may test and compare glass thermometers, digital electronic thermometers, and disposable paper thermometers. These products are evaluated for safety, accuracy, and efficiency. The purchasing agent reviews the recommendations from the nursing staff and considers other factors, such as cost, need, and means of storage before deciding which items to purchase. Other duties of the purchasing agent include the inspection of delivered goods, payment approval, and storage and distribution of materials.

A high school education and five years purchasing experience are required for this position. However, a college degree in business administration is a requirement for employment as a purchasing agent in many large institutions.

The purchasing agent is assisted by a storekeeper or a stockroom manager whose duties include the receiving, handling, and storing of all goods, supplies, and equipment used by the institution (**Fig. 7–4**). The store clerk delivers the supplies to the various departments within the institution. High school graduates are employed to work in the storeroom. Courses in business mathematics, bookkeeping, and computer keyboarding are useful in this type of work.

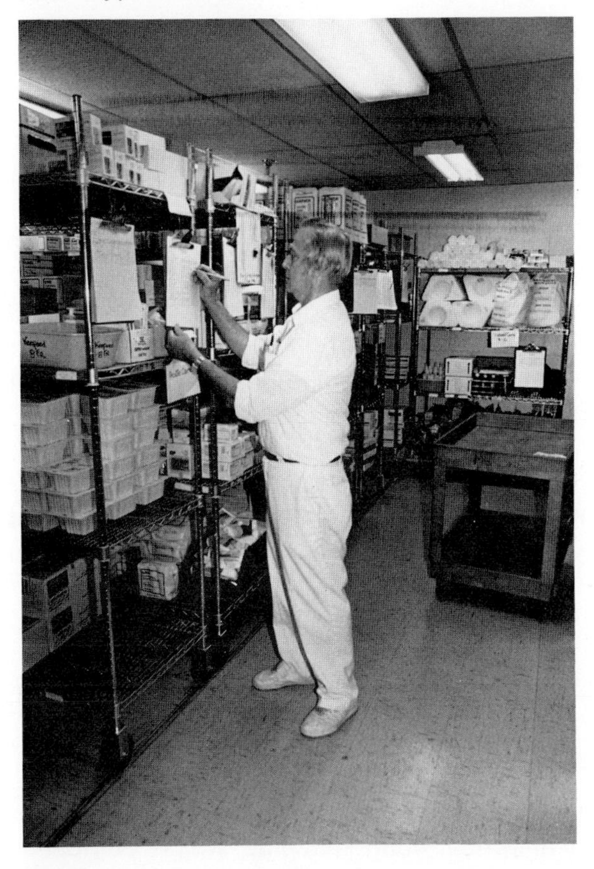

Figure 7–4. Storekeeper checks inventory of necessary supplies. (Courtesy of St. Mary Hospital, Langhorne, Pa.)

Additional information about careers in materials management may be obtained from:

American Health Care Association
1200 15th Street, N.W.
Washington, D.C. 20005

American Hospital Association
840 N. Lake Shore Drive
Chicago, Illinois 60611

Hospital Engineer and Maintenance Workers

Hospitals are large institutions that require special repairs and daily maintenance. A corps of workers is employed for the upkeep of buildings, grounds, and equipment: plumbers, stationary engineers (who operate the boilers), carpenters, painters, and electricians. They are supervised by the chief hospital engineer who is responsible for assigning specific duties and evaluating work performance. The institutional plant is inspected daily to determine the need for immediate repairs and scheduled maintenance. Lighting, heating, plumbing, and air conditioning are the responsibility of the maintenance department.

The chief hospital engineer holds a degree in mechanical or electrical engineering. In small hospitals or nursing homes, a high school education may be substituted for an engineering degree. Some hospital engineers have completed apprenticeship training in one of the building trades, such as carpentry, plumbing, or electricity (**Fig. 7–5**).

More information may be obtained from your local hospital.

Biomedical Engineer and Biomedical Engineering Technician

There was a time when open heart surgery was not feasible or practical, but today the heart-lung machine which pumps and oxygenates blood, has made it a common procedure. This machine is one of the devices developed by biomedical engineers in conjunction with cardiac surgeons. Others include various monitoring machines and equipment for cardiac diagnostic studies.

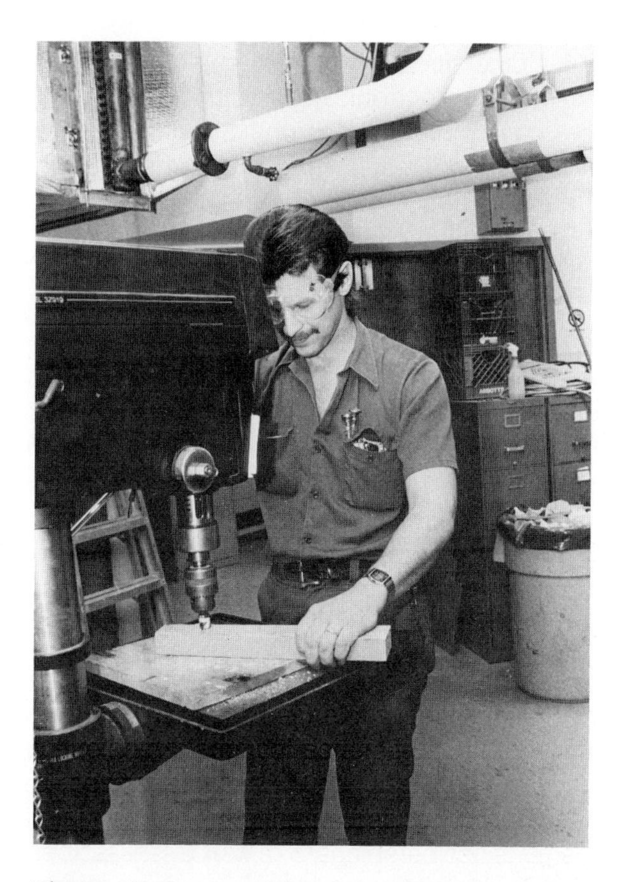

Figure 7–5. It takes many skilled workers to keep an institution running smoothly. (Courtesy of Bridgeton Hospital, Bridgeton, N.J. Photo by Gary F. Cooper.)

Biomedical engineers apply theories from chemistry, physics, and geology to solve medical problems. They use modern technology such as computers and electronics to put these theories to practical use in the development of medical instruments, machines, monitors, and replacement parts. Some examples are **noninvasive** imaging equipment, artificial kidney machines, and the heart-lung machine.

Biomedical engineering is a new, young career. The minimum educational requirement is a four-year bachelor's degree program in engineering, physics, or a related biological science. A graduate degree may be required for some positions.

The biomedical engineering technician constructs new instruments and machines in collaboration with the biomedical engineer. Since these products are highly diversified, other personnel (**orthotists, prosthetists,** opticians, glassblowers, electronic technicians, watchmakers, and computer technicians) have a hand in designing and manufacturing them.

Biomedical engineering technician programs are located in universities and four-year colleges.

Biomedical Equipment Technician

The equipment used in diagnosis, treatment, and patient monitoring must be kept in working order at all times. This is the job of biomedical equipment technicians. They also install, maintain, and sometimes operate equipment such as the heart-lung machine, artificial kidney, vital sign monitors, and automated laboratory equipment (**Fig. 7–6**).

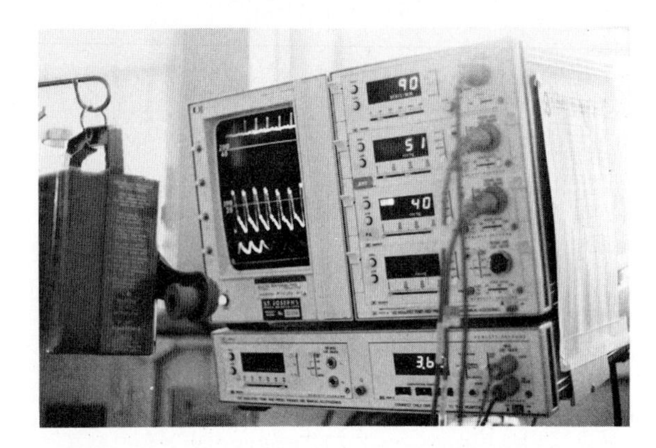

Figure 7–6. Biomedical equipment technicians install and maintain complex electronic equipment. (Courtesy of New Jersey Hospital Association. Photo by Cliff Moore.)

Two-year community college programs in biomedical equipment technology, biomedical engineering technology, electronic technology, or instrument technology prepare the graduate for employment.

More information on the above careers may be obtained from:

Alliance for Engineering in Medicine and Biology
1101 Connecticut Avenue, N.W.
Suite 700
Washington, D.C. 20036

Biomedical Engineering Society
P.O. Box 2399
Culver, California 90231

Unit Clerk, Unit Manager

Nurses have traditionally been required to do considerable paperwork; sometimes this has kept them at the desk instead of at the patient's bedside. Today, unit clerks (formerly called ward clerks) perform most of the clerical duties in a nursing unit. Their responsibilities vary but typically include: answering telephones and relaying messages; assembling charts and recording routine information (temperature, pulse, respiration); handling diet, laboratory, x-ray, and drug requisitions; stocking and ordering supplies; and assisting visitors and patients with non-nursing matters (**Fig. 7–7**).

High school graduates are employed in these jobs. A beginning knowledge of medical terminology and keyboarding skills are most helpful. Some vocational schools offer educational programs for unit clerks although most clerks are trained on the job.

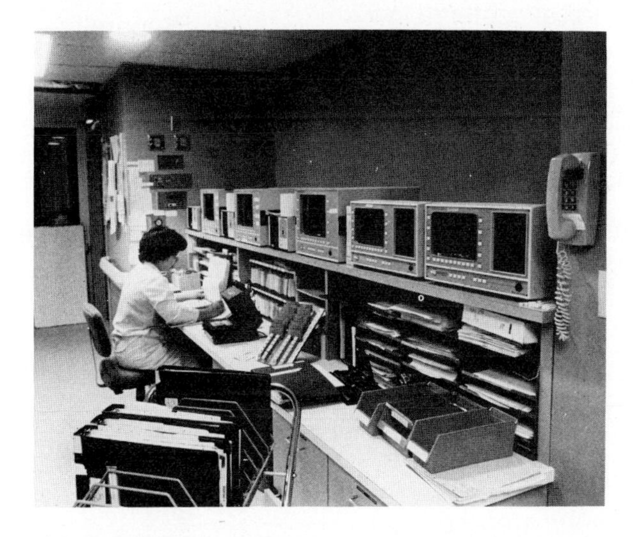

Figure 7–7. Institutional staff rely on the expertise of the unit clerk, or secretary, to handle clerical responsibilities. (Courtesy of Bridgeton Hospital, Bridgeton, N.J. Photo by Gary F. Cooper.)

Unit managers supervise the work of the unit clerks, conduct on-the-job training, make assignments, and evaluate job performance. Some unit managers are promoted from among the unit clerks, while some are college graduates with business administration degrees.

For more information, contact the human resources director of your local hospital.

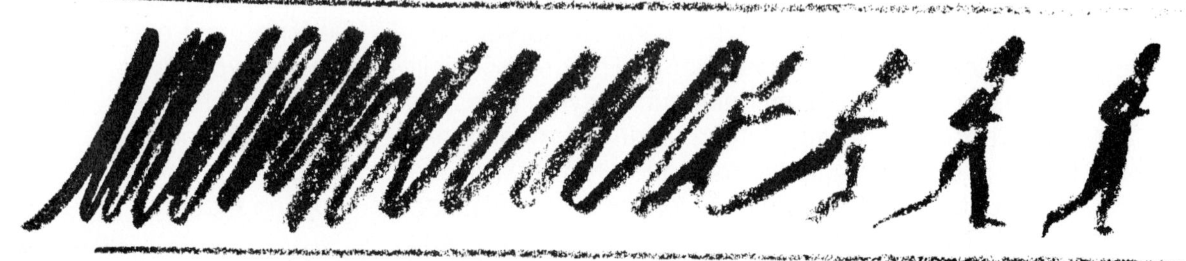

S·T·U·D·E·N·T A·C·T·I·V·I·T·I·E·S

1. Is the hospital in your community a general, specialized, or teaching hospital? Is it a medical center? How many beds does it have? How many buildings? Does it provide laundry, housekeeping, and food service, or are these services contracted to outside companies?
2. List as many items as possible that might be ordered by the purchasing agent in a medical center and/or nursing home.
3. List the various department managers with whom the health care administrator works (e.g., the chief laboratory technologist).
4. What schools in your area conduct educational programs in Institutional Careers?
5. Identify the hospital employee who would perform the following activity:
   a. Prepare microfilms of medical records
   b. Abstract statistics from medical records
   c. Manage the institution's finances
   d. Recruit new employees
   e. Purchase institutional equipment and supplies
   f. Store institutional equipment and supplies
   g. Scrub and polish floors
   h. Repair leaky faucets
   i. Record temperature, pulse, and respiration on a patient's/resident's chart.
   j. Maintain biomedical equipment.

Chapter 8

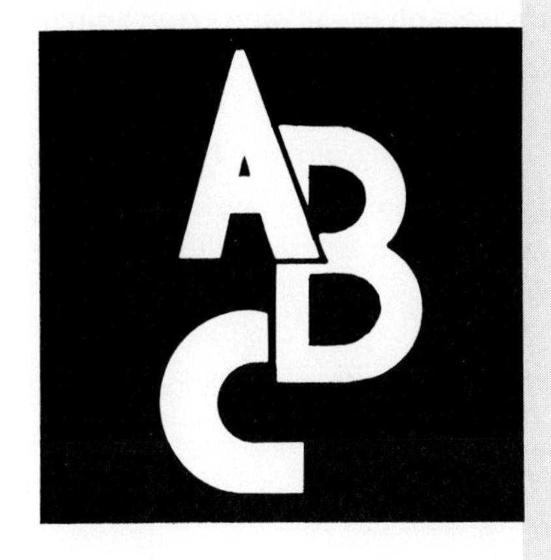

Health Career ABCs

Objectives

After completing this chapter, you should be able to:

- Discuss at least five personal characteristics and/or qualities needed by health workers.
- Describe ethical behavior of health workers.
- Discuss the "Patient's Bill of Rights."
- Discuss ethical and legal considerations for those health workers who have access to the patient's chart.
- Explain how health workers can protect the patient's right to privacy.
- Define 70 percent of the key terms listed for this chapter.

Key Terms

- **behavior** The way in which one acts
- **civil law** Law concerned with private rights and relationships between people, also known as private law

- **confidential** Private or secret
- **consent** Approval or acceptance of something done or proposed by another
- **controlled substances** Drugs that are regulated by federal law. The degree of regulation depends upon the potential for drug abuse, physical and psychologic dependence, and accepted medical use in the United States
- **communication** The sharing of thoughts, opinions, and information
- **criminal law** Laws concerned with offenses against the public or society as a whole, also known as public law
- **ethics** Standards dealing with good and evil and moral conduct
- **habit** An act or behavior that is performed so regularly that it becomes practically automatic
- **law** Rules of conduct established and enforced by a governing body
- **lawsuit** An action in court to recover a right or claim involving civil law
- **liable** Legally responsible for one's actions
- **malpractice** Unprofessional behavior that results in injury, loss, or damage to another person
- **negligence** Unintentional wrong in which a person does not act in careful and/or reasonable manner thereby causing injury or harm to another person
- **nonverbal communication** Communication without the use of words
- **personal hygiene** Care of the body by following rules for good health
- **privileged communication** Confidential information given by the patient to the person authorized to provide medical care
- **verbal communication** Communication using the spoken or written word

BEGINNING YOUR HEALTH CAREER

No matter what health career you choose, you will find that there are certain expectations and responsibilities common to all of these careers. They can be thought of as the "ABCs" of beginning a career: Appearance, Behavior, and Communication.

Appearance

Clothing

A is for appearance. Many people working in the health field will be expected to wear uniforms to work. Some, however, will wear street clothes or what is generally called business attire. In some instances, health care workers will wear laboratory coats over their street clothes. Whatever you wear to work, you will be expected to present a suitable appearance (**Fig. 8–1**).

Clothing should fit properly, being neither too large nor too small. Clean clothes should be worn every day. Inspect your clothes and make sure that they have been cleaned, ironed, and mended. If you will be having direct patient contact, you will appreciate comfortable, washable clothing which will allow you to move easily. Jeans are usually considered inappropriate attire for most health workers.

Identification

Most employers will require their employees to wear identification pins that state the employee's name and title (**Fig. 8–2**). These should always be worn when on duty so that the clients and staff members from other departments will be able to identify you and your department. In some work settings, identification badges are worn—all the time or at specific

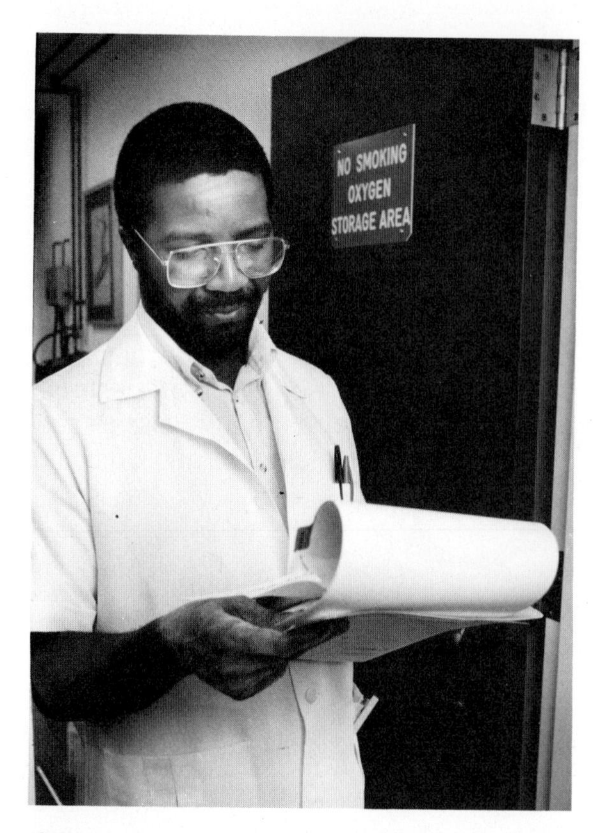

Figure 8–1. A neat appearance conveys a professional image. (Courtesy of Henry J. Austin Health Center, Trenton, N.J. Photo by Michael Mancuso.)

times during the day — in order to regulate who is allowed to enter certain areas and buildings. For instance, only those working in a hospital newborn nursery are permitted entrance. Usually, those staff members wear special identification badges in addition to specific types of clothing. Also, after certain hours most hospitals and nursing homes are closed to visitors. The security officers will admit only those persons wearing the proper identification badges. This is done to protect both the patients and staff from intruders.

Shoes, socks, and stockings

Shoes should be comfortable. Low heels provide a good base of support and help to prevent fatigue and accidents. If you wear white

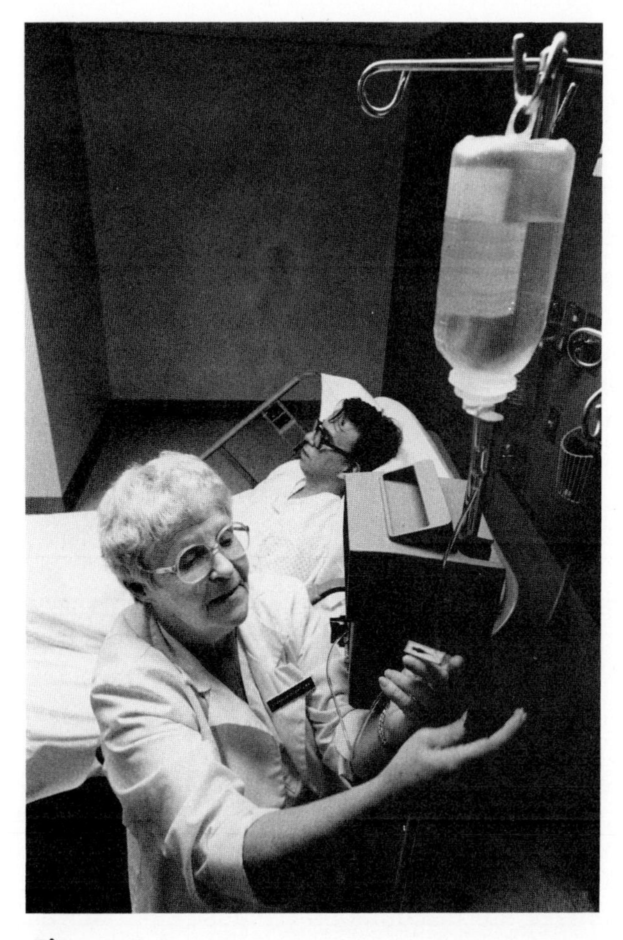

Figure 8–2. This nurse has a neat appearance and is wearing an appropriate identification pin. (Courtesy of Bridgeton Hospital, Bridgeton, N.J. Photo by Gary F. Cooper.)

shoes, they should **be** white. This means you will need to polish your shoes and wash your shoe laces every day. Run down, poorly fitting shoes are uncomfortable and hazardous. Buy the best shoes you can afford and keep them in good repair. They are an important investment, not only in how you look, but how you feel.

Wear clean socks or stockings every day. They should fit properly, without wrinkles, not too tight or constricting. Females wear white stockings only if these are considered a part of the uniform. If white is this year's fashionable color, wear it in your private life, not at work. White stockings are usually reserved for those staff members who wear white uniforms and perform direct patient care.

Underwear

Underneath it all, clean undergarments are essential. These, too, must be changed daily; in hot, humid weather, they should be changed more often. Underclothes should be comfortable and fit properly. They should not be obvious by being a darker color than the outergarments. Black or figured undergarments under a white uniform are totally inappropriate and do not create the appearance of dressing for business or success.

Jewelry, hair, and cosmetics

If you are caring for patients, you will not be able to wear jewelry on duty, although most institutions will allow you to wear a wedding band and a watch with a sweep second hand. In other areas, there may be no restrictions regarding jewelry. Check your agency policy, and be conservative in your choice of jewelry.

When working with patients, your hair should be off your collar, clean, in an easy to care for style. If a beard and/or moustache is worn, it should be trimmed and kept immaculately clean. Otherwise, daily shaving is essential. Short fingernails will prevent injury to patients and yourself. Long, polished fingernails are discouraged because both act as sites for bacteria to accumulate and grow. In other areas of health care, common sense should rule the length and color of nails. A conservative approach is always recommended.

If you wear make-up, again, be conservative in the amount and colors you select. You wish to be attractive not an attraction. Many fragrances cause allergic reactions and can actually cause nausea in sick people. Therefore, heavy perfumes, strong colognes, and after-shave lotions should be worn after work.

Daily hygiene

Daily bathing is the basis of proper hygiene. The skin is the largest organ in the entire body, and it acts as the body's first line of defense against infection. Proper care and cleansing of the skin will remove dirt and microorganisms and help to prevent odors and infection. Your teeth should be brushed when you wake up, before coming to work and, ideally, after every meal. If you are working closely with patients, you need to avoid foods (garlic, onions, peppers, etc.) that may give you bad breath.

An underarm deodorant/antiperspirant is most effective when used immediately after bathing and reapplied before coming to work.

Behavior

B stands for behavior. Webster defines behavior as personal conduct. In other words, it is the way you act, the habits you have, your attitudes, characteristics, and qualities.

Habits

Let's take a look at your habits. These are behavior patterns acquired by frequent repetition. Some habits are desirable while others are undesirable; in fact, some habits can be quite dangerous.

Personal health does not "just happen," it is gained by developing personal habits that promote the physical and mental wellness of the human being. As a health worker, other people will naturally look to you as an example of good health and hygiene. Your personal habits will help you to maintain health and promote wellness.

Proper diet

The proper balance of food, exercise, and rest are important factors in good health. Most of us are expected to work at our highest levels early in the day, usually before lunch. In fact, most people do experience their highest energy level in the morning. Therefore, the first meal of the day should provide adequate amounts of food to support that peak period of energy. A cup of coffee and a glass of orange juice does not provide the caloric or nutritional content necessary for an active work day. (For information on proper diet, see Chapter 14.) Those who work on evening or night shifts have energy peaks at different hours. They may be eating a bedtime snack for the traditional early morning meal while dinner or a late supper will provide the nutrition to get through the night.

Proper rest

Anyone working in a health career needs to be alert and "tuned in" to what is going on in the work place. In order to do this, you need to have an adequate amount of sleep. You cannot spend all day at the beach, dance until 10 P.M. and then go to work at 11:30 P.M. and expect to do your very best. After a day of such vigorous activity, your entire body (especially your brain) will want to sleep — at the very time when you most need to be able to function at your fullest. A regular pattern of sleep is necessary to refresh you and to restore the energy needed each day.

Proper exercise

Some health careers (physical therapy, recreation therapy, nursing) may involve strenuous physical activity — lifting, moving, walking. Other careers — such as dental laboratory technology, speech pathology, medical records coding — can be quite sedentary.

Workers in several health careers were clocked for their daily mileage. Dental hygienists walked 1.2 miles, interns walked 3.5 miles, and nurses walked 5.4 miles. Therefore, it is impossible to recommend any type of exercise that is appropriate for all health wokers. This will vary according to age, health status, and, of course, activity on the job. Almost everyone can benefit from rapid walking three times a week for 20 minutes. This exercises the long muscles, increases the metabolic rate, stimulates the heart and lungs, and promotes healthful sleep. Walking is an excellent way to exercise, anyone can do it, no special training or equipment is necessary, and the price is right.

Other types of exercise are so varied that the activity is limited only by your own interest, needs, available time, and physical abilities. Biking, swimming, running, skating, jogging, and skiing are among the many activities that provide exercise, entertainment, and relaxation.

Smoking

Certain habits are insults to the body and are factors which promote illness. Tobacco in any form — smoking, chewing, or inhaling (snuff) — is extremely irritating to the tissues of the human body and is a causative agent in cancer of the lung, lip, mouth, tongue, and throat. Tobacco smoke affects the lung and heart function, blood pressure, circulation, and digestive process. Secondhand smoke — smoke that is inhaled by a person who does not smoke but who works or lives in a smoky environment — will cause the same effects in the nonsmoker. There is nothing positive that can be said about the use of tobacco. In fact, any use of tobacco is an abuse of your body. Furthermore, most health care employers prohibit (often this is required by state law) smoking at work. If you smoke only on your off-duty hours, others can smell the odor of smoke because tobacco smoke permeates your clothing and hair. Not only are you harming your own physical health, but you are setting a poor example for others to follow.

Alcohol

In today's drug-oriented society, alcohol is the most popular and the most often abused drug. Many people say, alcohol's not a drug. A brief look at how it affects the body may convince you otherwise.

Alcohol is a central nervous system depressant that reduces the blood pressure, decreases the respiratory rate, reduces the protective reflexes (gagging and choking), diminishes reaction time, and eliminates the ability to think clearly and rationally. Alcohol can also cause death since it is a toxic substance. Too much alcohol will cause acute alcohol poisoning and death. Alcohol is detoxified by the liver — too much alcohol over a period of time can destroy the liver and cause death.

Even a little alcohol, one drink, can dull the senses, reduce judgment, and turn a valuable employee into a dangerous person who is not awake or alert enough to do his/her job. Alcohol and a health career do not mix. For example, the operating room team (the surgeon, the circulating nurse, the surgical technician) who is "on call" for the evening and night shifts cannot have a drink because they could be called into emergency surgery at 4 A.M.. They cannot afford to be under the influence of anything that can alter their ability to function at their very best.

Drug abuse

Drug abuse is a serious medical and social problem in the United States. Many of our young people — the future of our country — are being destroyed by the abuse of legal and illegal drugs. The medical term for these drugs is **controlled substances**; their control, storage, use, and possession is regulated by the Controlled Substances Act. This federal legislation was passed in 1970 and established the Drug Enforcement Agency (DEA) which enforces the Act.

Recent research indicates that health workers are especially susceptible to drug abuse and that they usually have their first experience with drugs when they are students. Drug abuse is a serious occupational hazard especially for those employed in health care facilities. It is not uncommon to hear of a physician who is addicted to drugs report that the first dose was taken from the locked drug supply in the hospital while still in medical school. Stealing drugs and replacing them with ineffective substitutes is standard practice for the health care worker who abuses drugs. Pity the patient who is depending on the "look-alike" substitute to provide relief from pain and discomfort.

Doctors, nurses, pharmacists, and other licensed health personnel may have their licenses to practice suspended or revoked due to drug abuse. Because health workers often have direct or indirect access to controlled substances, they have a special trust and responsibility to protect the drug supply so that it is available for patient use when prescribed within the confines of the law. You must never take a drug that has not been prescribed for you or give your prescribed drug to another person.

Because of the nature of your career, you can never illegally possess a controlled substance without threat of losing your job. Certainly, you will be subject to the full punishment under the law. In addition, you will be under scrutiny from your employer and, if you are licensed, by the licensing board in your state. Drug abuse can cost you your job and license/certification, not to mention your life.

If you use drugs, you are drugged. If you say that it is not so, then you are expressing denial of the true facts — a symptom of drug addiction. If you use drugs now, get help to stop. REMEMBER: You are always expected to be awake, alert, and "tuned-in." REMEMBER: The phrase is "tuned-in," not turned on.

If you have a problem, you can always find help without turning to drugs. Your teacher, guidance counselor, parents, minister, priest, or rabbi can help you or refer you to someone who can help you look at your problems objectively and find some options for dealing with the difficulties encountered in life. There are no magic pills to make life easy. Those in the health occupations, particularly, must take life and death as it comes and use their own internal coping resources without the use of drugs. Many times counseling can help us to realize that we are stronger and more competent than we ever thought and that we are indeed quite capable of dealing with our own problems in a constructive manner.

Ethical considerations

As you work in a health career, you will be faced with decisions about what is right and what is wrong, what is correct behavior and what is not. Many times you will need to decide what you can do and what you cannot do — the behavior that is appropriate for you within the scope of your education, experience, and legal responsibilities.

Many professional groups have established codes of ethics which are guidelines for judgment when moral decisions have to be made. Ethics is concerned with judgments about what is right and what is wrong conduct. Some say that ethics is what someone ought to do when there is no law or rule that says what one must or should do in a given situation. For example, the decision to remove life-support systems from a patient who is "brain dead" is an ethical issue that requires a serious decision on the part of the physician and the family. There are no easy answers, no specific existing rules to govern the behavior that may be decided.

As you gain more education and experience in your occupational area, you will learn more about the ethical issues involved in your specific career. There are no guaranteed ways to solve ethical problems. However, there are some things to be considered when faced with such a problem.

1. Gather as much information about the problem and all involved in the situation.
2. Study the possible consequences of each proposed action in the situation. Examine carefully the "worst possible" thing that could occur as a result of your behavior.
3. Think about who should make the final decision in the matter.
4. Talk to others who — by virtue of their position, education, and experience — can help you.
5. Always act as a responsible citizen.
6. Always know the limitations of your role and knowledge.
7. Be loyal to yourself and your employer.
8. Follow agency policies.

Suppose you observe a nursing supervisor, Mr. Johnson, opening the locked medication closet. You see him slip several medication containers into his pocket. What would you do? Could you use the suggestions listed above to reach a solution to this dilemma?

Legal considerations

Laws are rules of conduct or action established and enforced by a governing body. They are designed to protect the rights of the public. There are two types of laws — civil law and criminal law. Civil laws involve relationships between people (e.g., contracts and wills). Criminal laws involve wrongs against a person, property, or society in general. Rape, murder, and blackmail are examples of crimes.

Torts, Negligence, Malpractice. A tort is a wrongful act performed against another person. Torts may be intentional or unintentional. Wrongdoings common to the health care industry are listed below.

Negligence is an unintentional wrong. A person who does not act in a reasonable or careful manner is negligent and, thereby, is responsible for the wrongful consequences that may occur (e.g., leaving a confused patient alone on an x-ray table and the patient falls off). A negligent person may have to pay damages to the injured person.

Malpractice is a more serious form of negligence, usually on the part of professional persons. The court decides the difference between negligence and malpractice. Nurses, physicians, pharmacists, dentists, and physical and occupational therapists are all considered professional practitioners. Most professional persons carry malpractice insurance.

As a health worker, you are legally responsible (liable) for your own actions at all times. What you do can lead to a lawsuit if others are harmed or injured. At times, you may be directed to do something that is not within the scope of your responsibility. Your supervisor may tell you that it is "OK" to do what is asked because he or she will assume the responsibility for your actions. If something goes wrong, your supervisor may indeed be held responsible, but you will not be relieved of any personal liability. YOU ARE ALWAYS LIABLE FOR YOUR OWN ACTIONS AT ALL TIMES — NO MATTER WHAT ANYONE MAY TELL YOU, AND NO MATTER WHAT POSITION YOU MAY HOLD.

Communications

Finally, the C in the ABCs of beginning your career is communication. This involves the process of sharing thoughts, opinions, and information.

This may be done through speech, writing, or other methods. There is always a sender of the information and a receiver of the information (**Fig. 8–3**). An important part of the process is understanding the meaning of the information.

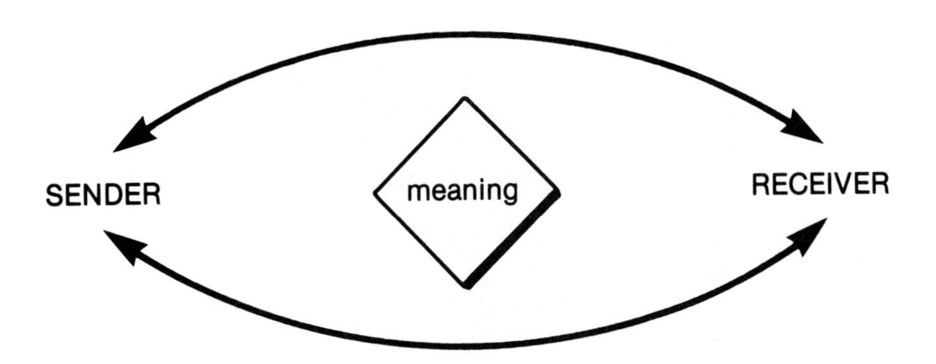

Figure 8–3.

For example, if you are in a strange city and ask someone for directions to the post office, you would expect the receiver of the message to understand what kind of information you require. However, if the receiver does not speak or understand English, you probably will be unable to communicate your problem or needs.

We are constantly surrounded by attempts to get our attention and our response. The telephone, television, radio, newspapers, books, gestures, body language, and sign language act as a means for senders to transmit information, opinions, and ideas. Some communications will be verbal and others will be nonverbal.

Verbal communication

Verbal communication involves the use of words, usually by speaking. However, the use of the written word is also considered a form of verbal communication. The use of written communications in health careers will be discussed in Chapter 10.

Nonverbal communication

Nonverbal communication involves the exchange of information without the use of words. You can send both positive and negative messages through nonverbal communication. Many times, what is not said — even silence — becomes the message. Actions sometimes do speak "louder than words" (**Fig. 8–4**).

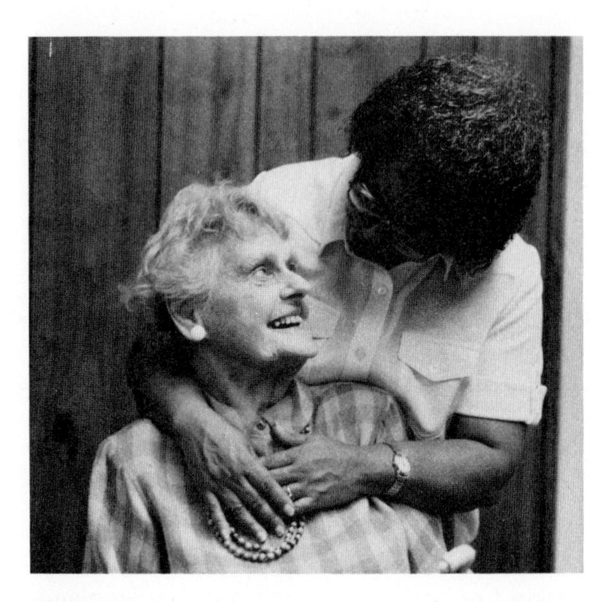

Figure 8–4. Sometimes a hug is better than any words. (Courtesy of Mercer Street Friends Center, Trenton, N.J.)

Eye contact. Most communication begins with eye contact. When you wish to speak to someone, you usually first "get their eye" and then continue with the conversation. However, when you arrive late for work, and your employer gets your eye by looking over his/her eyeglasses, this is not merely gaining your attention, a powerful nonverbal message is being sent.

Facial expression. Consider the effect of a smile, scowl, or a frown on communication. Facial expression really gets a message across, even without words. Posture, too, can convey a message. Try to visualize the posture of a person who is tired, bored, and defensive. Compare this with your mental image of a person who is happy, energetic, and healthy. Crying, laughing, sighing, and groaning all are audible — but nonverbal — means of communication.

Both types of communication can occur at the same time. For example, your friend tells you that "Everything is OK," when it is obvious to you that she has been crying. Her verbal communication tells you something quite different from the message you are getting from her nonverbal communication. It can be confusing to get two messages at the same time — there is no understanding and no communication.

When you begin your health career, you will need to be aware of your communications skills and the messages you are sending. Some examples of nonverbal communications are listed elsewhere in this chapter. Most of these actions are unconscious signals you give to others. Try to be aware of the effect that nonverbal communications can have on your employer and also in relationships with clients, coworkers, supervisors, and others.

Guidelines for communicating

Pay particular attention to your verbal communications. You can't be certain that you will always say the right thing, but there are some basic rules to consider. You should speak in a moderate tone, no shouting or screaming. Use proper English, avoid slang phrases, and NEVER use obscene language. Be courteous and polite. Instead of speaking out in anger, think things over before you speak. Always treat others as you would like to be treated. Listen carefully, don't turn people off, or listen with "half an ear."

Communication blocks

There are many blocks to communication, including preconceived ideas, snap judgment, **biases,** and **prejudice.** When you make up your mind that there is only one way to do something, you close your mind to communication. You will stick by your preconceived idea, and nothing that another person says or does will change your mind.

If you only see the color of another person, and do not hear their ideas, thoughts, or opinions, there can be no communication. It's equally hard to communicate when you are the object of prejudice — when all someone sees is your age, color, sex, handicaps, etc. — and automatically assigns you to a group, instead of seeing you as an individual.

The first woman doctor, Elizabeth Blackwell, had to face unbelievable prejudice both in medical school and when she began her private practice. But we can see by her example that she dealt with the needs of her patients and not their prejudice.

Certainly, prejudice should not be tolerated to excess, but you should not take it personally either. It is a good idea to discuss any problems of this nature with your teacher and/or supervisor.

Privileged Communications

Health workers often are the recipients of privileged communications. The information that you have access to is private and confidential (**Fig. 8–5**).

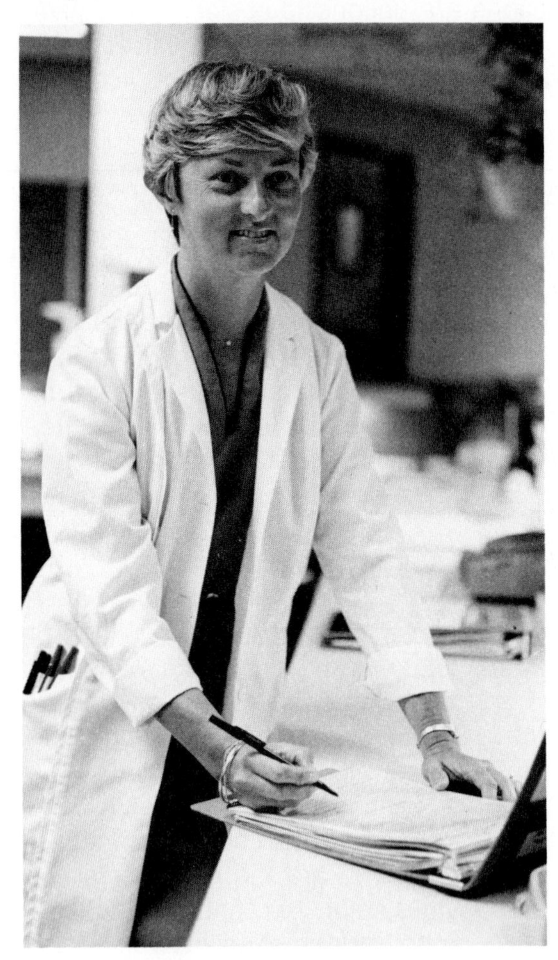

Figure 8–5. The hospital chart contains confidential information. (Courtesy of St. Lawrence Rehabilitation Center, Lawrenceville, N.J.)

This information should be guarded. It is for you to know because of your special position in the health care community. A client's diagnosis, laboratory test results, and chart contents are private and are not to be discussed anywhere at any time other than as a part of your specific job assignment. It is your responsibility always to guard the patient's right to privacy.

Patient's Bill of Rights

The "Patient's Bill of Rights" (**Fig. 8–6**), developed and distributed by the American Hospital Association in 1973, has an ethical and legal basis. It clearly spells out the right to privacy and informed consent. The patient has the right to decide who will perform any procedure, treatment, or other act that involves touching the body. This consent is usually written but involves more than just signing a name to a form. The patient must understand the nature of the procedure, the risks involved, and probable consequences.

While the Patient's Bill of Rights emphasizes the relationship between the doctor and patient, there are many implications for all health workers. Whether or not you have direct patient contact, you may have some access to confidential material. You may never see the patient, but you may prepare the bill and have access to confidential financial information. You may review the chart to document the diagnosis, **treatment protocol**, and length of stay in order to bill a third-party payer, such as an insurance company. In both instances, you have the obligation to provide complete privacy. This information should only be released to those individuals and companies which the client has designated. If a friend or a neighbor is a patient in a health care facility where you work or is a client of a physician who is your employer, you do not have the right to read that medical record. This would be unethical and would violate your friend's right to privacy. Many records are computerized and the health care worker may have an access code that will make all private information available at the push of the appropriate keys. Again, you should not look for information which you have no right to have.

The chart as a legal document

Medical records are legal documents which may be **subpoenaed** and used as evidence in court cases. They are extremely important and must be handled and stored properly. You will learn proper documentation techniques as you continue to learn and prepare for a specific health career.

Figure 8–6. The Patient's Bill of Rights

1. The patient has the right to considerate and respectful care.
2. The patient has the right to obtain from his physician complete current information concerning his diagnosis, treatment and prognosis in terms the patient can be reasonably expected to understand.
3. The patient has a right to receive from his physician information necessary to give informed consent prior to the start of any procedure and/or treatment . . . Where medically significant alternatives for care or treatment exist, or when the patient requests information concerning medical alternatives, the patient has the right to such information (and) to know the name of the person responsible for the procedures and/or treatment.
4. The patient has the right to refuse treatment to the extent permitted by law, and to be informed of the medical consequences of his action.
5. The patient has the right to every consideration of privacy concerning his own medical care program.
6. The patient has the right to expect that all communications and records pertaining to his care should be treated as confidential.
7. The patient has the right to expect that within its capacity a hospital must make reasonable response to the request of a patient for services.
8. The patient has the right to obtain information as to any relationship of his hospital to other health care and educational institutions insofar as his care is concerned (and) any professional relationships among individuals, by name, who are treating him.
9. The patient has the right to be advised if the hospital proposes to engage in or perform human experimentation affecting his care or treatment (and) has the right to refuse to participate.
10. The patient has the right to expect reasonable continuity of care.
11. The patient has the right to examine and receive an explanation of his bill regardless of the source of payment.
12. The patient has the right to know what hospital rules and regulations apply to his conduct as a patient.

This chapter has presented many concepts important for beginning your health career. They are just the start. As you prepare for a specific health occupation or profession, you will study detailed information relating to that particular career. This material provides a general overview and a foundation on which you can build new information.

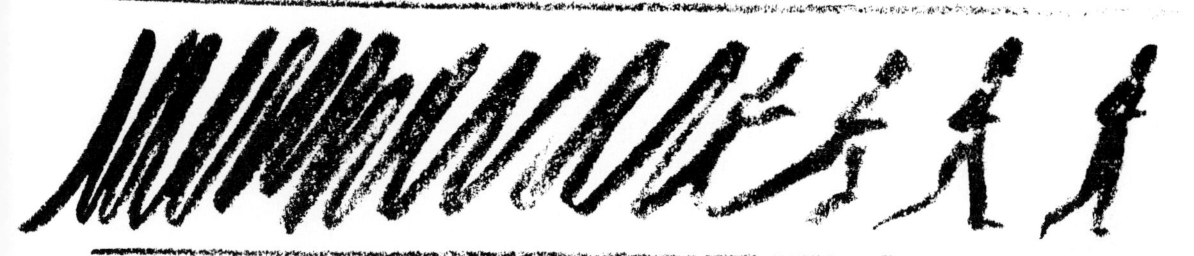

S·T·U·D·E·N·T A·C·T·I·V·I·T·I·E·S

1. Act out the following nonverbal communication signals. Ask a classmate to describe the meaning of your nonverbal activity:
   a. Standing erect with hands on hips
   b. Tapping fingers, cracking knuckles
   c. Twisting hair
   d. Hands covering eyes
   e. Pacing the floor — back and forth, back and forth — many, many times.
2. How would you handle the following ethical problems?
   a. Your mother asks you to find out what's wrong with her coworker who is a patient on your unit.
   b. You see a hospital employee taking money from a patient's bedside table.
   c. While working in the Clinical Laboratory you find out that a prominent politician has a venereal disease.
3. Read the Patient's Bill of Rights. Discuss each point. Do you agree or disagree with each? How can you respect the patient's rights?

Chapter 9

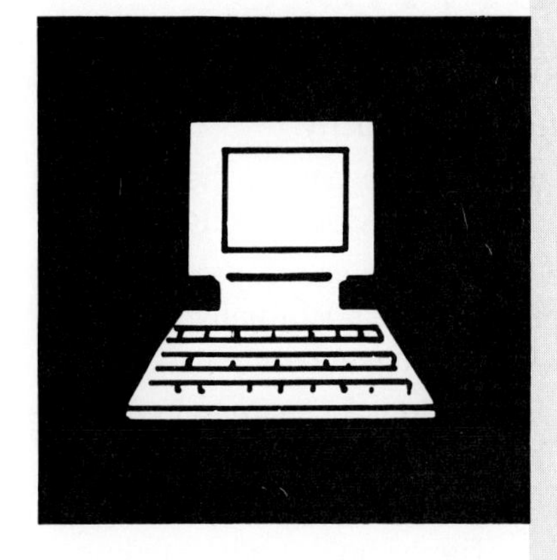

Computers in Health Care

Objectives

After completing this chapter, you should be able to:

- Describe at least three ways the computer has influenced the health care field.
- Distinguish between computer literacy and computer preparedness.
- Describe the three main parts to a computer system.
- Distinguish between hardware and software.
- Identify five health careers and how each utilizes the computer in everyday work activities.
- Discuss three ways the use of the computer by a health care practitioner could include some legal, ethical, or moral questions.
- Describe the advantages of a nursing documentation system.
- Explain why it is important for all computer users to have keyboarding skill.
- Define computer-assisted instruction and computer-aided design.

- Define the term GIGO. What does it describe?
- Define 70 percent of the key terms listed for this chapter.

Key Terms

- **bug** An error in a computer program that causes the processing to not function properly
- **central processing unit** The part of the computer that processes the information provided through input
- **computer** An electronic device capable of handling information at great speeds. It is usually comprised of three units — input, processing, and output
- **computer-assisted instruction** Learning with the help of the computer. Software programs are designed to allow the computer user to progress at a reasonable pace
- **computer literacy** The simple understanding of how the computer works and its strengths as well as its limitations
- **computer preparedness** Knowing how to operate the computer to perform a specific job function
- **data** Processed words, letters, or numbers that produce information to be used for a specific purpose
- **disk drive** The part of the computer hardware that accepts the software diskettes. Most computers have one or two disk drives
- **diskette** A floppy (flexible) magnetic storage device that is usually 3 1/2, 5 1/4, or 8 inches in diameter
- **GIGO** Acronym for Garbage In, Garbage Out. This means that the output from a computer system can only be as valid as the input to the system
- **hard disk drive** The part of the computer hardware that stores programs to be used for the processing of information. The hard drive is stationary and holds much more information than a diskette
- **hardware** The computer equipment that uses software to operate

- **input** The term used to describe data entered into the computer. Input is provided through a keyboard, from another computer or from storage
- **nursing documentation system** A computer system designed to assist nurses in performing their record-keeping tasks involving hygiene, vital signs, intravenous treatment, and diet
- **output** The term used to describe the form that information takes after being processed by the computer. Output could be data in storage, a paper report, a chart, or information on a computer screen
- **software** The program used to make the computer operate. These may be purchased from a supply house or prepared by a programmer
- **video display terminal (VDT)** The computer screen used for the displaying of information

BECOMING COMPUTER FRIENDLY

The term computer can be frightening or enlightening depending upon one's frame of mind and exposure to the computer and its uses. The health care field has made great strides in the implementation of the computer into almost every facet of each career group.

This chapter is designed to familiarize you with the computer and relate some of its uses in specific health careers. You will not be a computer expert after completing this chapter, but you will certainly have more information about the computer — what it can and what it cannot do — than you had before. With this information you will be, at least, computer literate as you enter your chosen career and, hopefully, have an understanding of the importance of learning how to keyboard and to use software in career preparation. The simple understanding of how the computer works, its strengths, and its limitations is called computer literacy. Knowing how to operate the computer — i.e., to provide input and receive output — is called computer preparedness.

Data

Data can be letters, numbers, or words which are processed to produce information that can be used for a purpose (**Fig. 9–1**). Information processing is the orderly arrangement of data into a purposeful, readable format serving a specified purpose.

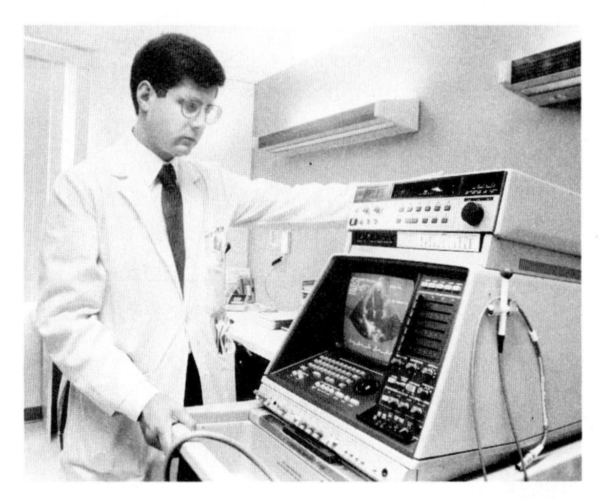

Figure 9–1. This cardiac ultrasound imaging unit displays data to monitor client's blood flow. (Courtesy of Bridgeton Hospital, Bridgeton, N.J.)

The Computer

Any computer or computer system is divided into three parts: input, the central processing unit (CPU), and output. Each part is usually dependent on the other two when processing information. Storage is sometimes considered a fourth part of the system.

Input can be provided by a keyboard, an optical scanner, information transferred over the phone lines, or other ways (**Fig. 9–2**). The input stage is necessary before any processing of data can occur. In addition, if the input is not appropriate, the computer cannot process the information appropriately. The term GIGO (Garbage In, Garbage Out) is used to describe the entering of incorrect data.

The CPU is the part of the computer that processes the instructions provided through the program, which generally is booted (loaded) on the

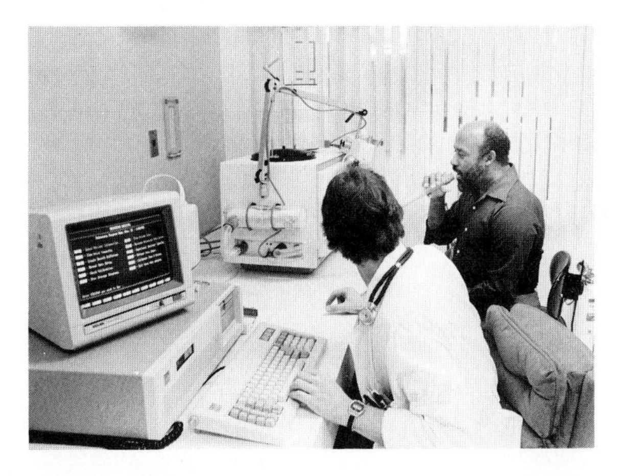

Figure 9–2. Input is provided by the patient during a lung capacity test. (Courtesy of Bridgeton Hospital, Bridgeton, N.J. Photo by Gary F. Cooper.)

computer through the diskette (software). The CPU contains the main computer memory where the processing takes place. The functions performed by the CPU cannot be seen by the computer user. The CPU performs the operations of the computer and will do whatever the software tells it to do. Software is the computer program that is used to operate the computer. The computer equipment itself is usually called hardware.

The final product delivered by the CPU is called output. The output could be a document which lists information, a letter which has been produced by the computer user, information transmitted to another user, or information sent to the storage device.

Storage is the place where the data resides ready for use by processing. Storage can be internal to the equipment or can be on removable diskettes.

COMPUTERS AS INSTRUCTIONAL AIDS

Some health career specialists believe that the computer will have the same impact on medicine that the microscope did in the nineteenth century. The computer is being used for computer-assisted instruction (CAI) — textbook material provided to students on diskettes. CAI is available for students in all aspects of health careers, including direct care (the dental, nursing, medical, mental health, and social work clusters), diagnostic (the radiology, optical, and medical laboratory clusters), therapeutic/restorative (physical therapy, occupational therapy, respiratory therapy, specialized rehabilitation, reconstructive and replacement, dietetic, and pharmacy clusters), and community and institutional health (**Fig. 9–3**).

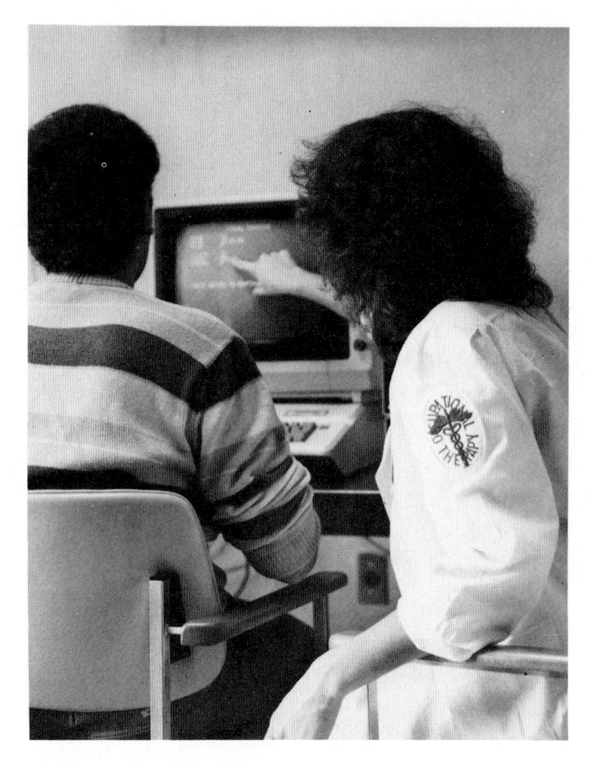

Figure 9–3. An occupational therapist teaches a client to use a computer. (Courtesy of St. Lawrence Rehabilitation Center, Lawrenceville, N.J.)

COMPUTERS IN THE WORK PLACE

In addition, the computer is used as a tool with which people perform their jobs within those related clusters. Many health career personnel should have the ability to use word processing, data base management, spreadsheet applications, and graphics to perform their tasks and duties. This need necessitates the acquisition of keyboarding skill.

There are a variety of software programs available that have been designed for direct care personnel. For example, some information systems allow health occupations personnel to input data, such as nurse's notes, directly into the computer. Through this process direct care personnel can document patient care, diagnostic data, and bedside services. Reports can then be generated on all phases of care, by sorting the information and presenting different perspectives on the data.

Some medical centers have installed input devices at the patient's bedside for nursing documentation. These devices link patient information such as hygiene, vital signs, intravenous treatment, and diet with a system located at a centralized nursing station. These data input stations permit the recording of detailed notes, which allow the nurses to spend more time with patients, and reduce the after-shift paperwork process. Each station costs approximately $1700 for a two-bed device, and can only be accessed with passwords given to the nurses. This system saves nurses a great deal of time and proves to be cost effective. Other software enables the health care worker to process reports through a data base management program. When a financial worksheet is needed, a spreadsheet program provides it. For most job clusters, the computer's ability to process information at great speed is a major advantage. Data can also be sorted and presented in different formats for interpretation and analysis.

The computer has become crucial to health care. By visiting a health care agency, you can see that the computer has many uses: when the patient is being admitted, when the patient is receiving care and treatment, and when the patient is released (**Fig. 9–4**).

When a patient is admitted, the personal data are entered into the system. This includes the patient's name, address, phone number, medical notes, and insurance policy numbers. Then, it is not necessary for the information to be repeated at other steps along the way. As diagnostic tests are performed, an informational data base is built and sorted as needed.

The output generated from the computer can also be used by personnel to analyze the level of patient care being administered. Things like time management, efficiency (of service or treatment), graphic comparisons of total patients, and billing to insurance carriers and patients can be generated from the same data.

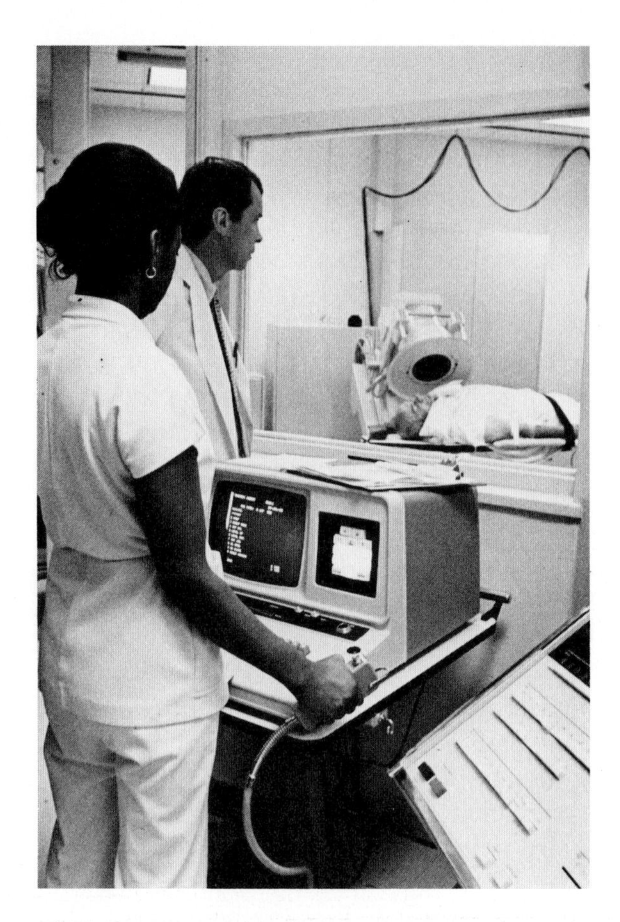

Figure 9–4. Noninvasive imaging techniques are possible with the use of computers. (Courtesy of New Jersey Hospital Association. Photo by David Greenfield.)

Because of the speed at which a computer can function and process information, medical/dental practitioners are utilizing software programs that allow them the flexibility of seeing the effect of decisions before administering to the patient. For instance, there are some programs available that show the probable effects of administering different kinds of drugs to different patients. The software leads the practitioner through a series of questions about the patient, the diagnosis, and the anticipated drug to be used. Almost immediately, the practitioner is told the probable effects of administering the drug.

The software also provides a drug record — when prescribed and when administered — and the patient's progress. The computer allows large volumes of data about previous patients and their medical histories to be instantly used in the analysis of a new patient, greatly enhancing the health care practitioner's ability to use all the data available.

As software continues to be developed, the computer is becoming more widely accepted by health care practitioners. Some practitioners, however, still do not care to use the computer for their work. Others express an interest in using technology, but don't exactly know when it will be implemented. So, although computers are showing up in the health care work place, the extent to which diagnostic software will be used is still questionable. But as the software improves, more and more uses will be adapted and adopted. Some dental practitioners are using computer-aided drafting (CAD) equipment and dental design software to build caps, bridges, and crowns to patient specifications *before* actually designing the dental work. This ability has enabled dental practitioners the freedom to try different compounds, design, and structural work, prior to preparing the work for use by the patient. Hours of work can be saved by using these software programs.

LEGAL QUESTIONS

While the available software programs can make patient care easier and provide the health care practitioner with a comprehensive tool with which to perform specific tasks, there are legal, ethical, and moral questions that come into consideration. If, because of an error (known as a bug) in the program, a drug is administered and a patient suffers great injury, or dies, who is accountable? If a diagnosis is made that is faulty based upon the software program, who is accountable? If inappropriate input has caused incorrect output and a care decision is based on that information, who is responsible if someone is injured or dies? The health care practitioner? The software firm that sold the product? The retail establishment that carried the product? The computer operator who processed the input and output? The programmer who wrote the program? All these questions must be considered as computers are developed for and used in the health care field.

SUMMARY

One thing is certain: The computer has streamlined many mundane, routine tasks for persons employed in the health care industry. The speed with which a computer can process data into usable information has assisted many persons to be more effective and efficient in their respective roles within the health care industry. The hardware and software has improved, decreased in price, and become more specific to health care applications. Once a system is used successfully in a particular aspect of one's job, the usage grows as the computer operator becomes more proficient. The health care industry has just begun to enter the computer field (**Fig. 9–5**).

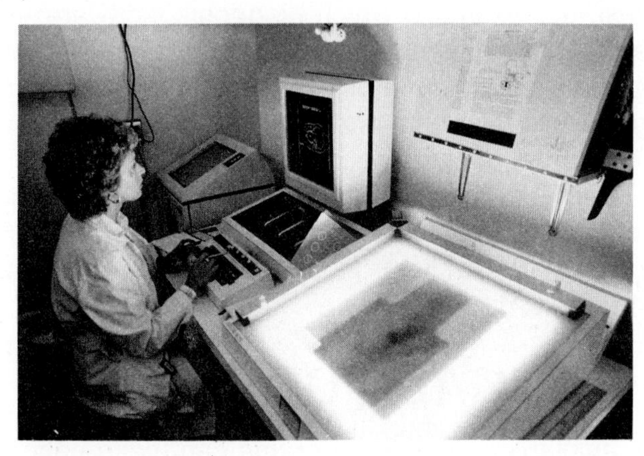

Figure 9–5. Computers, such as this one displaying a cross-section image of the body, will have great impact on the field of health care. (Courtesy of New Jersey Hospital Association. Photo by Cliff Moore.)

S·T·U·D·E·N·T A·C·T·I·V·I·T·I·E·S

1. Contact a local health care agency and arrange a visit to see how the computer is being used in the agency. Make a list of the occupations of the persons using the computer system, what their job tasks are, what kind of input is provided, and what kind of output is produced.
2. Visit a local computer store and ask to see the kinds of software packages available for the health care field. Request additional information from the manufacturers of the software.
3. Arrange a conversation, discussion, or visit to a local attorney's office to discuss the legal, ethical, and moral questions of using computers and software in the health care field.
4. Describe three ways that the computer has influenced the health care field.
5. Visit a health care agency and view the computer systems in use. Describe the input, processing, output, and storage phases.
6. Interview a nurse and discuss a nursing documentation system. List the major advantages and disadvantages of the system.

Chapter 10

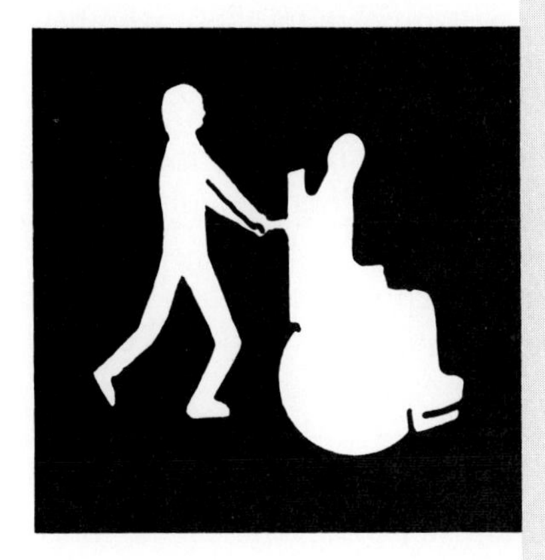

The Health Care System, The Patient, and You

Objectives

After completing this chapter, you should be able to:

- List at least five types of agencies and institutions that provide patient care.
- Explain the differences between at least five types of agencies and institutions that provide health services.
- Discuss the effects of illness on the patient and family.
- Define 70 percent of the key terms for this chapter.

Key Terms

- **acute illness** An illness with a rapid onset, severe symptoms, and of short, not chronic duration

- **chronic illness** A disease showing little change, slow progress, and of long duration, not an acute illness
- **dignity** The quality of being worthy or esteemed
- **disease** An abnormal process which interferes with a person's functioning; the state of being sick; illness
- **extended care** Long-term care for those who have chronic health conditions but do not require the services of a hospital
- **health** A state of complete physical, mental, and social well-being, not merely the absence of disease
- **health care delivery system** The agencies, institutions, and programs which provide health care and health maintenance. Also known as the health care industry
- **illness** Disease
- **nursing home** A facility which provides care at different levels for chronically ill people who can no longer live independently because of physical or mental debilitation, emotional trauma, or chronic illness
- **respect** To care about, to value, to hold in high esteem
- **skilled nursing facility (SNF)** A nursing home that provides 24-hour care, rehabilitation, and other specialized services under the supervision of a registered professional nurse

DEFINITION OF HEALTH

If you had a choice between being sick or being well, certainly you would not choose being sick. And so it is for most people. What, then, is health? In 1970, The World Health Organization (WHO) defined health as "a state of complete physical, mental, and social well-being, not merely the absence of disease."

This definition is complicated because it is not absolutely specific. You know that 2 + 2 always equals 4. However, we cannot state clearly what equals health. For example, many people who have chronic diseases, such as epilepsy or diabetes, take daily medication or follow a special diet, yet they are considered to be healthy because they are able to go about their day-to-day routine without any problems.

DEFINITION OF ILLNESS

Is illness then the absence of health? It is defined as an abnormal process which interferes with a person's functioning — i.e., the state of being sick. The synonym for illness is disease. Many terms are used to further clarify the meaning of the word disease. An acute illness has a rapid onset and a relatively short duration. A chronic illness has a slow onset and lasts for a long time. Congenital disease is present at birth, and a communicable disease can be spread from one person to another.

SEEKING HEALTH CARE

When a person feels sick, their first thought may be, "I don't feel so well today." That feeling is expressed in some way. "I can't go to work today. I'm as sick as a dog with a fever, coughing, stuffy nose, and a lousy headache." What happens next depends on an individual's attitude about that illness. Is it a serious illness? Or does the person decide that rest, drinking plenty of fluids, and letting the illness take its course is the proper thing to do. After all, "It's just a cold, and there is no real treatment for a cold." However, if the illness is severe and does not respond to usual home treatment, the person should seek medical assistance for diagnosis and treatment.

HEALTH CARE DELIVERY SYSTEM

In recent years, the focus in the health care industry has shifted from care of the sick to the promotion of health and disease prevention. Certainly, diagnosis, treatment, and rehabilitation are still essential elements of the health care delivery system, but no longer are these the only services available to clients. In fact, the health care delivery system is very complex. It serves many people in many different locations ranging from huge medical centers to small storefront neighborhood health centers.

Outpatient Facilities

Most sick people first visit an outpatient facility in order to obtain medical assistance. They may go to a private office to visit the doctor, nurse, or dentist, or they may see a health professional in a hospital or freestanding clinic. Ambulatory care centers are similar to clinics and provide walk-in services for sick persons.

Some clinics and ambulatory care centers are highly specialized. They are alternatives to hospital admission for minor surgery and some diagnostic and treatment procedures. Outpatient (same-day) surgery is becoming routine in the treatment of specific diseases, such as cataracts and hernias (**Fig. 10–1**).

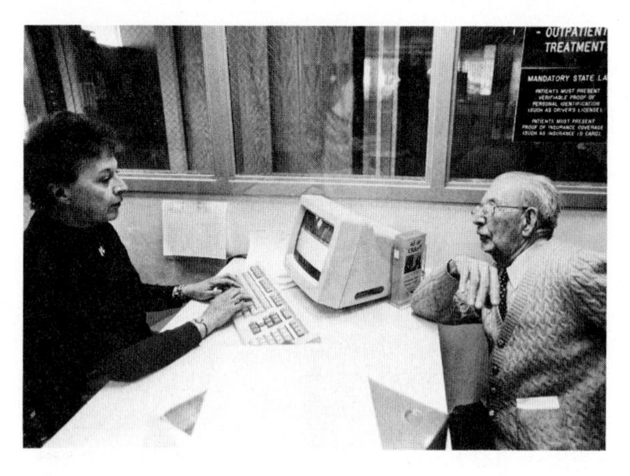

Figure 10–1. Outpatient clinics are an alternative to hospital admissions for minor surgery and some diagnostic and treatment procedures. (Courtesy of Bridgeton Hospital, Bridgeton, N.J. Photo by Gary F. Cooper.)

Community Agencies

Each community has outpatient health agencies that meet the special needs of its population. Home health agencies offer health care to persons who are at home and in need of nursing, homemaking, and rehabilitative services (**Fig. 10–2**). Women's Health Centers, crisis intervention centers, and mental health clinics are examples of agencies that exist within communities and are unique to that geographic area. For

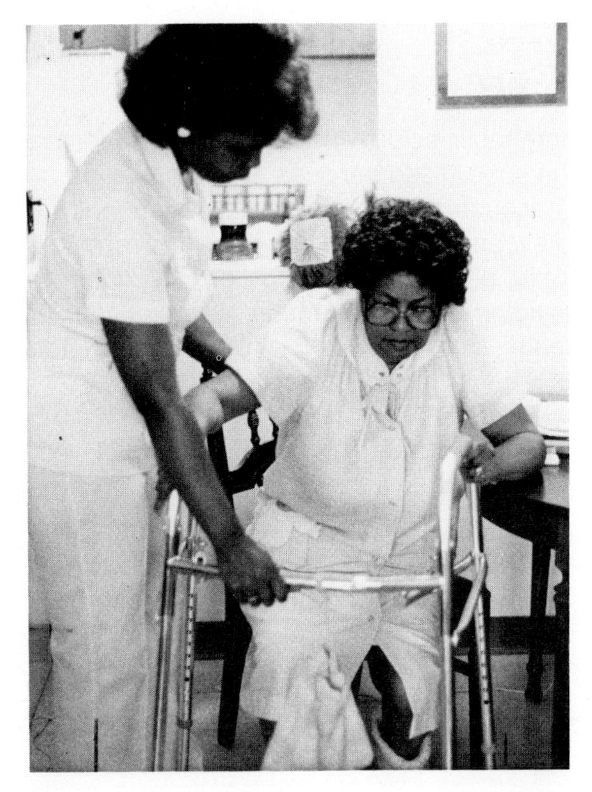

Figure 10–2. A home health aide helps a client to walk. (Courtesy of Mercer Street Friends Center, Trenton, N.J.)

example, a prenatal clinic would be useless in a senior citizen's village, but a home-delivered meals program could offer an appropriate and useful service to homebound older adults.

Inpatient Facilities

Hospitals are facilities that admit patients for diagnosis, treatment, and rehabilitation on an overnight basis. Hospitals also have outpatient and emergency room services. In recent years, hospitals have expanded their focus to offer additional services, including geriatric day care, speaker's bureau, support groups, and specialized clinics. Patients usually stay in hospitals for a short period of time.

Extended Care Facilities

Extended care facilities provide long-term care for those persons who do not require the specialized services of a hospital but are unable to care for themselves because they require some treatment, rehabilitation, or a period of convalescence. Nursing homes, long-term care facilities, and skilled nursing units all provide this type of care. Many types of services are available including nursing, nutrition, pastoral care, and rehabilitation (**Fig. 10–3**).

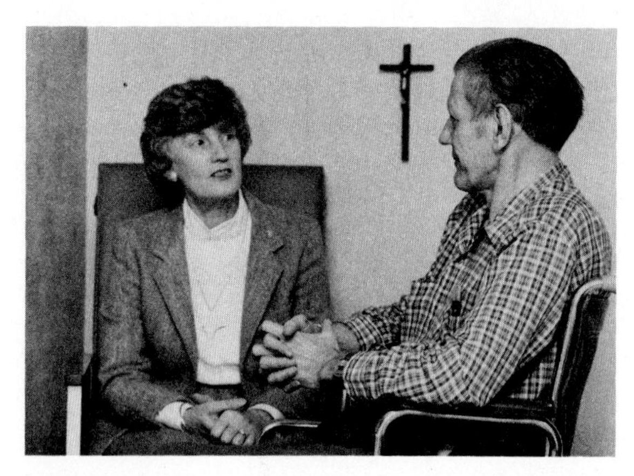

Figure 10–3. Pastoral care is available from many health care agencies. (Courtesy of St. Lawrence Rehabilitation Center, Lawrenceville, N.J.)

Specialized Institutions

Rehabilitation centers teach patients to return to the activities of daily living, such as bathing, grooming, and dressing, within the limits of their handicap. The length of stay is determined by the extent of the rehabilitation required.

Psychiatric hospitals provide treatment for patients on an inpatient basis — particularly during the acute phase of an emotional illness.

Hospices

Agencies that care for terminally ill persons are called hospices. Initially developed in England, the hospice movement spread to the United States as an alternative to hospitalization of the dying patient. Patients and families choose hospice care so that the patient may die with dignity within the family setting. In some locations, a hospice is a building with a homelike atmosphere where the patient resides and the family participates in care. In other areas, a hospice is a program, rather than a facility, which provides care for the patient who remains at home. The needs and concerns of the family are a vital part of the hospice movement.

Continuing Care Retirement Communities

The continuing care retirement community (CCRC), sometimes called "life care," is a lifestyle option for older adults. The nonprofit continuing care retirement community has as its aim the provision of a continuum of care. These communities offer their residents privacy in one's own apartment or cottage, with one's own belongings. There is no need to worry about maintenance or housekeeping chores. There is independence and access to health care for the rest of the resident's life. Of course, residents who want to live there for the rest of their lives must make a financial investment. Many services are available, including medical, nursing, various therapies, and special diets.

PAYING FOR HEALTH CARE

Insurance Plans

Everyone knows that health care is very costly. Those who have been hospitalized will joke that they could have gone on a world cruise or stayed in a luxury hotel for less money than it cost to stay in the hospital. Therefore, most people have some type of health insurance plan — either privately purchased or through a group plan. These insurance plans, called "third-party payers," meet the costs of medical care. While they do pay some or all of the bills, the cost eventually is paid by the subscriber through the increasing costs of the insurance premium.

Health maintenance organizations (HMOs) provide health maintenance and illness care services for a specific fee. The subscriber pays a monthly or quarterly payment whether or not any services are required. The client must use the personnel and facilities of the HMO. If the client wishes to seek medical care from someone outside of the HMO group, the HMO staff must institute a referral. If this procedure is not followed, the client may be responsible for all expenses incurred by visiting the non-HMO personnel.

Preferred provider organizations (PPOs) are groups of physicians who affiliate with a hospital. Both the physicians and the hospital agree to provide comprehensive health services at a discount to companies under contract.

Dental care is also available through third-party payers, such as dental insurance plans and dental HMOs.

Prescription drugs, too, may be covered by some health insurance, HMO, or PPO plans.

Medicaid

The federal and state governments support this health insurance program. Benefits and eligibility vary from state to state. The program provides hospitalization and many other services to those who are blind, disabled, or have a low income.

Medicare

Medicare, the health insurance program for older adults, is administered by the Social Security Administration. Monthly premiums are paid by those over 65 who are recipients of social security payments. Hospitalization, long-term care, home care, and other types of services are reimbursed on a deductible basis. The benefits are always under constant review and revision. Current information can be obtained from the local Social Security Administration office.

Diagnostic Related Groups

In 1983, Congress passed legislation to institute diagnostic related groups (DRGs) as a means of paying hospital bills. A DRG is a list of specific diagnoses. The government has determined the typical length of stay and the cost of treatment allowed for this particular group of illnesses. The hospital is paid this specific amount for Medicare and Medicaid patients. If the hospital's costs for care are less than the predetermined amount, the hospital gets to keep the excess funds. If the costs are more than the reimbursement, the hospital must assume the loss.

While the purpose of DRGs — cost cutting — is admirable, the effect has been that many patients, especially older ones, are still sick when they go home. Home health agencies and long-term care facilities have seen a tremendous increase in the number of very sick patients in their care.

EFFECTS OF ILLNESS

Dependency

Perhaps the most obvious effect of illness is that of dependency. When you are sick at home with a miserable cold, it's nice to have another person nearby to bring you a cup of tea, adjust the TV, and fluff your pillow. The dependent role is pleasant and tolerable for a short period of time.

When one has an acute, brief illness which requires admission to a health care facility, there may be complete dependency as one undergoes diagnostic and treatment procedures. A prolonged illness, requiring extensive rehabilitation, will result in a lengthy period of dependency. Most people will find this a very difficult adjustment, especially those who are seeking independence as a part of their normal development — such as adolescents and older adults. Fathers, mothers, husbands, and wives are also affected by this dependency because their roles and responsibilities may be changed.

Anxiety

Anxiety is a troubled feeling — a sense of apprehension and concern for what might happen. Everyone has felt anxious from time to time; it is a normal part of living. "Will I pass my driver's test?" "How will the job interview go?" "What questions will the interviewer ask?" "What shall I wear?" "How do I look?" All these questions reflect the usual anxieties in everyday life.

Illness itself does not cause anxiety. The threat of illness and its possible effect on the future and on one's health is indeed anxiety-producing. The amount of anxiety varies from person to person, family to family. It depends on many factors, including cultural background and life experience. Some persons would choose to tolerate the most uncomfortable toothache rather than go to the dentist. They are afraid of the drill; they are afraid that the tooth may have to be extracted; they are afraid of the pain that they "think" might occur in the dental office. Another individual with a toothache would visit the dentist as soon as possible to have the diseased tooth properly treated.

Anxiety can be so severe that it may interfere with treatment. Sometimes the fear of "what the disease could be" is so profound that the sick person will not seek medical assistance. "It might be cancer." "It might be AIDS." "What would I do?" Some people choose to live in fear of the possibility rather than identify and treat the reality.

Denial

Denial is a refusal to admit the truth. This will reduce the discomfort that is felt by uncomfortable facts. It is common for people to deny the fact that chest pain might indicate a heart attack. "Oh, it's a little indigestion." "I'll take something for it." "It'll go away." Comments like these are typical of denial. The client does not want to face the fact that he or she may have a life-threatening illness. "Oh no, it can't possibly be, not me." We all use denial, and, at times, it may be effective and may help persons to cope with illness. At other times, it may interfere and even be dangerous.

Anger

Another emotion that we all experience is anger. This may be even more pronounced in sick persons. "Why did this have to happen to me?" "Why did God do this to me?" "If you kept the floor cleaned up, I wouldn't have fallen and fractured my leg. It's all your fault. I'm furious with you." "Why did you put me in this nursing home? You just wanted to get rid of me and get my money. I'm your mother, or don't you remember that!"

Patients who are unable to express their anger may be extremely hostile to the staff. "How can you be so incompetent? This is no way to run a place. I'm paying plenty for this room, and I demand service immediately." "This is the most inefficient office I have ever been to — can't you people ever get anything right?" Angry words for angry feelings — probably toward one's family, situation, dependency, illness, and who knows what else may all be dumped on the staff of the health care agency.

Withdrawal

When an illness is prolonged or extremely severe, the patient may avoid contact with others. Visitors may be turned away, the person may retreat to the bedroom and choose to be alone as much as possible. This may be due to the nature of the illness — the person may be too sick to tolerate other persons. Other causes might include the side effects of treatment or depression caused by the illness.

Role Change

People have various roles in life — mother, father, student, employer, employee. Illness causes a role change for the sick person who becomes a patient, thereby assuming a dependent, "sick role." It also causes changes within the family since other persons must step in and assume the responsibilities of the sick person. This may be done by another family member in the household or by a relative outside the immediate family. Sometimes a helper, such as a homemaker, will be employed by the family to assist during a time of sickness.

A great shift in family roles and responsibilities may occur if the sick person is the sole wage earner, and the income is discontinued. When the husband/father becomes so handicapped that he is unable to work, rehabilitation may prepare him to function as a homemaker while the wife/mother becomes the sole wage earner.

Decisions causing major changes in family roles must always be decided by the entire family including the patient (if capable). Sickness should not eliminate a person from the decision-making process unless they are totally unable to function.

Growth and Development

Illness can severely affect the progress of growth and development. A child with a chronic illness may be unable to run, play, and socialize with other children because of restrictions that may be a part of the treatment program. Some children may be institutionalized for long periods of time for specialized treatment of severe problems. Instead of going to school, they will go to a classroom in the institution. Instead of going home at night, they will return to their room — their exercise and activity will be learning to walk in a physical therapy department. Can you imagine how this can affect their growth and social development?

How do eating disorders affect the growth and development of young adults? What effect do illnesses like anorexia and bulemia have on college students — their adjustments, their relationships, their grades, their self-images?

Body Image

Body image — how we think we look to others — is very often affected by illness. The woman who must have breast surgery is anxious about her appearance. The child who has no hair as a result of cancer therapy will not want to go to school. The amputee will not go swimming for fear of being seen without a prosthesis.

Our culture tells us that we must be perfect. We must have teeth that are shiny white and perfectly straight. We are not allowed to have pimples or to perspire. Always, always we must be perfect like models in magazines. But we are not perfect, and we can never be. Certain illnesses can cause obvious handicaps that will alter a person's body image.

INTERACTING WITH PATIENTS

Patients are people — they are feeling some or all of the emotional effects of illness that were discussed earlier in this chapter. In addition, these people are sick — they are in pain; they are bleeding; they are facing surgery. All of these factors must be considered when interacting with patients.

Cheerfulness

You have heard the old sayings, "You get more flies with honey than you do with vinegar," or "It's nice to be nice." These are basic guidelines for working with patients. A smile goes a long way to make people feel comfortable and is really appreciated by patients. It makes them feel like you are "on their side."

Be cheerful and friendly. Let patients know you are there to help them. Don't be silly or act foolishly — a certain amount of seriousness must always blend with the cheerfulness. There will be times, when patients are very sad, that a calm, quiet approach would be more appropriate. At these times, silence or a touch of the hand may be the most effective response — for some patients, a hug (**Fig. 10–4**).

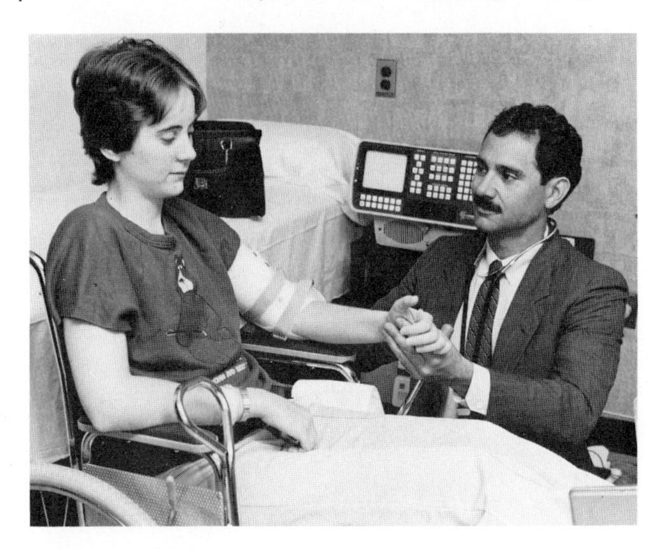

Figure 10–4. A calm, quiet approach helps to put the patient at ease. (Courtesy of St. Lawrence Rehabilitation Center, Lawrenceville, N.J.)

Respect and Dignity

Each person must be treated with respect (**Fig. 10–5**). While someone's lifestyle, dress, politics, or creed may not be acceptable to the health care worker, we must respect the person as an individual with specific rights and needs. Prison inmates have the right to quality health care. Persons with acquired immune deficiency syndrome (AIDS) have the right to quality health care. Homeless persons have the right to quality health care. All of these people have the right to expect to be treated with dignity, as persons of worth, no matter what the health care worker thinks.

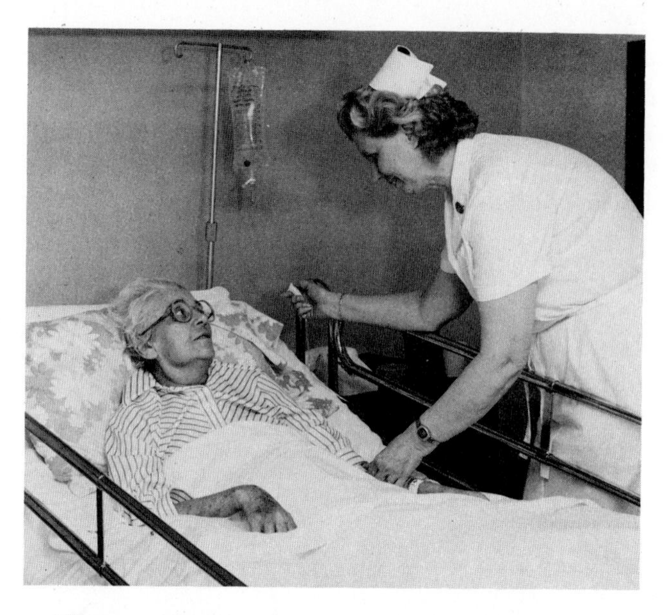

Figure 10–5. Showing patients care, kindness, and respect are part of the health care worker's job. (Courtesy of St. Lawrence Rehabilitation Center, Lawrenceville, N.J.)

Answering Questions

No one has all the answers, especially a beginning health worker. Sometimes even if you know the answer to a patient's question, it might be inappropriate for you to respond. Some answers are best provided by the physician, social worker, or the nurse. Don't be afraid to say, "I don't know, but I'll ask the social worker to discuss that with you," or "That's a really tough question, perhaps you should ask your doctor."

Certainly, you can answer questions about rules and regulations regarding routine matters. Questions you should be able to answer: "What time is lunch?" "When are visiting hours?" If you work in the billing office, you would be expected to be knowledgeable about patient's bills.

You should know your limitations regarding patient's questions. If you do not know what to say or do, tell the patient that you must ask your supervisor to help you with that question. And do so — always consult your teacher and your supervisor.

Sticky Issues

Certain topics of discussion should always be avoided, in particular, partisan politics and religion. These are always sticky issues, ones where people have firm and fast opinions. Our business is to promote health and prevent illness, not to discuss the relative merits of one political party over another.

Also, avoid discussing intimate details of your personal life. Leave your problems at home. Your paycheck, your dissatisfaction with your supervisor, and other types of griping will not help sick people to feel better. Remember that the problems, conditions, and diagnoses of other patients are private. Lastly, gossip about the staff is not your business and definitely not the patient's business. "I really don't know anything about that" is a good response in these situations.

Silence

At times it is best not to say anything. This may cause you to feel quite awkward, but there are times when just nothing you can say will be appropriate. When a patient is very angry and "lets you have it" because the "food is always cold" or the "service is lousy," it is best to respond with silence. You cannot change the situation and you may not be able to correct it. Listen in silence. When the patient has finished you may respond by saying, "I'm sorry you feel that way," "I understand how you feel," or "I'll ask my supervisor to come in and talk with you to see if anything can be done."

You will find that there are times when no words will help the situation, and you may sit quietly with the patient or family. A fearful, crying child may be comforted by hand-holding. It may be more appropriate to recognize the child's need to express fear and discomfort in this manner. Talking may be useless.

Difficult Patients

Sometime, somewhere in your health career you will meet a difficult patient. What is a difficult patient? It is a patient you do not like or do not choose to work with. It may be a complaining patient, an abusive patient, or a patient who makes overt sexual advances. Whenever you feel that a patient is "difficult" for any reason, you must discuss this with your supervisor and your instructor. If the entire staff feels that the patient is "difficult," then this attitude will most certainly interfere with patient care. A group conference to discuss this matter and to develop some strategies to solve the problem is in order. If you are the only person experiencing difficulties with the patient, perhaps your assignment could be changed. Nevertheless, you should try to further understand your feelings and clarify just why you feel that way about a particular patient.

Interacting with patients is a complicated part of health care, but it is the important part. If your health career involves working with people rather than equipment and supplies, hopefully you will find this the most satisfying and challenging part of your work (**Fig. 10–6**).

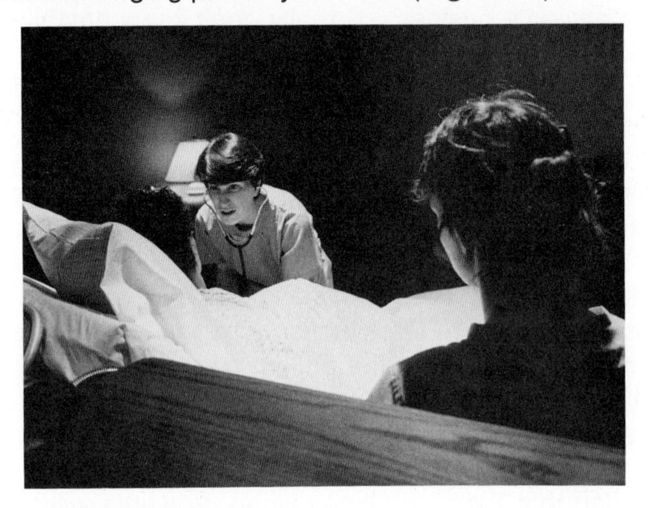

Figure 10–6. Working with people can be a satisfying experience. (Courtesy of Bridgeton Hospital, Bridgeton, N.J. Photo by Gary F. Cooper.)

S·T·U·D·E·N·T A·C·T·I·V·I·T·I·E·S

1. Identify one home health agency that serves your community. What kind of services does this agency provide for its clients? How does one obtain services from this agency?
2. Is there a hospice or hospice program in your community? How many health workers are employed by the hospice, and how many health careers are represented? How does one obtain the services of a hospice?
3. Prepare a poster, chart, or booklet illustrating five types of agencies and/or institutions that provide patient care within your community or nearby area.
4. Discuss the effects of an acute illness upon an individual and family members. Compare these with the possible effects of a chronic illness. Consider physical, emotional, social, and economic impact.
5. Prepare a chart showing the difference in cost between nursing home care and acute hospital care. How much does it cost for home health care if the client has home health aide services? What is the rate for a visiting nurse, occupational therapist, speech therapist, and physical therapist?

Chapter 11

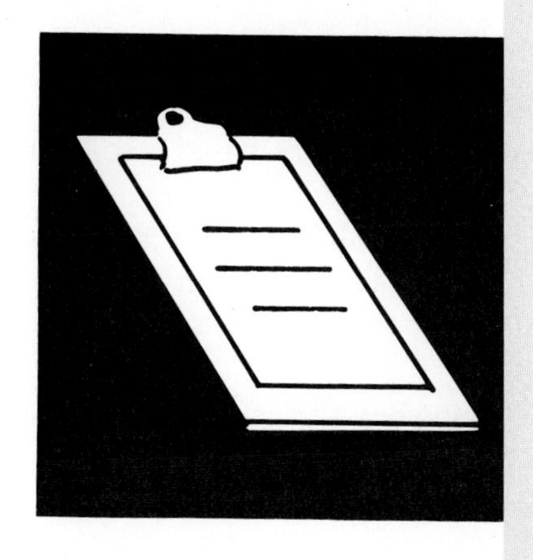

Observing and Recording

Objectives

After completing this chapter, you should be able to:

- Identify the basic components or parts of a client/patient record.
- Differentiate between objective and subjective symptoms.
- Explain the basic components of medical terminology — prefixes, root words, suffixes, and abbreviations.
- Demonstrate the use of prefixes, root words, and suffixes by completing the student activities.
- Define 70 percent of the key terms listed for this chapter.

Key Terms

- **cardinal symptoms** Measurement of the body temperature, pulse, and respirations (sometimes includes the blood pressure)

- **flow sheet** A form designed for recording information specific to a particular area. For example, graphic sheets to record temperature, pulse, and respiration
- **Kardex** A system of file cards that are used as a quick reference for obtaining information found on a patient record
- **nursing care plan** The statement of goals and activities for providing nursing care for clients. This is developed by the professional nurse based upon the nursing assessment
- **objective symptoms** Information that can be measured or observed by the staff. Changes in skin color, vomiting, breathing difficulty, and rapid pulse are examples of objective symptoms
- **prefix** A word beginning; that component of a word which precedes the root word
- **regimen** A systematic course of treatment
- **root word** Foundation of the word; that component of a word to which prefixes and suffixes may be attached
- **subjective symptom** Symptom perceived by and apparent to the patient only. For example, pain, numbness, nausea, dizziness
- **suffix** A word ending; that component of a word which follows the root word
- **symptom** Any perceptible change in the body or bodily functions that indicates disease

AN IMPORTANT DUTY
OBSERVING AND RECORDING

For some health workers it will be necessary to observe patient symptoms and to record these on the chart. Dental assistants, nursing assistants, nurses, physicians, emergency medical technicians, respiratory therapists, medical assistants, and many other health workers have some responsibility for observing patients and documenting their observations.

The Types of Symptoms

Objective Symptoms

Changes in the body or its function that indicate disease which are apparent to the observer are called objective symptoms. Examples are: vomiting, bleeding, swelling, pallor, coughing, and hyperactivity. All of these may be observed by the health worker and are recorded on the appropriate sheet in the patient's record.

Cardinal Symptoms

Cardinal symptoms are those that relate to the temperature, pulse, and respirations. Difficult breathing, rapid pulse, and elevated temperature (fever) are examples of cardinal symptoms. Observations of these symptoms are usually recorded on the patient's Clinical or Graphic Sheet. This sheet is used to record daily observations of the cardinal symptoms for institutionalized patients.

Subjective Symptoms

Those symptoms apparent only to the patient are known as subjective symptoms. Examples include: pain, nausea, dizziness, ringing in the ears, blurred vision, and anxiety. These are important observations and can be a vital part of diagnosis or evaluation of the therapy regimen. Therefore, subjective symptoms must be recorded accurately and completely.

PATIENT RECORDS

Patient records will vary from agency to agency, institution to institution, and many will be computerized. However, there are some basic components that will be found on all charts, whether in the dental office, medical office, or other facility.

Information Sheet

The Information Sheet, sometimes called the front sheet, contains all the essential information about the patient — e.g., name, address, age, marital status, religion, insurance company, group or individual membership number, etc. In a hospital, this sheet is completed upon admission. In a private office, it is updated regularly for change of address and other pertinent information. When patients are too sick to complete this sheet, a relative may be asked to do so. Parents will complete this information for minor children (**Fig. 11–1**).

History and Physical

A record of the patient's objective and subjective symptoms and vital signs will be found in the patient's chart. This may be done as a part of the diagnostic process or to have a record of what is normal for a client who is not sick but who is participating in a health maintenance or wellness program.

In the dental office, this will include a chart showing all of a patient's teeth and detailing those which are missing, diseased, or restored.

A patient's history may be recorded by the medical assistant, nurse, dental assistant, and others according to the specific questions on a history form (**Fig. 11–2**). It includes family disease history, the patient's health record and other past relevant information. All this information is used to assist in making a diagnosis as well as maintaining a person's health. The physical examination is always performed by the professional who has specialized education in assessment techniques.

Laboratory/X-ray/Diagnostic Records

Reports of all diagnostic procedures and the findings will also be a part of the patient's record. For example, urinalysis report, complete blood count, chest x-ray, etc.

PATIENT NO.	ADMIT DATE	TIME	N. STA.	BED	TYPE	SERV	F/C	#INS	ADM SRC	ADM PRI	SEX	RACE	DISC. DATE	M.R. NO.

PATIENT: PATIENT NAME LAST, FIRST, MI; ADDRESS; CITY/STATE/ZIP; PHONE; SS#

ADMITTING PHYSICIAN; REFERRING/PERSONAL PHYSICIAN

DATE OF BIRTH; BIRTH PLACE; AGE; M.S.; SMOKE; PREV. SMH DATE/NAME

EMPLOYER: EMPLOYER NAME; ADDRESS; CITY/STATE/ZIP; PHONE; OCCUP

PREV. FACILITY; PREV. FAC. ADMIT DATE

ACCIDENT DATE; TIME; ACCD TYPE; RELIGION; CHURCH; NEWBORN RELIGION

RELATIVE: NEAREST RELATIVE NAME; ADDRESS; CITY/STATE/ZIP; RELATION; HOME PHONE; WORK PHONE; EMPLOYER NAME

GUAR NAME; ADDRESS; ADDRESS; RELATION; CITY/STATE/ZIP; PHONE; SS#

EMERGENCY: EMERGENCY CONTACT; ADDRESS; CITY/STATE/ZIP; RELATION; HOME PHONE; WORK PHONE; EMPLOYER NAME

GUAR EMPLOYER; ADDRESS; CITY/STATE/ZIP; PHONE; REG BY

INSURANCE:

INS 1; POL NO; GRP NO; BC PLAN CODE; SUBSC NAME; ADDR; REL

INS 1; POL NO; GRP NO; BC PLAN CODE; SUBSC NAME; ADDR; REL

MA INS; EXP DATE; CARD NAME; COUNTY CODE; RECORD NO; CAT NO; CONTROL DIGIT; LINE NO; RES CODE; STATE

ADD INS; POL NO; GRP NO; BS PLAN CODE; SUBSC NAME; ADDR; REL

ADMITTING DIAGNOSIS/PROCEDURE

PRINCIPAL DIAGNOSIS (CONDITION ESTABLISHED AFTER STUDY TO BE RESPONSIBLE FOR HOSPITALIZATION) DO NOT ABBREVIATE — DICTATIONS: SUMMARY | OR

CODE

1.

OTHER DIAGNOSES OR COMPLICATIONS (LIST ALL DIAGNOSES AND COMPLICATIONS INCLUDING INFECTION & DRUG REACTION)

OPERATIONS OR PROCEDURES (LIST PRINCIPAL FIRST) — DATE

DISCHARGE STATUS: ☐ RECOVERED ☐ IMPROVED ☐ NOT IMPROVED ☐ EXPIRED ☐ RELEASED AGAINST ADVICE ☐ NEWBORN ☐ TRANSFER

I CERTIFY THAT THE NARRATIVE DESCRIPTIONS OF THE PRINCIPAL AND SECONDARY DIAGNOSES AND MAJOR PROCEDURES PERFORMED ARE ACCURATE AND COMPLETE TO THE BEST OF MY KNOWLEDGE.

SIGNATURE OF ATTENDING PHYSICIAN — DATE

CHART

Figure 11–1. Admission record form. (Courtesy of St. Mary Hospital, Langhorne, Pa.)

CHIEF COMPLAINT

HISTORY OF PRESENT ILLNESS

PAST MEDICAL HISTORY

FAMILY HISTORY

REVIEW OF SYSTEMS

PHYSICAL EXAMINATION

OUT-PATIENT STUDIES

HISTORY AND PHYSICAL

Figure 11–2. A History and Physical form provides essential information about a patient. (Courtesy of St. Mary Hospital, Langhorne, Pa.)

Progress Records

Observations of the patient's progress by the physician, therapist, nurse, etc. will be posted on the progress record (**Fig. 11–3**). In a patient care facility, certain professionals may record the patient's treatment and observation on separate, individual sheets, e.g., nurses' notes, physical therapy notes, etc. In other agencies, all professionals will record on the same document. In still other areas, all information will be placed in the computer terminal located in the specific department (occupational therapy, operating room, radiology, etc.). Some hospitals have computer keyboards at the patient's bedside and observations are charted and recorded instantly.

Flow Sheets

Flow sheets are forms for observing and recording symptoms specific to a special area. They are check sheets and may be a part of a computerized system of recording certain basic symptoms. For example, in a newborn nursery, the staff observes a baby's eating, sleeping, elimination, reflexes, breathing, crying, etc. These observations are common to all normal newborn infants and the use of a checksheet (flow sheet) ensures that everyone documents the essential information quickly and properly (**Fig. 11–4**).

Other Records

Social Service evaluation, consultant reports, surgical reports, medication records, and other documents may be found within the patient record. There are many different forms depending upon the setting and the patient's condition (**Figs. 11–5, 11–6,** and **11–7**).

Kardex

In institutions that provide nursing care, a system of file cards, the Kardex, is used as a quick reference to the nursing care plan and the daily activities for the patient. You may see this device in departments that provide various therapies — speech, physical, occupational. The unit secretary usually keeps the Kardex up to date. This makes it easy to find pertinent information without digging through an enormous chart (**Fig. 11–8** and **Fig. 11–9**).

DATE							
HT-WT							
HYGIENE:							
Bedbath							
Partial							
Self							
Shower/tub							
Oral							
H.S.							
ACTIVITY:							
Bedrest							
BRP							
BR$\bar{c}$BRP							
Dangle							
Chair/W.C.							
Amb							
Other							
Rails	7-3-11	7-3-11	7-3-11	7-3-11	7-3-11	7-3-11	7-3-11
DIET:	8-12-5	8-12-5	8-12-5	8-12-5	8-12-5	8-12-5	8-12-5
NPO							
Liquid							
Soft							
Regular							
Spec.							
HOLD							
OTHER:							

Intake	11-7	7-3	3-11	11-7	7-3	3-11	11-7	7-3	3-11	11-7	7-3	3-11	11-7	7-3	3-11	11-7	7-3	3-11	11-7	7-3	3-11
Oral																					
I.V. or Subq.																					
Blood																					
Other																					
Total 24 Hr. (cc)																					
Output Urine																					
Total 24 hr. (cc) Urine																					
Emesis																					
Other																					
Total 24 Hr. (cc)																					
Stool																					
Signature																					

Figure 11–3. A patient care record charts a variety of activities.

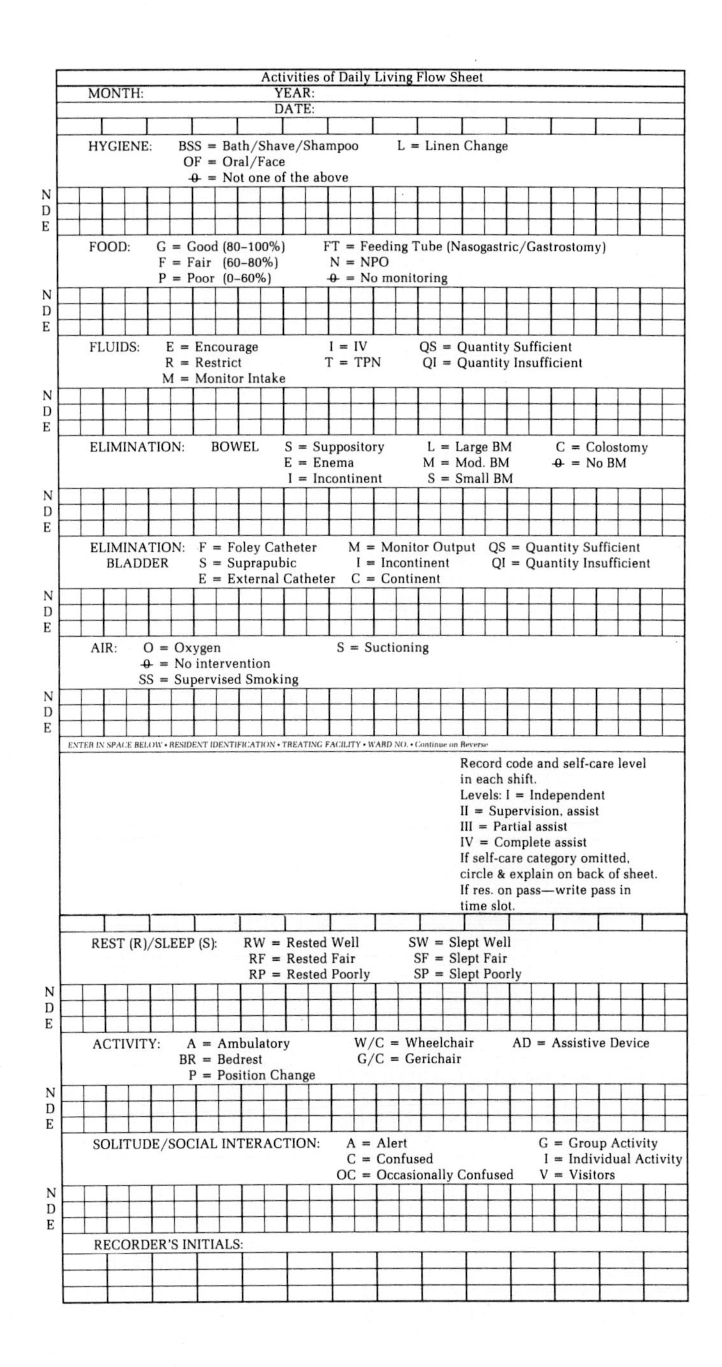

Activities of Daily Living Flow Sheet

MONTH: YEAR:

DATE:

HYGIENE: BSS = Bath/Shave/Shampoo L = Linen Change
OF = Oral/Face
Ø = Not one of the above

N
D
E

FOOD: G = Good (80–100%) FT = Feeding Tube (Nasogastric/Gastrostomy)
F = Fair (60–80%) N = NPO
P = Poor (0–60%) Ø = No monitoring

N
D
E

FLUIDS: E = Encourage I = IV QS = Quantity Sufficient
R = Restrict T = TPN QI = Quantity Insufficient
M = Monitor Intake

N
D
E

ELIMINATION: BOWEL S = Suppository L = Large BM C = Colostomy
E = Enema M = Mod. BM Ø = No BM
I = Incontinent S = Small BM

N
D
E

ELIMINATION: BLADDER F = Foley Catheter M = Monitor Output QS = Quantity Sufficient
S = Suprapubic I = Incontinent QI = Quantity Insufficient
E = External Catheter C = Continent

N
D
E

AIR: O = Oxygen S = Suctioning
Ø = No intervention
SS = Supervised Smoking

N
D
E

ENTER IN SPACE BELOW • RESIDENT IDENTIFICATION • TREATING FACILITY • WARD NO. • Continue on Reverse

Record code and self-care level in each shift.
Levels: I = Independent
II = Supervision, assist
III = Partial assist
IV = Complete assist
If self-care category omitted, circle & explain on back of sheet.
If res. on pass—write pass in time slot.

REST (R)/SLEEP (S): RW = Rested Well SW = Slept Well
RF = Rested Fair SF = Slept Fair
RP = Rested Poorly SP = Slept Poorly

N
D
E

ACTIVITY: A = Ambulatory W/C = Wheelchair AD = Assistive Device
BR = Bedrest G/C = Gerichair
P = Position Change

N
D
E

SOLITUDE/SOCIAL INTERACTION: A = Alert G = Group Activity
C = Confused I = Individual Activity
OC = Occasionally Confused V = Visitors

N
D
E

RECORDER'S INITIALS:

Figure 11–4. ADL flow sheet. (From Hogan, Sorrentino: Mosby's Textbook for Long-Term Care Assistants, St. Louis, 1988, The C.V. Mosby Co.)

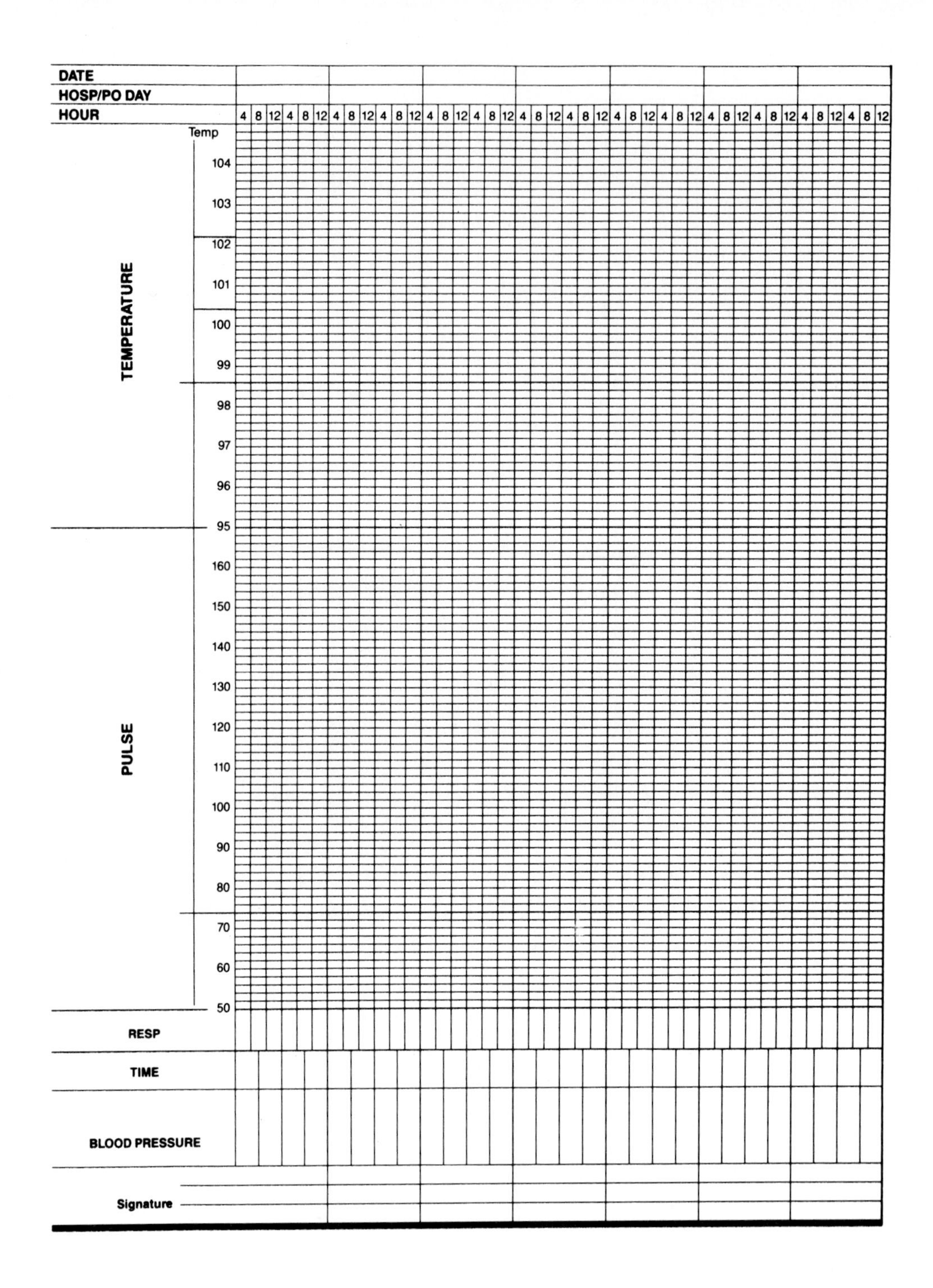

DATE

HOSP/PO DAY

HOUR 4 8 12 4 8 12 4 8 12 4 8 12 4 8 12 4 8 12 4 8 12 4 8 12 4 8 12 4 8 12 4 8 12 4 8 12 4 8 12 4 8 12

TEMPERATURE

Temp

104

103

102

101

100

99

98

97

96

95

PULSE

160

150

140

130

120

110

100

90

80

70

60

50

RESP

TIME

BLOOD PRESSURE

Signature

Figure 11–5. Sample graphic sheet for recording vital signs.

TOTAL INTAKE AND OUTPUT SHEET

INTAKE DATE ______________ **OUTPUT**

	ORAL	I.V.		TOTAL
7:30-3:30				
3:30-11:30				
11:30-7:30				
TOTALS				

24 hr. Intake __________ cc

URINE	EMESIS			TOTAL

24 hr. Output __________ cc

DATE ______________

	ORAL	I.V.		TOTAL
7:30-3:30				
3:30-11:30				
11:30-7:30				
TOTALS				

24 hr. Intake __________ cc

URINE	EMESIS			TOTAL

24 hr. Output __________ cc

DATE ______________

	ORAL	I.V.		TOTAL
7:30-3:30				
3:30-11:30				
11:30-7:30				
TOTALS				

24 hr. Intake __________ cc

URINE	EMESIS			TOTAL

24 hr. Output __________ cc

DATE ______________

	ORAL	I.V.		TOTAL
7:30-3:30				
3:30-11:30				
11:30-7:30				
TOTALS				

24 hr. Intake __________ cc

URINE	EMESIS			TOTAL

24 hr. Output __________ cc

DATE ______________

	ORAL	I.V.		TOTAL
7:30-3:30				
3:30-11:30				
11:30-7:30				
TOTALS				

24 hr. Intake __________ cc

URINE	EMESIS			TOTAL

24 hr. Output __________ cc

DATE ______________

	ORAL	I.V.		TOTAL
7:30-3:30				
3:30-11:30				
11:30-7:30				
TOTALS				

24 hr. Intake __________ cc

URINE	EMESIS			TOTAL

24 hr. Output __________ cc

Figure 11–6. Sample Intake and Output sheet.

815-25-7119
Lorenzo Jeffries
418 Frost Avenue
Dorset, NY 11588
Dr. Walter Hurst
Unit 7E

DOCTOR'S ORDER SHEET

DATE	TIME	PROB. NO.	ORDERS	DOCTOR	NOTED BY	TIME	CODE NO.
1/18/89	3 P.M.	6	ERYTHROMYCIN 250 mg.	W. Hurst	B.A.		
			p.o. q. 6 hr.				

Figure 11–7. A sample of the various hospital forms used for recording a patient's care.

Diet:

Activities:	Bath:	Travel:	Position:
___ Complete bed rest ___ Bed rest ___ Bathroom privileges ✓ Up ad lib	___ Bed bath ___ Partial ✓ Bathe self ___ Tub ___ Shower	___ Wheelchair ___ Stretcher ✓ Ambulatory ___ Walker ___ Cane ___ Crutches	

Side rails:	Oxygen:	Special equipment:
___ Constantly ___ Nights only ✓ Side rail release	___ Liters per minute ___ PRN ___ Constantly ___ Tent ___ Catheter ___ Mask ___ Cannula	

Prosthesis:	Special privileges:	Allergies:
___ Dentures ✓ Eye glasses ___ Contact lenses ___ Hearing aid ___ Limb ___ Other	May shampoo hair as desired	None known

Date	Medications	Date	Treatments
8/21	Tagamet 300 mg qid – 9-1-5-9 – po	8/21	Vital signs – qid
8/21	Mylanta 10 ml po 90 min pc + HS		Fluids
		8/21	Intake and output
		8/21	Hematest stools for occult blood
8/22	HS Med Dalmane 30 mg po		
PRN 8/22	Tylenol tabs 2 po q4h – headache		IVs
		8/21	D5W 1000 ml q8h

Room	Name	Age	Diagnosis	Doctor
333-1	Bailey, Laura	46	Duodenal ulcer	J. Wilson

Figure 11–8. A sample Kardex. (From Sorrentino: Mosby's Textbook for Nursing Assistants, ed. 2, St. Louis, 1987, The C.V. Mosby Co.)

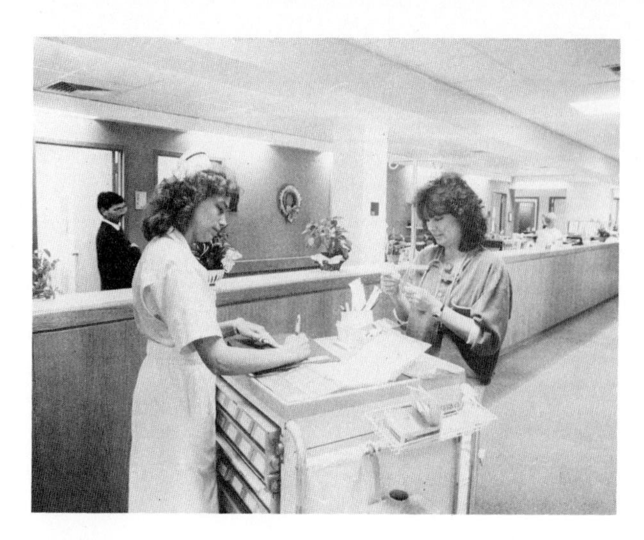

Figure 11–9. Information on the Kardex is essential for preparing and giving medications. (Courtesy of Bridgeton Hospital, Bridgeton, N.J. Photo by Gary F. Cooper.)

With computerized records, the staff has quick access to essential information. However, the Kardex continues to be the method used by most institutions, even if the computer is in use.

Rules for Recording

The following basic rules for recording are adapted from *Mosby's Textbook for Nursing Assistants*. They apply to anyone who will be recording on patient charts. NOTE: The policy of your employer determines who will chart and who will not. In some areas, an assistant may not be permitted or expected to chart.

Basic Guidelines for Charting

1. Always use ink.
2. Include time and date whenever a recording is made.
3. Make sure writing is legible and neat.
4. Use only abbreviations approved by your employer.
5. Make sure spelling, grammar, and punctuation are correct.
6. Never erase or use correction fluid to cover an error. Draw a line through your mistake. Write "error" above it. Place your initials and the date next to the word "error." Rewrite the entry.

7. Sign all entries with your name and title, according to employer policy.
8. Record only what you have observed or performed yourself.
9. Be accurate and factual. Be descriptive, do not interpret. Record what the patient says, not what you think the patient meant.
10. Make sure each form is dated and includes the patient's name and other required data.

TERMINOLOGY AND ABBREVIATIONS

In order to read and understand patient records, you must understand the special language of medicine — medical terminology. Just as any occupation has its own language, so do the health occupations. So as you begin your health career, you start to learn this new language.

Word Roots

Most medical words are made up of several components. One section of the word that is *always present* is the root. This is the word base to which other parts are attached. The root also gives the basic meaning of the word. For example, in the word microscope, the root is scope. A scope is an instrument for viewing. Try it yourself. What is the root in the word arthritis? Did you say *arthr*? That is correct. *Arthr* is the word root — it means joint.

Suffixes

There may be a suffix attached to the word root. The suffix modifies the meaning of the word root. In the example above, the suffix, *itis*, modifies the word root *arthr*. The suffix *itis* means inflammation. Therefore, *arthr* + *itis* = inflammation of the joints.

Prefixes

Other words may have a prefix attached to the beginning of a root word which will also modify the meaning of the word root. In the example, microscope, the word root *scope* is modified by the prefix *micro*. The prefix *micro* means very small. Therefore, *micro* + *scope* = an instrument for viewing something that is very small. In the word hemocyte, the prefix, *hemo*, means blood and the root word, *cyte*, means cell. Therefore, *hemo* + *cyte* = blood cell.

Combining Vowels

Some words will require a combining vowel between two root words or a root word and a suffix to make the word easier to pronounce. In order to combine the root word *arthr* and suffix *scope*, it is necessary to add the vowel "o." Therefore, *arthro* + *scope* = an instrument for examining (looking into) the joints. Generally, if a suffix begins with a vowel, it will not be necessary to add another vowel to make a combining form. Look at arthritis and arthroscope, and you can see how this general rule can be applied.

The list below is a small sample of medical word components that, when combined, form the terms used in the health industry. As you progress in your health career, you will learn words that are specific to your occupational specialty.

Prefixes	**Meaning**
a, an-	without, absence of
ab-	away from
ad-	toward
ante-	before
anti-	against
auto-	self
bi-	two
circum-	around
contra-	against
dys-	painful, difficult
ecto-	outside
en-	in, into
endo-	inside
epi-	upon
erythro-	red
ex-	out, away from
hemi-	half
hyper-	above, over, excessive
hypo-	under, below normal

inter-	between
intra-	within
leuk-	white
lymph-	lymph
macro-	large
mal-	bad
meso-	middle
micro-	small
mono-	one, single
olig-	scanty
para-	near, beside,around, abnormal
per-	through
peri-	surrounding
poly-	many
post-	after
pre-	before
retro-	behind
semi-	half
supra-	above
trans-	across
uni-	one

Suffixes	**Meaning**
-algia	pain
-asis	condition (abnormal)
-blast	embroyonic, immature
-cele	pouch, hernia
-centesis	surgical puncture to remove fluid from a cavity
-coccus	type of bacteria
-cyte	cell
-dynia	pain
-ectasis	stretching
-ectomy	surgical removal
-emesis	vomiting
-emia	blood condition
-genic	producing or causing
-gram	record of
-graph	instrument for recording
-graphy	process of recording

-iasis	condition of
-itis	inflammation
-logy	study of
-lysis	breakdown
-megaly	enlargement of
-meter	measuring instrument
-metry	measurement
-oid	resembling
-oma	tumor
-opia	vision
-opsy	to view
-osis	abnormal condition
-partum	birth or labor
-pathy	disease
-penia	deficiency, lack of
-phagia	swallowing
-phasia	speaking
-phobia	fear
-plasty	surgical repair
-plegia	paralysis
-pena	breathing
-ptosis	sagging, drooping
-rrhage, rrhagia	excessive flow
-rrhaphy	suture, surgical repair
-rrhea	profuse flow, discharge
-scope	instrument for examining
-scopy	process of using a scope
-stasis	stopping
-stomy, ostomy	new opening
-tomy	cutting, incision
-trophy	development, nourishment into
-uria	urine, urination
-y	condition or process

Root (combining vowel)	**Meaning**
abdomin (o)	abdomen
aden(o)	gland
adren (o)	adrenal gland

apex (apico)	summit or peak; such as the tip of the root of a tooth
arteri(o)	artery
arthr(o)	joint
ather(o)	yellowish plaque; fatty substance
audi (o)	ear
broncho	bronchial tubes
bucc (o)	cheek
card, cardi (o)	heart
cephal (o)	head
chem (o)	drug; chemical
chol (e, o)	bile
col (o)	bowel
crani (o)	skull
cusp	point or crown of a tooth; part of a valve of the heart
cyan (o)	bluish color
cyst(o)	cyst, bladder
cyt (o)	cell
dent (i, o)	tooth
dist (o)	far
encephal (o)	brain
enter (o)	intestines
fibr (o)	fiber
gastr (o)	stomach
gingiv (o)	gums
gloss (o)	tongue
gluc (o)	sugar
glyc (o)	sugar
gynec (o)	woman, female
hemo, hema, hemat (o)	blood
hepat (o)	liver
herni (o)	hernia
hydr (o)	water
ile (o), ili (o)	ileum
labi (o)	lips
lapar (o)	abdomen
laryng (o)	larynx, voice box

lingu (o)	tongue
mamm (o)	breast
mandibul (o)	lower jaw bone
mast (o)	breast
maxill (o)	upper jaw bone
medi (o)	middle
men (o)	menses
my (o)	muscle
myc (o)	fungus, mold
myel (o)	spinal cord, bone marrow
nas (o)	nose
necr (o)	death
nephr (o)	kidney
neur (o)	nerve
ocul (o)	eye
odont (o)	tooth
ocul (o)	eye
ophthalm (o)	eye
orth (o)	straight, normal
oste (o)	bone
ot (o)	ear
pedi (o)	child
pharyng (o)	pharynx
phleb (o)	vein
pnea	breathing
pneum (o)	lung, air, gas
proct (o)	rectum
psych (o)	mind
pulmo	lung
py (o)	pus
rect (o)	rectum
rhin (o)	nose
splen (o)	spleen
sten (o)	narrow
stern (o)	breastbone
stomat (o)	mouth
submaxill (o)	lower jaw bone
therm (o)	heat
thoraco	chest

thrombo	clot
thyr (o)	thyroid
toxo	poison
trache (o)	trachea
uro	urine, urinary tract, voiding
urethr (o)	urethra
urin (o)	urine
uter (o)	uterus
vas (o)	blood vessel, vas deferens
ven (o)	vein
vertebr (o)	spine, vertebrae

ABBREVIATIONS

Many medical phrases and word combinations are used repeatedly. In order to save time and space in written communications, abbreviations are used. Some abbreviations are standard, that is, in common use and understood by medical personnel in the United States. Examples of these are listed below. Some employing agencies will use abbreviations that are exclusive to that facility only. You will be given a list of those abbreviations when you start your job. It is wise to ask your employing agency for a listing of these abbreviations.

If you do not know whether an abbreviation is acceptable, you should write the complete phrase so the record will be accurate and easily understood.

Abbreviation	Meaning
abd	abdomen
a.c.	before meals
ADL	activities of daily living
ad lib	as desired
b.i.d.	twice a day
BM or bm	bowel movement
BP	blood pressure
c̄	with
Ca	cancer
CAT	computerized axial tomography
CBC	complete blood count
cc	cubic centimeter

CCU	coronary care unit
c/o	complains of
COPD	chronic obstructive pulmonary disease
CPR	cardiopulmonary resuscitation
CT	computerized tomography
CVA	cerebral vascular accident (stroke)
d/c	discontinue
DOA	dead on arrival
DON	director of nursing
dx	diagnosis
ECG/EKG	electrocardiogram
EEG	electroencephalogram
ENT	ear, nose, and throat
ER	emergency room
F	Fahrenheit
FBS	fasting blood sugar
FF	force fluids
F/u	follow up
GB	gallbladder
GI	gastrointestinal
GU	genitourinary
Gyn	gynecology
h or hr.	hour
Hg or Hgb	hemoglobin
H_2O	water
H.S. or h.s.	hour of sleep, bedtime
ht	height
ICU	intensive care unit
I&O	intake and output
IPPB	intermittent positive pressure breathing
IV	intravenous
L	liter or left
Lab	laboratory
lb.	pound
LLQ	lower left quadrant
LMP	last menstrual period
LUQ	left upper quadrant
L&W	living and well
meds	medications

min	minute
ml	milliliter
neg	negative
nil	none
noc	night
NPO	nothing by mouth
O_2	oxygen
OB	obstetrics
OOB	out of bed
OD	right eye
OJ	orange juice
OR	operating room
OS	left eye
os	mouth
OT	occupational therapy
OU	each eye
OV	office visit
oz.	ounce
p.c.	after meals
PDR	*Physicians' Desk Reference*
Peds	pediatrics
per	by, through
p.o.	by mouth
postop	postoperative
preop	preoperative
p.r.n.	as required, when necessary
PT	physical therapy
pt.	patient
q	every
q.d.	every day
q.h.	every hour
q.2h., q.3h., q.4h., etc.	every two hours, every three hours, every four hours, etc.
q.i.d.	four times daily
q.o.d.	every other day
q.s.	sufficient quantity, as much as necessary
R	rectal, right
RLQ	right lower quadrant
ROM	range of motion

RR	recovery room
rt.	right
RUQ	right upper quadrant
Rx	treatment
s̄	without
SOB	shortness of breath
spec	specimen
stat	immediately
Surg	surgery
Sx	symptoms
Tbsp.	tablespoon
t.i.d.	three times a day
TLC	tender loving care
TPR	temperature, pulse, and respiration
tsp.	teaspoon
WBC	white blood count
w/c	wheelchair
wt	weight

Study the abbreviations, prefixes, suffixes, and root words found in this chapter. They are part of the special language that is used in health careers. You must know and understand these words and be able to use them in order to communicate within the health care delivery system.

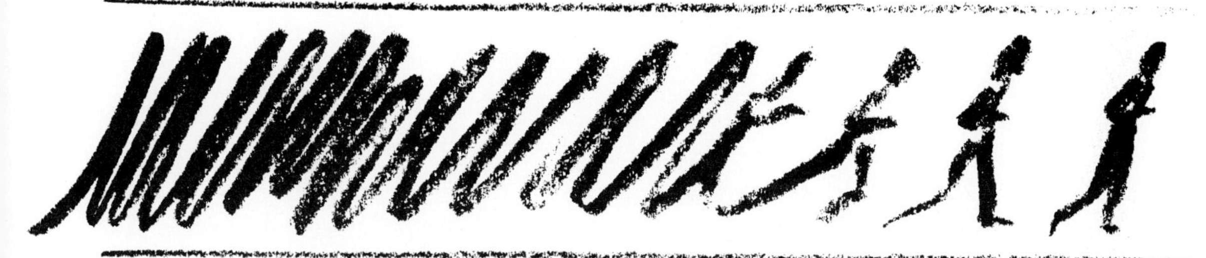

STUDENT ACTIVITIES

Identify the prefix, root, and suffix in each of the following words.

1. Osteoarthritis
2. Hypoglycemia
3. Hypertension
4. Colostomy
5. Odontalgia
6. Hyperplagia
7. Dentition
8. Periapical
9. Bicuspid
10. Psychology
11. Appendectomy
12. Gastritis
13. Glossitis
14. Osteoporosis
15. Leukocyte
16. Mononeucleocyte
17. Dentalgia
18. Gingivitis
19. Glycosuria
20. Hemiplegia

Write the meaning of the following abbreviations:

21. OOB t.i.d. ____________________

22. pt. complains of pain in the RUQ and is SOB ____________________

____

23. NPO from midnight, to OR in AM

____

24. dx CVA ____________________

25. DOA in ER ____________________

____

26. Complete admission forms and history forms by interviewing classmates. Obtain appropriate forms from your instructor.

Chapter 12

Safety On — and Off — the Job

Objectives

After completing this chapter, you should be able to:

- Identify at least seven common occupational hazards to which the health worker is exposed.
- Identify at least five common hazards to which clients are exposed.
- Discuss three methods to prevent infection.
- Demonstrate handwashing technique.
- Discuss safety precautions to prevent accidents to staff and clients.
- Identify at least five safety measures to prevent accidents at home.
- List three signs of choking.
- Describe the first aid for choking.
- Describe the steps to be taken in an emergency.
- List the steps to be taken in case of a fire.
- Define at least 70 percent of the key terms for this chapter.

Key Terms

- **accident** An event occurring by chance or unintentionally
- **asepsis** Sterile; a condition free from germs, from infection, or any form of life
- **autoclave** Apparatus for sterilization, using steam under pressure
- **biohazard** Any pathogenic organism, disease vector, or physical chemical agent, that produces adverse health effects in humans or other species who may inhale, ingest, or absorb the pathogenic organism or toxic agent
- **body alignment** The way body parts are lined up with each other; posture
- **body mechanics** The use of body movements in an efficient manner
- **carrier** A person who spreads a specific pathogenic organism without contracting the disease
- **emergency** An unexpected serious occurrence which demands immediate attention
- **infection** The state or condition in which the body is invaded by a disease-producing organism
- **medical asepsis** Clean; free from germs
- **microbe** A living plant or animal that can only be seen by a microscope
- **nosocomial infection** Infection acquired in a hospital
- **pathogen** A microorganism or substance capable of producing disease
- **pathogenic** Disease-producing
- **sterile** Free of any form of living microorganisms
- **sterilization** The process of destruction of all living microorganisms on a substance by chemical or physical means
- **surgical asepsis** Elimination of all forms of microbial life

THINK SAFETY

You may be wondering why a book on health careers has a chapter on safety. After all, we don't think of health careers as being particularly dangerous or hazardous. In fact, most people would think that safety was a problem associated with heavy industries such as manufacturing and construction. Health workers do not usually operate manufacturing equipment, weld girders on 50-story buildings, or drive large combines to gather a harvest, but they do work in environments that are as dangerous as those described.

Perhaps you have heard the old joke — hospitals are dangerous places, after all, they are full of sick people. That is true, and one of the hazards of working with sick people is the danger of infection. You can pick up an infection in the work place, and your clients can, too. Therefore, it is vital that you learn to use the proper procedures for preventing the spread of infection. This will protect both you and your clients.

Since many sick people have difficulty moving, they will need assistance with turning, moving, and positioning for comfort and diagnostic studies. Other clients will need help with activities of daily living (ADL), using the toilet, bathing, walking, and eating. In addition, various types of equipment will have to be moved and positioned properly. Use of proper lifting and transfer techniques will help to prevent injury to you and your client. A note of caution — if you don't know the proper procedure, or if you are alone and unable to move a person or an object, call for help. NEVER ATTEMPT ANY PROCEDURE WHERE YOU OR ANOTHER PERSON COULD BE INJURED.

The leading cause of injury is falls. If you work in an office, storeroom, or in the housekeeping department it may be necessary for you to do some climbing to reach things on high shelves. Be cautious! Most falls can be prevented by using common sense. Chairs are for sitting, not climbing. Use the equipment that is designed for safe climbing. If you do not have what is necessary, don't climb.

Health care workers are surrounded with hazardous equipment and supplies. X-ray machines, dental drills, sharp knives and instruments, steam tables, elevators, electric beds, and sterilizers are a few examples. Electrical cords and telephone wires often cause people to trip and fall. Each particular supply item or piece of equipment requires special handling. You will learn about each in your particular area as you progress in your health career. Be sure that you understand how each machine works and that you know all of the necessary safety precautions before operating any equipment. Always read the directions and the operating manual. Never be afraid to ask for help. If you haven't been taught how to use or care for the equipment, leave it alone until you have been properly instructed (**Fig. 12–1**).

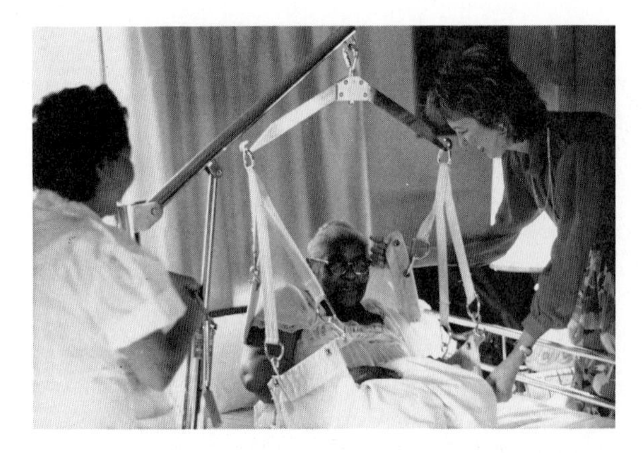

Figure 12–1. Proper use of equipment can prevent injury to the client and the caregiver. (Courtesy of Mercer Street Friends Center, Trenton, N.J.)

Dangerous chemicals are found in all work places and even at home. Some substances that are specific to the health industry include disinfectants, laboratory dyes and stains, radioactive isotopes, x-rays, and irritating drugs. Each and every health career, medical and dental specialty, and institutional department has its unique problems with specific types of chemicals. For example, oxygen is an essential element, vital for human life. It is basic to the treatment of patients with heart and lung conditions. However, premature babies who have been exposed to high concentrations of oxygen have developed blindness. Furthermore, oxygen supports combustion, and there is always an increased danger of fire when oxygen is in use. What is life-saving to one person can be hazardous to another. The storage and monitoring of the oxygen supply and maintenance of the delivery system are important factors in the proper handling of this medical gas.

As you learn more about your career, you will learn how to handle dangerous chemicals and how to protect yourself and your clients. You must always follow the precautions and the procedures exactly as you were taught. This is essential to ensure safety for you, your coworkers, and your clients.

BODY MECHANICS

This section of the chapter will discuss the proper use of your body as you perform work that requires lifting, moving, twisting, or reaching. A word of caution: **Basic concepts** will be covered, but your teacher and employer will provide guidelines for your specific health career.

Your body is a marvelously flexible mechanism that is able to bend, jump, lift, run, dance — in short, move in many directions for many different purposes. Your skeleton makes up the bony framework of your body. There are 206 bones in all. They are long, short, flat, and irregular in shape and size. The bones are hard and rigid. They are able to move only at the joints (places where they meet). Smooth tissue — cartilage — covers the ends of the long bones and acts as a cushion. A special membrane lines each joint and produces a lubricating fluid called **synovial fluid**. Strong bands of connective tissue, called ligaments, connect the bones at the joint.

There are several types of moveable joints. Ball and socket joints, located at the hips and shoulders, permit movement in all directions. Hinge joints, however, move in only one direction, as with the elbows and the knees. The pivotal joint allows turning from side to side; the joint between the skull and the spine is an example.

Muscles are attached to the bones by long, tough cords called tendons. Along with the muscles, they move the bones, much like the movement of a lever. If you hold your wrist with the opposite hand, you will be able to feel the tendons working as you move your fingers to open and close your hand to make a fist.

The muscles of the arms, legs, shoulders, and buttocks are long, strong muscles that are structured and used for work such as lifting and moving. The muscles of the back are large, flat, overlapping structures which allow for flexibility and protection of internal structures. The back muscles are not meant to sustain heavy lifting; they are too weak to be used for this purpose.

Some basic rules for lifting and moving persons or objects are provided below.

Always use good posture. This will help you to have good balance, conserve energy, and prevent strain. Good posture helps to maintain the natural curves of your spine. Do not arch your back or keep it abnormally stiff. Try to picture in your mind what good posture looks like. When standing, the head should be erect, chest up and forward, abdomen flat, feet parallel to each other with one foot slightly forward. Normal spinal curves at the neck, chest, and lower back should be maintained (**Fig. 12–2a, b**).

Good posture is essential for comfort when sitting. Again, the head should be erect, the chest up and forward, and the abdomen flat. The hips should be bent at right angles and the weight should be supported by the thighs. Also, the person should be sitting back in the chair with the feet resting on the floor. This is not always possible for persons with very short legs. They will be much more comfortable if they can rest their feet on a small stool.

Lifting is done from a standing position with the knees bent. Remember: The long, strong muscles of the legs and arms do the lifting — *NOT THE BACK*. If it is necessary for you to bend in order to do the lifting, it is the knees that are bent. *NEVER BEND YOUR BACK — ALWAYS KEEP IT STRAIGHT*. The muscles of the thighs and buttocks should be doing the work.

Body mechanics is a way of using your body so that the work is distributed over several groups of muscles with the stronger ones being used (**Fig. 12–3a and b**). The rules of good body mechanics include:

1. Stand with your feet comfortably apart, with one foot forward and your toes pointing in the direction of the movement.
2. Tighten your abdominal muscles when you lift — they help support your back.
3. Stand close to the object or person being moved and bend your hips and knees when stooping or bending.
4. Use your long, strong arm and leg muscles to do the work.
5. Carry heavy objects close to the body.

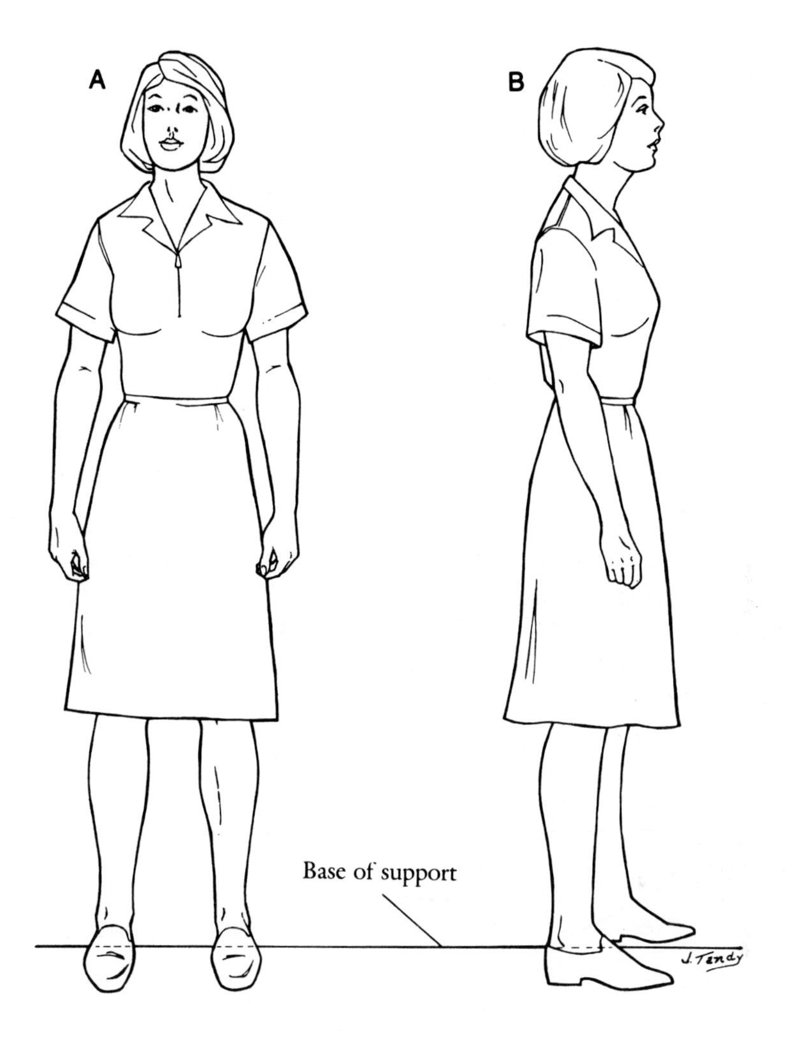

Figure 12–2. **A,** Front view of adult in good body alignment with feet apart for a wide base of support. **B,** Side view of adult with good posture and alignment. (From Sorrentino: Mosby's Textbook for Nursing Assistants, ed. 2, St. Louis, 1987, The C.V. Mosby Co.)

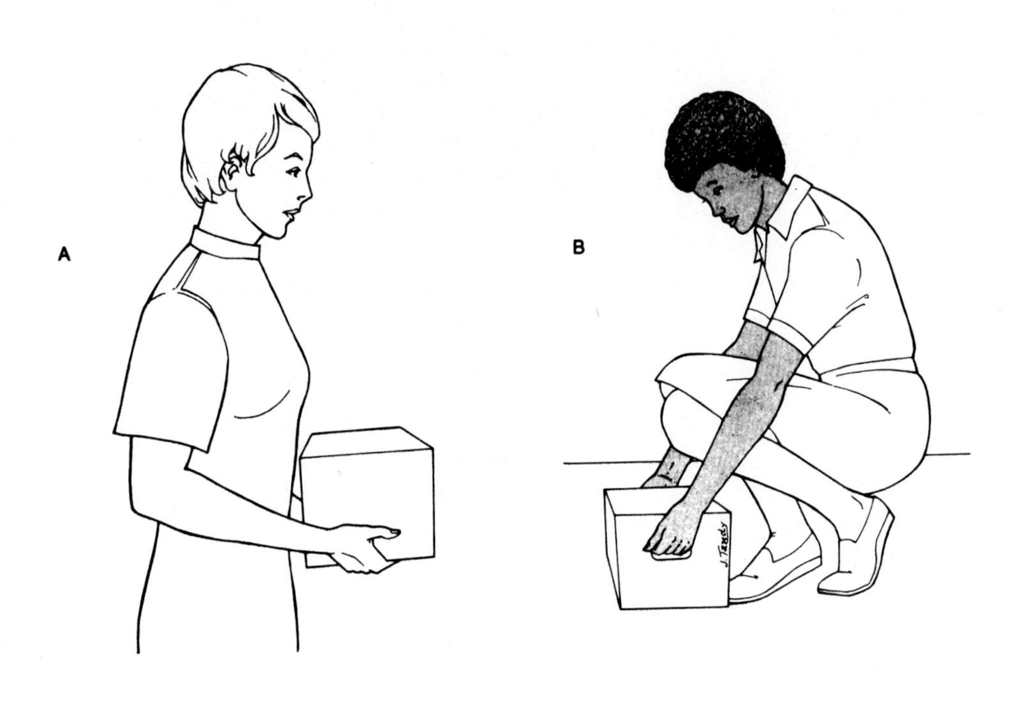

Figure 12–3. Picking up and carrying a box using proper body mechanics. (From Sorrentino: Mosby's Textbook for Nursing Assistants, ed. 2, St. Louis, 1987, The C.V. Mosby Co.)

6. Whenever possible, slide, roll, or turn the patient or object at hip level rather than lifting.
7. Maintain the natural curves of your back to keep your balance.
8. Always utilize any and all assistance that is available.
9. Push rather than pull.
10. Learn ways to strengthen your muscles and joints to prevent injury and promote wellness. Proper exercise helps to keep your muscles in good working condition.

PREVENTION OF DISEASE AND INFECTION

Infection is a condition caused by microorganisms entering the body and causing disease. Micro means small — not visible to the naked eye. A microbe is a living plant or animal that can be seen only by the microscope. Microorganisms are found everywhere. Those that are harmful and capable of producing disease are called pathogens. Other microbes are nonpathogens and do not produce disease in humans. They may be used to perform helpful functions. For example, yeasts are used to make bread or to cause fermentation in breweries.

Pathogens have distinct shapes and characteristics which can be observed in the medical laboratory. Bacteria are a type of plant life that multiply rapidly. Fungi live on other plants or animals. Examples are yeasts and molds which may be seen on old bread or fruit. Athlete's foot is an example of a disease caused by a fungus.

Protozoa are one-celled animals that are often found in water and have caused many serious diseases in third world countries where the water sources are contaminated by these organisms. Protozoa may infect the eye when proper disinfection and storage of soft contact lenses is not observed.

Rickettsiae are forms of microscopic life found on fleas, ticks, and insects. A disease caused by rickettsiae is Rocky Mountain Spotted Fever.

The smallest of all the known microorganisms are the viruses. They grow in living cells and are so tiny that they are called ultramicroscopic. Viruses cannot be seen through the ordinary laboratory microscope. An electron microscope is necessary to visualize these organisms. Many diseases are caused by viruses, ranging from the common cold to the more serious hepatitis and acquired immune deficiency syndrome (AIDS).

Growth of Microorganisms

In order to thrive, all microorganisms need a warm place to grow. Body temperature is about the ideal temperature to promote the growth of pathogens. As with all other living things, these organisms require moisture and food to flourish. Again, the human body proves to be an ideal host because it is an excellent source of both food and moisture. Lastly, all pathogens like to grow in dark places, such as body cells, tissues, and organs. Most microorganisms are oxygen-loving. These are called aerobic organisms. A few, however, flourish without the presence of any oxygen at all. These are known as anaerobic organisms. They are often found in foods that have been improperly canned, often at home. Botulism, a form of food poisoning, is an example of a serious — often fatal — illness caused by anaerobic bacteria.

Pathogenic microorganisms are "opportunistic," meaning that they seize the opportunity to infect the weakest and least resistant organism. So, a person who is already sick becomes an excellent host for a bacteria looking for a site to live and grow. This is an important reason to maintain excellent health! It is the very same reason to protect clients from the possibility of any type of infection. Many people have become sicker in the hospital than at home because they acquired a **nosocomial** infection while they were patients.

If you looked for microorganisms with the naked eye, you wouldn't see anything. But they are everywhere — on the skin, in the mouth, under the fingernails, in the lower digestive tract. Some stay in the places they belong without causing any trouble. These are known as normal flora. But when one of these organisms gets where it does not belong, a serious infection can occur. For example, the E. Coli is a bacteria that lives in the large colon and is not normally pathogenic. If it should get into the urinary tract, an infection could result.

The skin is the largest organ of the human body and our first line of defense against injury and infection. It is a wonderful envelope that protects our internal structures against all types of mishaps. Broken skin is particularly prone to invasion from pathogenic organisms. Once a wound becomes infected, it then becomes a source of infection to other parts of the body as well as to other persons.

Signs of Infection

When an infection develops, several classic symptoms can be observed. The affected area becomes red, swollen, hot, and sore. The client may experience nausea and vomiting, fever, and a decreased appetite. These symptoms will vary in intensity according to the site and severity of the infection.

Sources of Infection

There are many sources of pathogenic organisms. For instance, there may be a reservoir of infection in the environment. That is, there is a source of supply of an infectious agent or disease. This could be a person, animal, plant, or organic matter that allows an infectious agent to live. The reservoir for tuberculosis is usually a person. However, in some countries it could be found in the cow and her milk.

A carrier is a person who harbors a specific pathogenic organism without exhibiting any signs or symptoms of the disease. This person is capable of spreading the organism to others. The best known case of a human carrier was **"Typhoid Mary"** who never exhibited the disease whose causative agent she carried.

How do pathogens enter the body? They do so in a number of ways — broken skin, contaminated food and water, dirty utensils, poor hygiene, direct contact, contaminated dressings, insects, and animals. One of the best sources of infectious agents is our hands, which always handle dirty things such as money, door knobs, water faucets, books, pencils, newspapers. Therefore, a health worker must develop aseptic practices. Asepsis means free from germs. If you work in an area where surgery is performed you will apply surgical asepsis. This means to protect against infection before and during surgery by the use of **sterile technique**. For other areas of health work, medical asepsis will be sufficient because there will be no disease-producing organisms present. This is often known as clean technique.

Common Medical Aseptic Practices

1. Wash hands after using the bathroom.
2. Wash hands before handling or preparing food.
3. Wash raw fruit and vegetables before eating or serving.
4. Use individual hygiene items (towels, washcloths, toothbrushes, etc.) for each member of the family.
5. Cover nose and mouth when coughing, sneezing, and blowing. Never let anyone sneeze or cough on you.
6. Wash hands before, after, and between caring for clients.
7. Use regular hygiene and good grooming habits.

8. Use proper sanitation practices when handling or disposing of trash or sewage.
9. Keep clean things together and dirty things together. Never mix the two. Have a separate space for all used equipment and supplies. Discard contaminated objects immediately and properly.
10. Learn and follow all recommendations to reduce the risk of exposure to blood and body fluids in the health care setting. (Specifics follow.)

To Protect Yourself From Blood and Body Fluids

- **HANDS** should always be washed before and after contact with patients even when gloves have been used. If hands come in contact with blood, body fluids, or human tissue, they should be washed immediately with soap and water.
- **GLOVES** should be worn when contact with blood, body fluids, tissues, or contaminated surfaces is anticipated.
- **GOWNS** or plastic aprons are indicated if blood spattering is likely.
- **MASKS and PROTECTIVE GOGGLES** should be worn if spattering and misting are likely to occur as in dental and surgical procedures, wound irrigations, postmortem examinations, etc.
- **MOUTH PIECES,** resuscitation bags, or other devices should be used in the event of emergency mouth-to-mouth resuscitation.
- **SHARP OBJECTS** should be handled in a manner to prevent cuts and punctures. Follow the proper technique for handling and disposing of used syringes. All needle stick accidents, contaminations of wounds, and splashes with body fluids or blood must be reported immediately.
- **BLOOD SPILLS** should be cleaned up promptly according to the health agency's policy and procedure, using gloves and the proper disinfectant.
- **MOST IMPORTANT:** Consider all patients' blood specimens biohazardous.

Care of Hands

Look at your hands, examine your fingers and fingernails closely. What do you see? Nothing? That is exactly what you see when looking for bacteria on skin surfaces. But they are present in large numbers. Bacteria are found under the nails, around the nail beds, and in the chips and cracks found in nail polish. So, a general rule to remember is no nail polish on the job and certainly no false fingernails. Rings also offer bacteria a hiding place, and most health care facilities only permit you to wear a plain wedding band to work.

Handwashing

Purpose. To prevent the spread of infection by removing microorganisms from the hands.

Equipment. **Soap** — Liquid soap, since it is not constantly handled by other persons, is preferred to bar soap. When bar soap is used, it is held throughout the entire procedure.

Warm, running water — Homemaker/Home-Health aides, public health nurses, and others who work in community health may not always find warm, running water in the home and will develop ways that handwashing can be performed using the proper principles.

Paper towels — After completing the handwashing procedure, a paper towel is used to turn off hand-operated faucets. The faucets are considered to be contaminated, and your hands are clean (**Fig. 12–4**).

Orange wood sticks, nail file, or hand brush — These are used to thoroughly clean under the nails (**Fig. 12–5**).

Wastebasket

Hand lotion, if desired

Procedure:

1. Assemble all equipment at the sink.
2. Remove your wrist watch or push up onto your forearm about four to five inches.
3. Stand back from the sink so that your clothing does not become wet.
4. Turn on the faucet.
5. Adjust the water so that it is warm and comfortable.
6. Completely wet your wrists and hands under the running water. Always keep your fingers and hands below your elbows to prevent dirty water from contaminating your arms (**Fig. 12–6**).
7. Apply soap to your hands. If using bar soap, it should be rinsed before using.

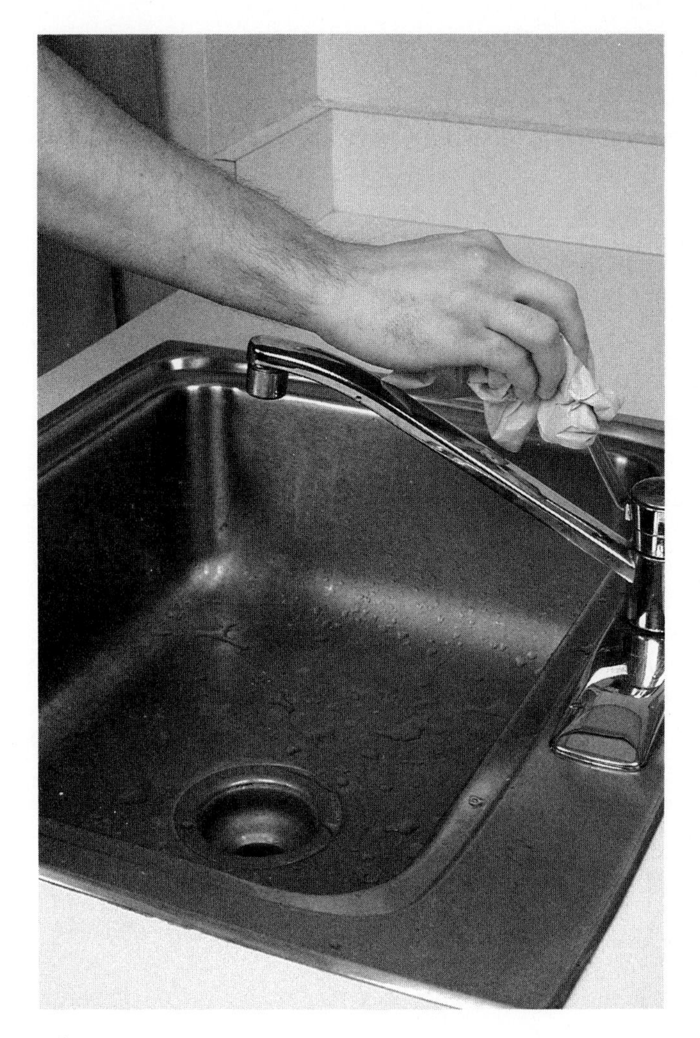

Figure 12–4. Use a paper towel to turn off the faucet. (From Sorrentino: Mosby's Textbook for Nursing Assistants, ed. 2, St. Louis, 1987, The C.V. Mosby Co.)

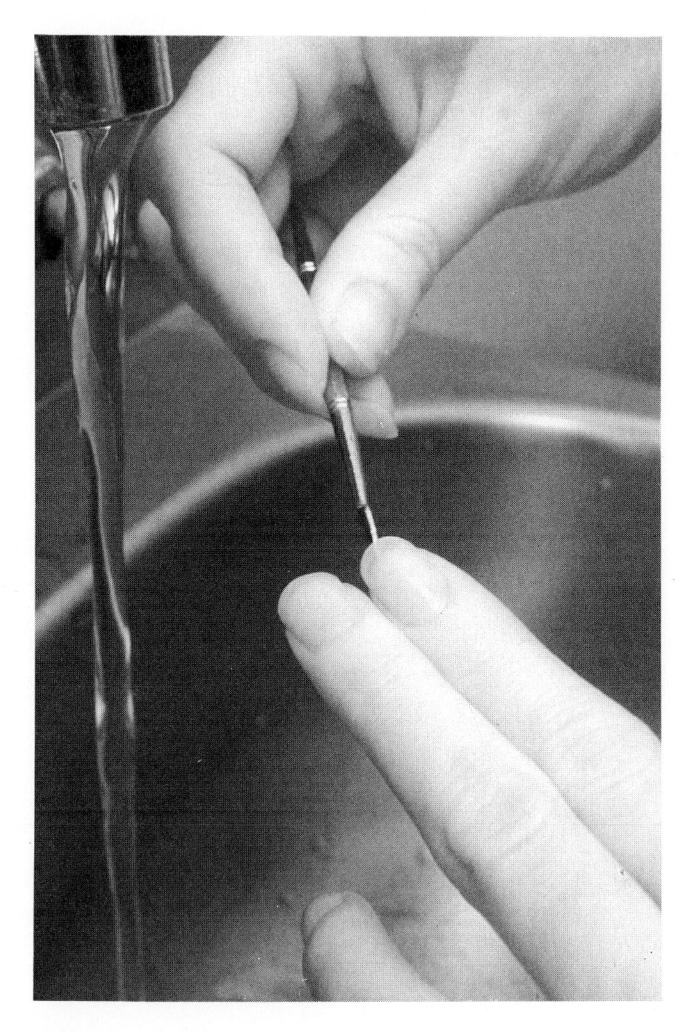

Figure 12–5. Clean under the fingernails with an orange stick. (From Sorrentino: Mosby's Textbook for Nursing Assistants, ed. 2, St. Louis, 1987, The C.V. Mosby Co.)

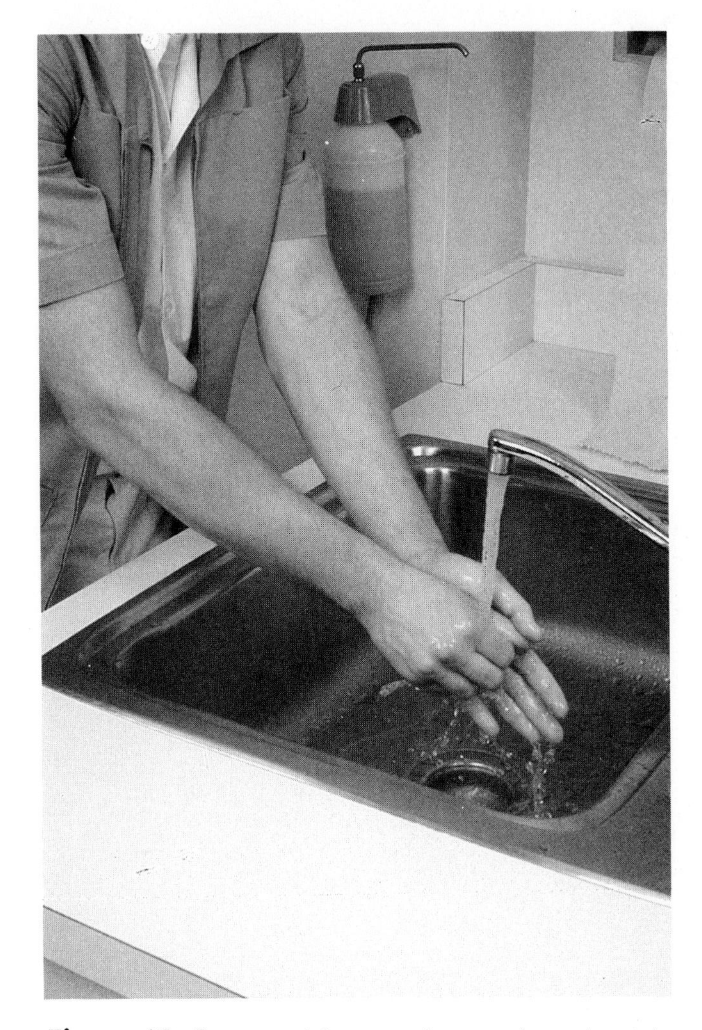

Figure 12–6. Stand far enough away from the sink so that the uniform does not touch the sink and keep hands lower than the elbows. (From Sorrentino: Mosby's Textbook for Nursing Assistants, ed. 2, St. Louis, 1987, The C.V. Mosby Co.)

8. Lather your hands well by rubbing the palms together (**Fig. 12–7**).
9. Wash hands and wrists thoroughly. Rub your fingernails against the palms of your hands to clean this area (**Fig. 12–8**).
10. Continue washing for a minute or two using rubbing and rotating motions.

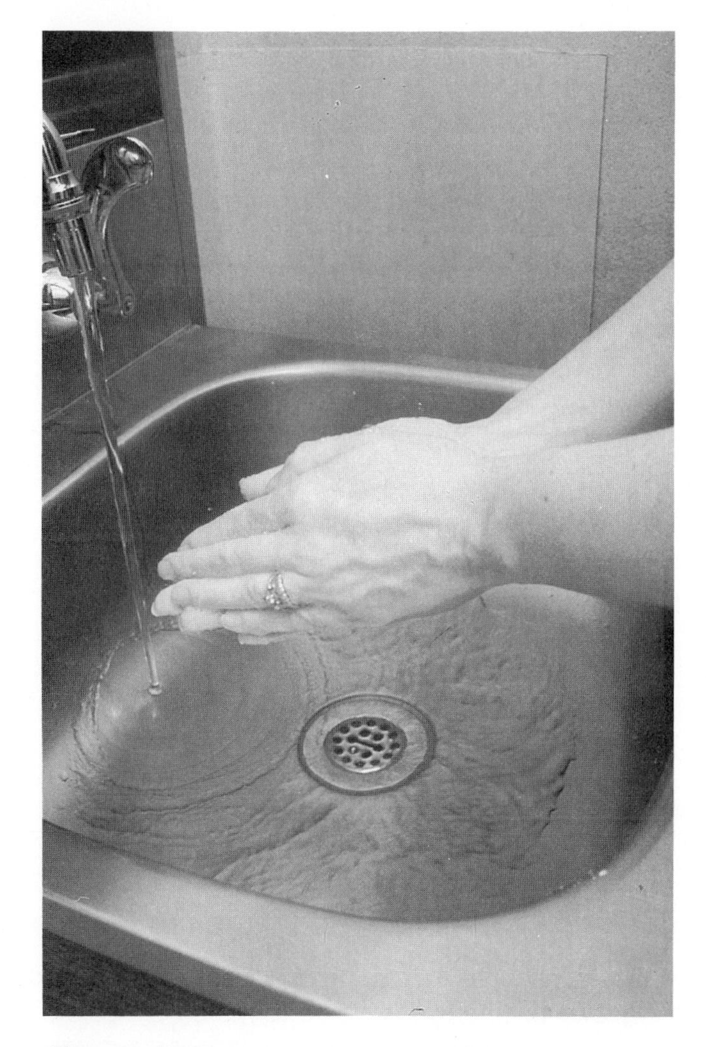

Figure 12–7. Rub palms together and work up good lather. (From Sorrentino: Mosby's Textbook for Nursing Assistants, ed. 2, St. Louis, 1987, The C.V. Mosby Co.)

11. Clean under your fingernails using an orange wood stick, nail file, or hand brush (refer to **Fig. 12–5**).
12. Rinse hands under the running water. Keep hands and fingers below the elbows so the water flows from the finger tips directly into the sink.
13. Repeat entire procedure from #6 to #12.
14. If you have been using bar soap, return it to the soap dish. DO NOT TOUCH THE SOAP DISH.

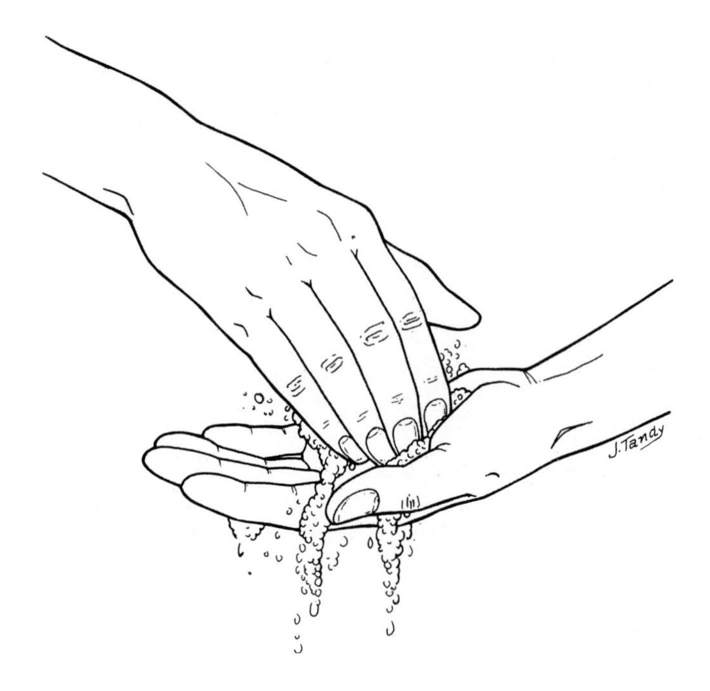

Figure 12–8. Rub tips of fingers against the palm to clean under the fingernails. (From Sorrentino: Mosby's Textbook for Nursing Assistants, ed. 2, St. Louis, 1987, The C.V. Mosby Co.)

15. Dry your hands and wrists with paper towels.
16. Drop the used paper towels into the wastebasket.
17. Turn off the faucets using another paper towel. Discard the towel (refer to **Fig. 12–4**).
18. Apply hand lotion if desired.

Points to Remember about Handwashing

1. Hand-operated faucets are considered contaminated. Always use a paper towel when turning off the water after you have finished washing your hands.
2. The inside of the sink is also considered contaminated. Do not touch this area when handwashing.
3. Always keep your hands below your elbows during the handwashing procedure.

4. Bar soap is washed before using and held during the entire procedure.
5. Use friction and vigorous motions during the handwashing procedure.
6. Handwashing is to be used:
   –when arriving at work
   –before you give patient care or have any direct personal contact with a client
   –after you give patient care or have any direct personal contact with a client
   –if patient care is interrupted
   –when you use the bathroom
   –when you cough or sneeze
   –before meals
   –before you leave work to go home
   –any time your hands become contaminated with body fluids.

Disinfection

Disinfection is the process by which pathogenic microorganisms are destroyed. There are several methods of disinfection including the use of moist heat and chemicals. Certain objects, such as silverware and dishes, may be boiled for 15 minutes. The lid must be kept on the pot so that the boiling process will be effective. This method of disinfection does not destroy all types of bacteria and is not usually used in health care facilities. However, this procedure is used at home. For instance, infant bottles and nipples can be disinfected prior to filling with formula.

Disinfectants are chemicals that kill bacteria. Chemical disinfection involves the application of a physical agent that kills vegetative growth of microorganisms. There are many types of disinfectants. Each has a specific purpose. Some, such as alcohol and iodine, are used for skin degerming. Chlorine is used to disinfect water and to clean and sanitize dishes and utensils. Others, such as Lysol, are used as general disinfectants. *BEFORE USING ANY DISINFECTANT, READ THE LABEL AND FOLLOW THE DIRECTIONS CAREFULLY.* Most products used for general cleaning and room disinfection are extremely irritating to the skin and gloves should be worn. Disinfectants should not be mixed together. (It's not a good idea to play "mad scientist" and mix chemicals together. You may create toxic vapors.) Good ventilation is necessary when you are using chemical disinfectants.

Sterilization

The process of killing microorganisms is called sterilization. This is done by exposing the object to be sterilized to chemical or physical agents that remove the microorganisms.

In the health care facility, the method most often used is autoclaving. An autoclave is a machine that uses steam pressure to sterilize medical instruments. This equipment can be very large, as for use in a large medical center, or small enough to be utilized in a medical or dental office (**Fig. 12–9**). In private homes, dry heat is used for sterilization. When sterile sheets, towels, or dressings are needed, the clean objects are wrapped in another sheet and then placed on a baking pan or cookie sheet. All this is placed in the oven and baked at 350°F for 2 hours. Be sure to use a pot holder to remove the sterile objects from the cookie sheet and let items cool before using.

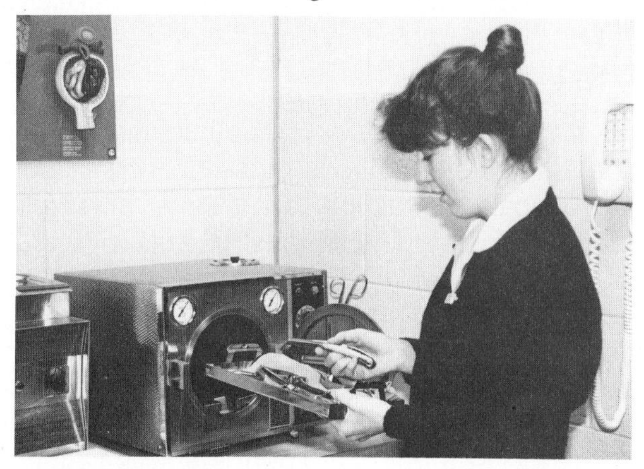

Figure 12–9. An autoclave is used to sterilize equipment. (Courtesy of Camden County Vocational Technical School, Sicklerville, N.J.)

General Considerations

Prevention of infection can be accomplished by learning and following all of the above rules and procedures. There are several other important points to remember.

Hold soiled equipment and linens away from your uniform. Do not shake linens. Shaking spreads lint, dust, and microorganisms. Always use a damp dust cloth and work from the cleanest to the dirtiest area to prevent additional soiling of the area. Wipe away from yourself when cleaning. Dispose of contaminated materials directly into the toilet, if appropriate. Do not sit on patients' beds. Do not come to work sick, and do not take personal items from one patient/client to another. Patients should have their own personal belongings as well as a drinking glass, thermometer, linens, etc. Offices should have enough instruments and equipment so that everything can be disinfected or sterilized between clients. Disposable equipment and supplies should be used once only and discarded in the appropriate manner.

FIRE PREVENTION

Always be alert to the possibility of fire. In the health care agency, one of the first topics discussed when orienting a new employee is fire prevention and procedures to follow in case of a fire. This includes following emergency procedures if you discover a fire, reporting the fire, and participating in the evacuation of the building if necessary.

The following precautions should be taken to prevent fires in the health care facility:

- Smoking is permitted in designated areas only — for employees, patients, and visitors. Because smoking is injurious to health, many health care agencies, medical, and dental offices do not permit smoking on the premises. Also, many states have legislation forbidding smoking in these public places, and failure to observe the law is punishable by fine or imprisonment.
- Electrical cords must be in good condition, not frayed. Electrical circuits and outlets should be properly grounded and not overloaded.
- Emergency exits are easily accessible. Nothing is stored in front of the doors nor are they blocked or locked.
- Fire extinguishers are in working condition. They are easily reached and properly labeled. Extinguishers are checked periodically to determine their condition. Once a fire extinguisher has been inspected it is tagged with the name of the inspector and the date. Check the fire extinguishers in your building to see if the information is available. It is essential that all staff know where the fire extinguishers are located and how to use them.
- All staff are instructed on the emergency procedures for containing a

fire, if possible. They are also instructed on how to report fires and participate in evacuation procedures. Unannounced fire drills are a regular part of the staff education program, including implementation of evacuation procedures. (Local fire and police departments participate with health care facilities in these fire drills.)

Fire Safety at Home

The following safety tips can help to prevent fires at home. But, you should always be prepared to act in case of a fire by knowing the telephone number of your local fire department. Keep the telephone number on or near the telephone for easy reference.

Install smoke alarms and test them periodically to assure proper working order. Keep extra batteries on hand for quick replacement when necessary. Do not smoke in bed. If a fireplace is used, make sure that the chimney is cleaned periodically. A screen will prevent hot sparks from flying out of the fireplace. Keep a fire extinguisher in the kitchen and other locations where a fire may occur — basement, garage, etc. Have the fire extinguisher checked periodically to assure proper working order. Follow the manufacturer's instructions regarding the maintenance schedule. Many local fire departments provide this service. In addition, make sure that all family members know how to use the fire extinguisher.

Flammable liquids (kerosene, gasoline) should be placed in suitable containers, labeled, and stored out of children's reach. These liquids should be stored away from any sources of sparks or heat.

Know the proper use and precautions in operating kerosene heaters, stoves, and other space heaters. Many communities have laws forbidding the use of kerosene heaters because of the great hazard involved. Check with your fire company to learn about your community's regulations.

Make sure that electrical appliances are in good working condition. Do not overload electrical circuits. Burned out fuses need proper replacements; there is no suitable substitute. Have major appliances and heating/air conditioning systems checked periodically to assure proper working order. Properly discard newspapers, rubbish, oily rags, etc.

Establish a fire evacuation procedure for the family and practice periodically. Local fire departments provide instruction on safe practices for evacuation.

Preventing Home Accidents

Accidents usually occur when we are distracted or not concentrating on the task at hand. How many times have we tripped over an object in our way when hurrying to answer the phone! The National Safety Council reports that most accidents occur in the home — where we *can* control the environment.

Listed below are some basic guidelines to follow in preventing accidents from occurring in the home.

- Clean up spills of liquid immediately.
- Keep toys, books, newspapers, etc., off the floor.
- Place electrical cords, telephone cords, etc., where they will not be obstacles.
- Install hand railings and safety treads on all steps and stairs. Install safety gates to prevent small children from falling down stairs.
- Discard frayed rugs. Discard "throw" rugs.
- Floors and stairs should not be highly waxed or polished.
- Do not operate electrical appliances near water.
- Store medicines out of children's reach.
- Store garden fertilizers, pesticides, etc., in marked containers in an area out of children's reach.
- Keep sharp objects (scissors, knives, etc.) out of reach of children.
- Instruct all family members about safety in the home.

Accident Reporting

When an accident or injury occurs in your home, use the first aid techniques you have learned to assist the injured and then call for help. The telephone number of the nearest police/first aid/rescue squad should be memorized or placed directly on the telephone for easy access. Also, you should know the telephone number of the nearest poison control center. Today, many large cities use the number 911 to request help in an emergency. Try to be calm as you provide the following information to the person taking your call:

- Where you are calling from: address and location (apartment number, if appropriate),
- Phone number, and
- Nature of the injury and number of people injured.

Answer questions and be as specific as you can. Wait for directions from the person taking the call. If there is no phone, stay with the victim and send someone for help. If you are alone, give first aid within your abilities, and then call for help. Go to the door and scream for help — if no one responds, yell, "Fire!" This always gets some kind of a response.

First Aid

As you progress in your health career, you will learn techniques of giving emergency care — first aid (**Fig. 12–10** and **Fig. 12–11**). If you do not know what to do, it is best to do nothing. You need to know your own abilities and your own limitations.

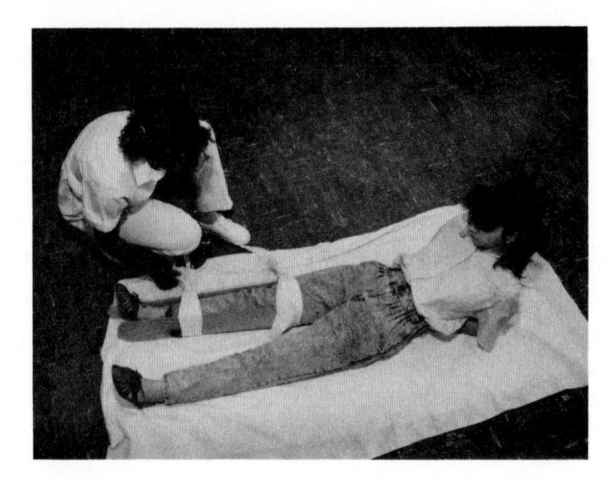

Figure 12–10. HOSA members participate in a First Aid/CPR regional competition. (Courtesy of Bridgeton High School HOSA Chapter, Bridgeton, N.J.)

Certainly, one technique that every one should know is the Heimlich Maneuver. This is used when a person is choking from an object that has become lodged in the airway. When this happens, it is impossible for the victim to speak or breathe. The victim will die of strangulation in four minutes if action is not taken.

Your instructor will teach you how to do the Heimlich Maneuver, in which you exert pressure that pushes the diaphragm upward and compresses the air in the lungs, causing the obstruction to be expelled from the airway. Signs that indicate choking are:

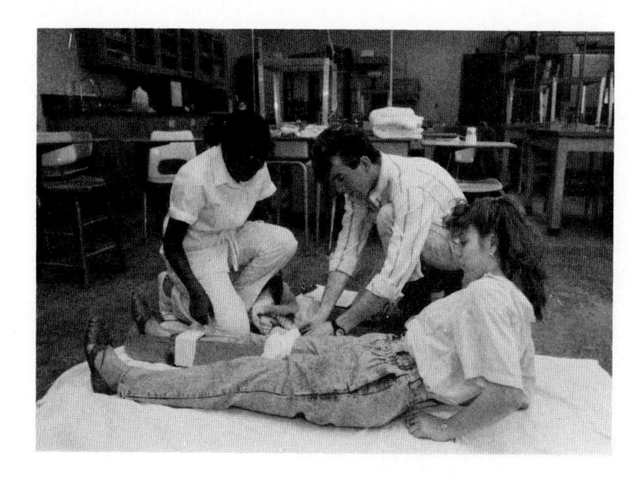

Figure 12–11. First aid instructor, acting as judge, evaluates the performance of a local HOSA chapter's first aid team member. (Courtesy of Bridgeton High School HOSA Chapter, Bridgeton, N.J.)

1. The victim cannot speak or breathe.
2. The victim turns blue and holds hand to neck as a signal of "I am choking." The blue color may be observed in the fingernails and lips.
3. The victim collapses.

It is important that the Heimlich Maneuver be used properly and immediately to save the victim's life. Be sure you know how to perform this emergency procedure.

Choking can be avoided by following some common sense rules. Don't eat and run, laugh, or talk at the same time. Eat small bites, chew thoroughly, and swallow solids before drinking liquids. Keep small objects away from small children who may inhale them. Check toys, especially stuffed animals, for buttons or other parts that might fall off or be bitten off by a small child.

"Safety is no accident." This old, often heard saying is true. Be aware of your surroundings. Always wear your seat belt. (It's the law in many states!) REMEMBER: Whatever you do, do it the SAFE way.

S·T·U·D·E·N·T A·C·T·I·V·I·T·I·E·S

1. Using a check list, evaluate each room in your home for safety hazards. What actions will you take to correct the deficiencies and why?
2. Develop a fire evacuation procedure for your home. Practice test this plan to determine its effectiveness. Evaluate the results of your test. Change the evacuation procedure as necessary, based upon your "test run" and its evaluation.
3. Where is the nearest fire extinguisher? Learn how to use it.
4. Prepare a list of phone numbers for the following:
   a. Rescue squad
   b. Fire department
   c. Police department
   d. Poison control center

   Post these numbers in a conspicuous place near your home telephone.
5. Locate newspaper or magazine articles on biohazards. Bring them to class and discuss.
6. Practice handwashing as discussed in this chapter. Teach a family member this technique.
7. Learn the universal nonverbal sign which can be used to indicate choking. Teach this to every member of your family.

Chapter 13

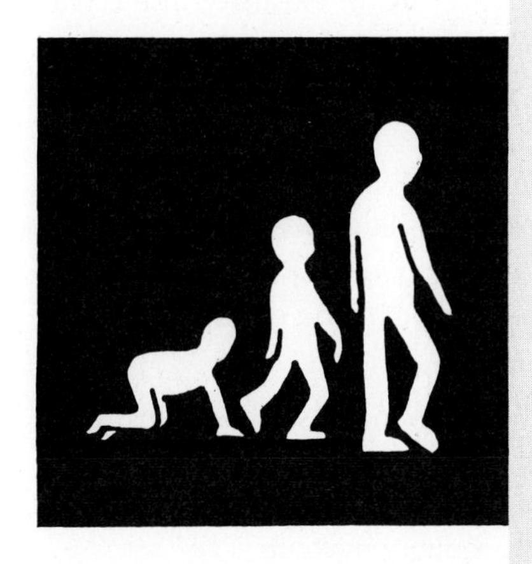

Human Growth and Development

Objectives

After completing this chapter, you should be able to:

- Discuss five of the basic concepts of growth and development.
- List all stages of growth and development.
- Discuss normal growth and development for each stage.
- Discuss three developmental tasks to be accomplished at each stage of development.
- Define at least 70 percent of the key terms for this chapter.

Key Terms

- **arteriosclerosis** Condition in which there is a thickening, hardening, and loss of elasticity in the walls of the blood vessels, especially the arteries
- **atherosclerosis** Deposits of fatty compounds on the lining of the arteries
- **development** Emotional and social changes that occur during various stages of life
- **developmental tasks** Activities which a person needs to accomplish during a specific period of development
- **egocentric** Self-centered
- **environment** The surroundings, conditions, or influences that surround a person
- **genes** Materials within the chromosome of the cell which determine our hereditary makeup
- **growth** The progressive development or increase in size of a living thing
- **peristalsis** Wave-like contractions that propel food along the digestive tract
- **physiological** Normal body functioning
- **puberty** The period of life at which one of either sex becomes capable of reproduction
- **ventricles** The lower chambers of the heart

UNDERSTANDING THE BASICS

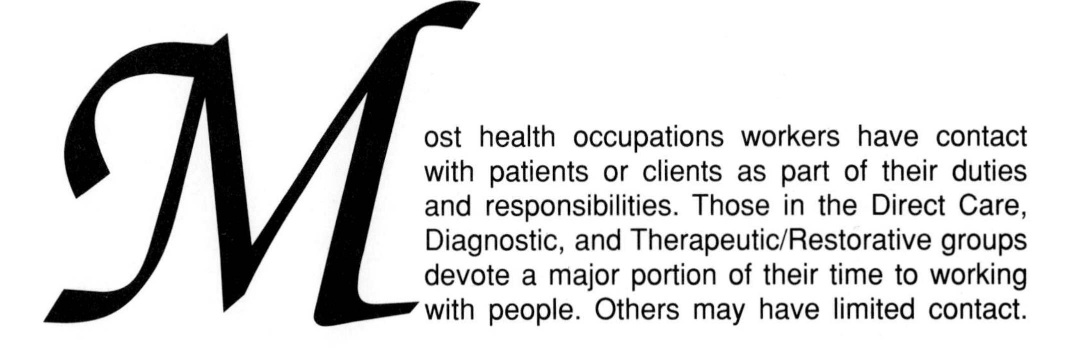

Most health occupations workers have contact with patients or clients as part of their duties and responsibilities. Those in the Direct Care, Diagnostic, and Therapeutic/Restorative groups devote a major portion of their time to working with people. Others may have limited contact.

Despite the percentage of time, health occupations workers will touch the lives of people of all ages — infants to older adults — all of them growing and developing at various stages in the life cycle. Therefore, a basic knowledge of how people grow and develop is important so that you can give intelligent care by modifying that care depending upon the person's stage in the life cycle. It's important to know what is normal for the various stages of development in order to understand how disease and illness are affecting your patient's or client's development.

This chapter, then, will discuss the factors which contribute to our development, how illness and disease affect an individual's growth and development, and implications for the health care worker. Throughout the chapter, you will find key terms which describe this field of knowledge. Therefore, it is important to understand the key terms listed above.

Each of us has perceptions of the way we grow and develop. Some commonly held notions about growth and development are listed below. Rate each statement true or false.

1. Our genes are the most important determinants of how we grow and develop as individuals.
2. What we experience early in our lives becomes unimportant as we grow and develop.
3. Physical growth occurs at our own individual rate, but we develop socially and emotionally according to an orderly plan.
4. Many of us skip a stage in our growth and development and go on to the next without any difficulty.

If you answered *FALSE* to each question, you were right. Let's look at each question and review why the statements are incorrect.

1. *Our genes are the most important determinants of how we grow and develop as individuals.*

There are many factors which play important roles in the way we grow and develop. Genes contain codes for determining our physical make-up (bone structure, facial features, color of eyes, hair, skin, hereditary diseases). However, they are not the ONLY factors.

Another important one in the process of growing and developing socially and emotionally is the role of the primary caregiver early in our lives. In the traditional family structure, the mother assumes this role as the principle person who gives both the physical care and loving emotional support to the infant and child. The mother, in many families today, continues to provide for the basic needs of the child. However, families are changing — sometimes the biological mother gives up the infant for adoption or she must get a job shortly after the child's birth. The infant may be cared for by the grandmother, aunt, other relative, or guardian. Sometimes, the family will hire a person to act as a substitute mother or "nanny." In other situations, the "family" becomes the staff of the institution caring for an abandoned child.

In our society today, the role of principle caregiver is provided by a variety of types of people. Nevertheless, the principle caregiver, the person who provides for the physical and emotional needs of the infant and child, is an extremely important person in our growth and development. As we grow older, peers, teachers, relatives, and other friends contribute to our development. But it is the primary caregiver, early in our lives, who plays the critical role.

The quality of nutrition given as we develop certainly influences our physical growth. And because physical growth is intertwined with social and emotional development, good nutrition becomes extremely important.

The overall environment is critical. Does the environment provide for the physical needs of the infant and child (**Fig. 13–1**)? Food, shelter, warmth — all living organisms need these basics. Does the environment show that there is a loving and caring relationship between members of the family? Are members accepted for who they are rather than what they can do for others? Does the environment allow for each person to make mistakes, be corrected or disciplined with love and learn from these mistakes? Does the environment permit the person to grow and develop as a unique human being who contributes those special talents to society?

2. *What we experience early in our lives becomes unimportant as we grow and develop.*

What we experience early in life lays the foundation for our growth and development during the succeeding stages of life. If the infant is poorly nourished, physical growth will be seriously affected. If emotional nourishment — love and affection in a caring environment is absent or severely lacking, emotional and social growth and development will also be seriously affected. Therefore, what happens early in our lives can have a profound influence on our future.

3. *Physical growth occurs at our own individual rate, but we develop socially and emotionally according to an orderly plan.*

There are several principles which guide our physical growth and development. They are:

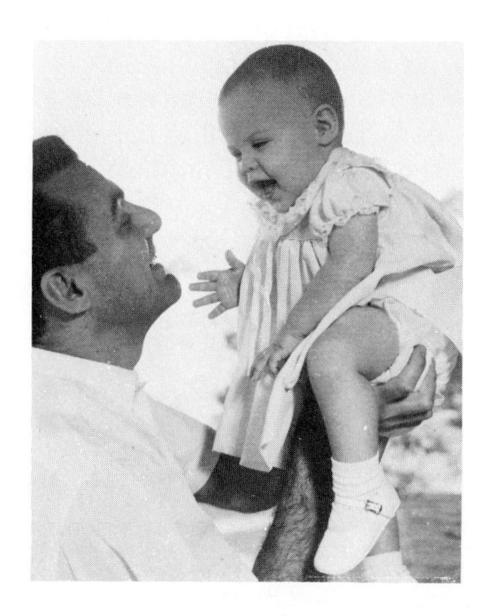

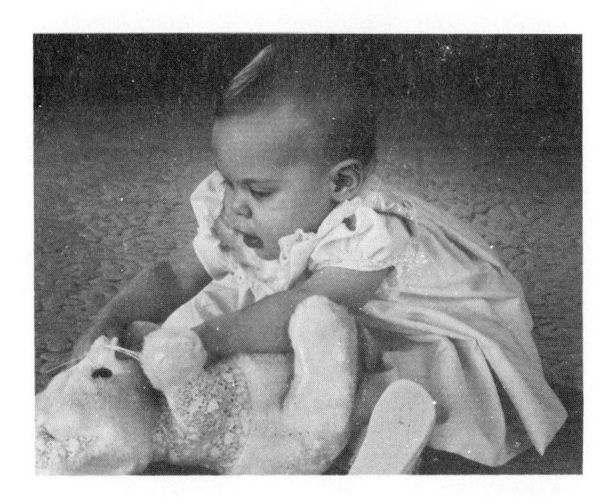

Figure 13–1. Affection and touch are extremely important to the developing newborn.

A. Infants begin to control movements in an orderly manner, starting from the head and progressing to the feet. The infant raises the head before controlling the shoulders and crawls before walking (**Fig. 13–2**). This is called the "head-to-toe principle." Growth, then, begins in the upper part of the body and progresses downward and from the middle of the body outward.

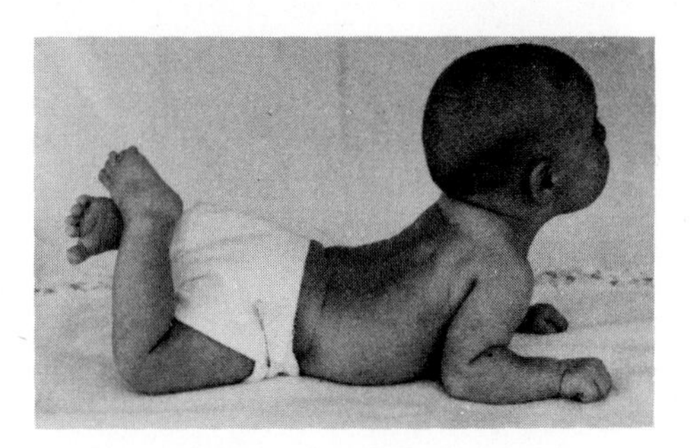

Figure 13–2. At three months, an infant can raise the head and shoulders. (From Sorrentino: Mosby's Textbook for Nursing Assistants, ed. 2, St. Louis, 1987, The C.V. Mosby Co.)

B. Growth is symmetrical, meaning that the right side of the body grows at the same time the left side grows. Growth is organized and proceeds in an orderly pattern. There is no such thing as skipping a phase and progressing to the next stage. One stage must be completed before proceeding to the next.

Developmental tasks are those activities which a person needs to accomplish during a specific period of development. For example, the child has to learn how to hold a pencil before learning how to write. Simple tasks must be mastered before the more complex.

C. The process of human development does not occur at an even, steady rate. If this were so, who knows how tall or heavy each of us would be! Rather, physical growth occurs at a rapid rate during infancy, then slows during childhood. There is another growth spurt during adolescence. Bone growth stops around age 21. The pattern of growth varies among people. Physical maturity also varies. Just as physical maturation occurs at different ages for different people, their emotional and social development varies as well. The rate and pattern of physical, emotional, and social development is dependent upon life experiences of the individual. Each of us grows and develops physically, emotionally, and socially in our own way. What makes us unique is caused by our hereditary and environmental influences. Each plays an important role in influencing our uniqueness.

Therefore, human development is very complex because it is comprised of many factors, many processes that interact with each other. While physical growth stops at a certain age, humans grow emotionally, socially, and intellectually throughout our lives.

The following charts show the progress of growth and development for the major stages of life. Each chart is preceded by a brief description of important aspects of each phase.

INFANCY — BIRTH TO ONE YEAR

This is a period of phenomenal physical growth as well as social and psychological growth and development. It is a stage where an infant learns how to survive outside the mother's protective uterus. Gradually, as the nervous system matures, the other body systems become more stabilized and coordinated. From uncoordinated movements of the arms and legs during early infancy, a baby learns to crawl and perhaps walk during this first year. An infant learns to take solid food and experiences a variety of new foods and textures. From its first cry to age one, a baby develops the ability to talk and perhaps even speaks its first word. By age one, an infant sleeps about 14 hours per day as opposed to 22 hours per day as a newborn. An infant's "world" widens as new experiences occur. If this "world" is dependable, consistent, loving, and comfortable, a sense of trust in the environment develops. Physical closeness to others without fear is a requirement necessary to provide a foundation for further personality development.

INFANCY *birth to 1 year*

Age	*Physical Growth*
3 months	Startle reflex disappears
6 months	Doubles birth weight Lower teeth begin to erupt
1 year	Triples birth weight Length increases 50% Lungs triple in weight Heart doubles in weight Brain grows almost to one-half adult size Body temperature stabilizes Head grows more slowly than rest of body

Age	*Activity Patterns*
Newborn	Sleeps 22 hours/day
1 month	Holds head up
2 months	Smiles and follows objects with eyes
4 months	Can sit for short time if supported
5 months	Grasps objects Eats solid foods
6 months	Sleeps 16 hours/day Sits alone for short time
9 months	Stands, holding on for support Crawls
11-12 months	First step
1 year	Sleeps 14 hours/day Naps once or twice daily Eats table foods

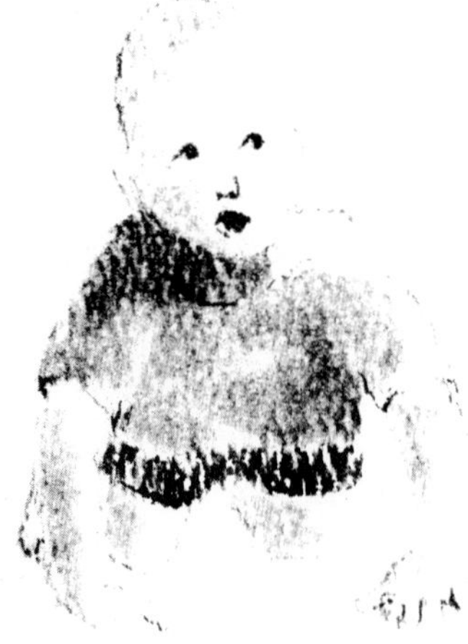

INFANCY *continued*

Age	*Psychosocial Development/ Developmental Tasks*
Newborns	Dislikes loud noises and bright lights Likes to be held, kissed, cuddled, and spoken to softly
5-6 months	Learns to take solid foods
8 months	Afraid of strangers
10 months	Learns to talk; understands words like "bye-bye" and "dada" Responds with smiling, cooing, laughing when satisfied
11 months	Learns to walk

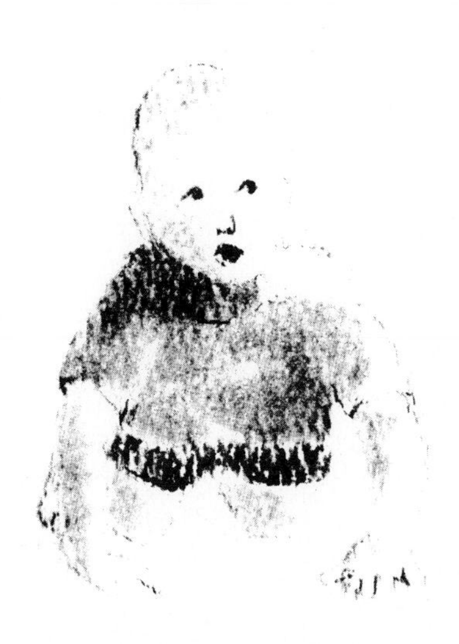

TODDLER — ONE TO THREE YEARS

The world of toddlers expands because they are physically more coordinated and more able to explore. New skills are being developed, based upon physical growth and those skills and knowledge acquired at an earlier stage of development.

They are becoming less dependent on their primary caregiver and begin to exert their independence (**Fig. 13–3**). However, when frightened or frustrated, they return for love and affection. Brief periods of separation from the primary caregiver are tolerated although this process of learning separation can be a difficult one for both caregiver and toddler.

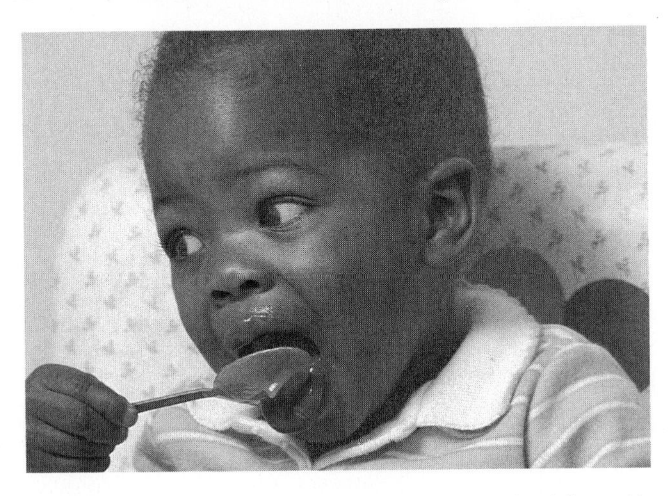

Figure 13–3. As the toddler learns to feed herself, she becomes more independent. (From Sorrentino: Mosby's Textbook for Nursing Assistants, ed. 2, St. Louis, 1987, The C.V. Mosby Co.)

This period is one of endless activity. The child is egocentric: "Mine" is a prominent word in a limited vocabulary. Temper tantrums occur as a reaction to discipline. Toddlers get into everything, and in this period of development, children are accident-prone due to their curiosity and their inability to understand danger.

TODDLER *1 to 3 years*

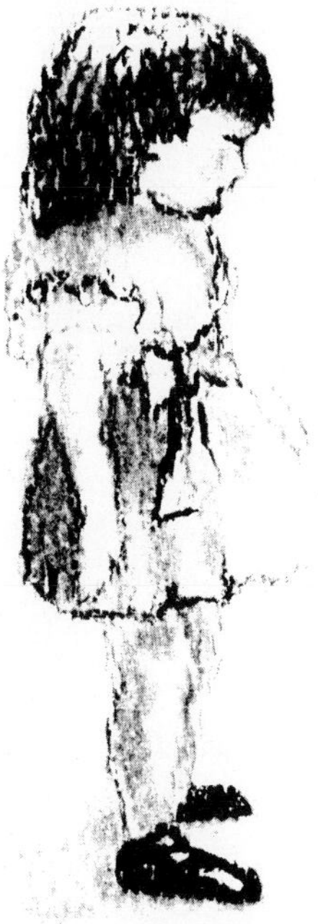

Age	Physical Growth
2 to 2½ years	Gastrointestinal system matures to allow for bowel control Chubby in appearance; pot belly Rapid muscle growth; gross and fine movements more controlled

Age	Activity Patterns
1 to 2 years	Sleeps 12 hours/day Takes naps Very active Learns to push and pull toys Can drink from a cup Uses a spoon Plays alongside other children, does not share toys; parallel play
3 years	Climbs Rides a tricycle Walks up and down stairs Can speak in short sentences

Age	Psychosocial Development/ Developmental Tasks
1½-2 years	Learns to control the elimination of body wastes
2 years	Has little fear of danger Frequent temper tantrums Begins to tolerate separation from primary caregiver
2-3 years	Vocabulary increases-"no" is an often-used word
3 years	Begins to form concepts and names them: chair, table, colder, warmer
2-6 years	Learns sex differences — begin to learn their sexual identity

PRESCHOOL — 3 TO 6 YEARS

This developmental period is characterized by an increase in the child's ability to control complex muscular movements — running, jumping, climbing, etc. The world of the home expands to include nursery school and other preschool programs. The child now is interacting with others and learning how to relate in a "give and take" way. They like to imitate and their eagerness to learn prepares them for entering the first grade (**Fig. 13–4**). Imaginary playmates are common. The development of initiative during this time also is an important preparation for school. Safety precautions and supervision are extremely important because a child still does not have a real concept of potentially dangerous situations.

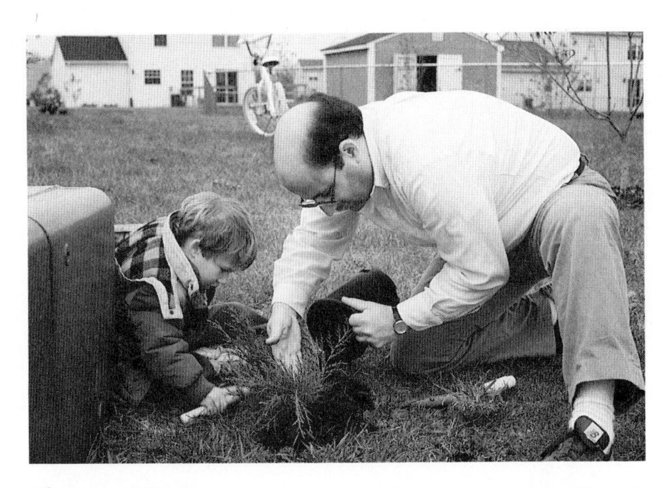

Figure 13–4. Pre-school children, such as this 5-year-old, imitate and learn from adults. (From Sorrentino: Mosby's Textbook for Nursing Assistants, ed. 2, St. Louis, 1987, The C.V. Mosby Co.)

PRESCHOOL *3 to 6 years*

Age	*Physical Growth*
3 years	Rapid muscle growth—gross and fine movements improve
5 years	Efficient kidney function Normal vision
by 6 years	20 deciduous (baby) teeth already present; begin to fall out Doubles weight of 1 year of age
6 years	Chubbiness disappears

Age	*Activity Patterns*
4 years	Skips, jumps, runs
5 years	Handles body movements with ease
3 to 6 years	Sleeps 12 hours/day Napping continues

Age	*Psychosocial Development/ Developmental Tasks*
3 years	Plays with peers Vivid imagination
3-4 years	Curious about sex differences
5 years	A sense of conscience begins to develop

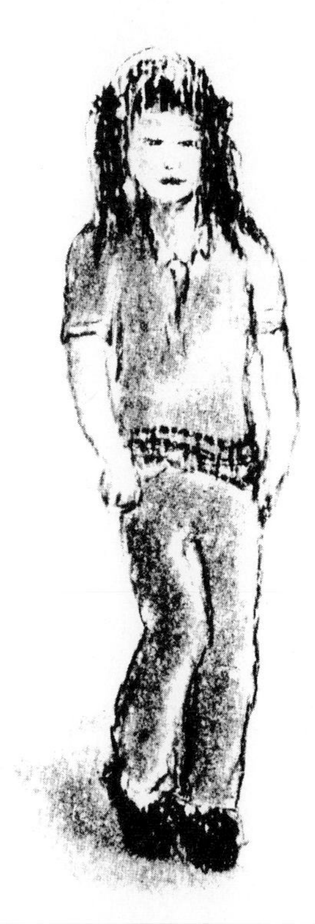

MIDDLE CHILDHOOD — 6 TO 12 YEARS

This is often called the school-age period since this is the time the child spends in elementary school. It is a period of slow but steady growth. Around the age of 12, there is a rapid growth spurt which begins the transition into the adolescent period. School-age children are active and physically strong. They enjoy being out of doors and playing with friends (**Fig. 13–5**).

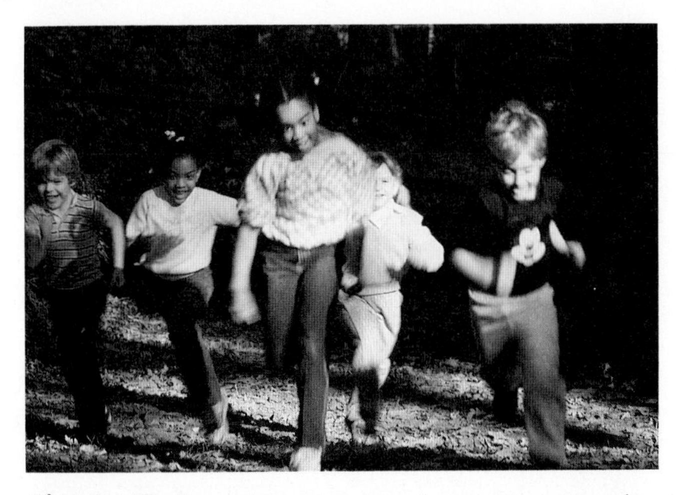

Figure 13–5. Physical activity is very important for children in the middle childhood years. (From Sorrentino: Mosby's Textbook for Nursing Assistants, ed. 2, St. Louis, 1987, The C.V. Mosby Co.)

MIDDLE CHILDHOOD *6 to 12 years*

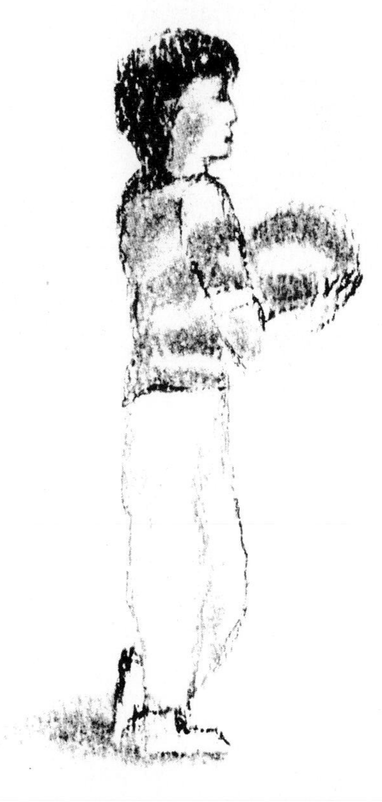

Physical Growth

Brain 95 percent of adult size
Nervous system is almost completely developed
Well-coordinated
Diet similar to adult
All body systems are approaching adult development

Activity Patterns

Sleeps 12 hours/day
Games involve great activity of large muscle groups—running, kicking, jumping, climbing
Likes outdoors
Moves out from family to seek other relationships
Enjoys playing in groups and working on group projects

Psychosocial Development/ Developmental Tasks

Learning physical skill for everyday games
Building good self-concept
Learning to get along with others the same age
Learning masculine/feminine social roles
Developing basic skills—reading, writing, mathematics
Developing concepts for daily living
Developing conscience, morality, sense of values
Becoming independent
Developing attitudes towards groups and organizations

ADOLESCENCE — 12 TO 18 YEARS

The period between childhood and adulthood is known as adolescence. It is sometimes called puberty. This is a period of rapid growth and development — a time when there are many physical, emotional, and social changes taking place (**Fig. 13–6**).

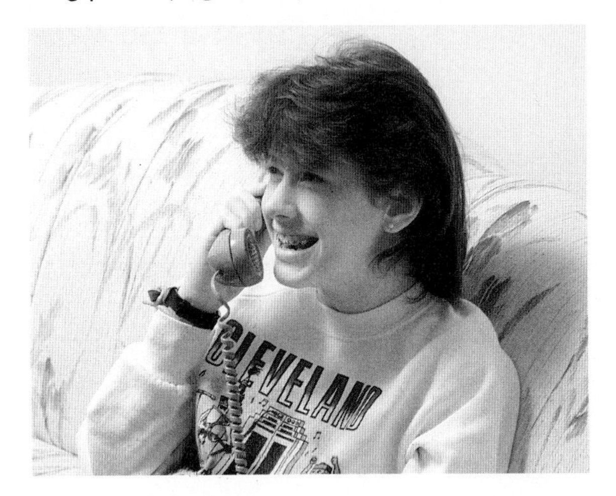

Figure 13–6. Socializing and peer acceptance become very important during puberty and adolescence. (From Sorrentino: Mosby's Textbook for Nursing Assistants, ed. 2, St. Louis, 1987, The C.V. Mosby Co.)

ADOLESCENCE *12 to 18 years*

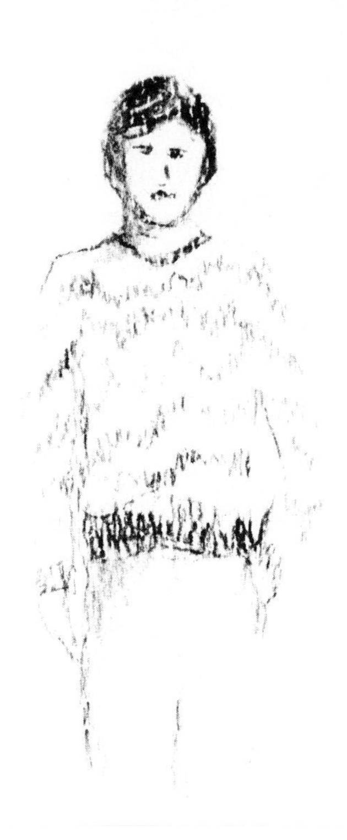

Physical Growth

Rapid physical growth
Must adjust to changing size and shape of body
Muscle growth continues—boys have twice the muscle mass of girls by age 17 (average)
Blood pressure and **blood values** same as an adult
Food requirements and calorie needs are high
Reproductive maturity occurs, able to conceive and bear children
Menstruation begins between the ages of 11 and 15
Full adult size—some males may to continue to grow even into early adulthood

Activity Pattern

Fatigue is common—sleep needs may be ignored
Overactivity
Expends a great deal of energy
Adequate nutrition and rest are essential because of rapid growth and tremendous activity level

ADOLESCENCE *continued*

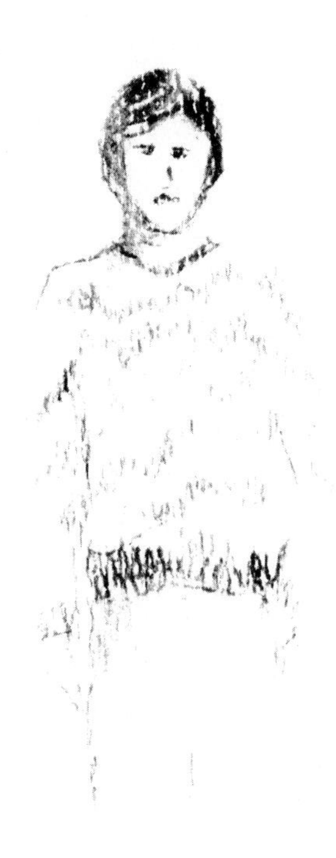

Psychosocial Development/ Developmental Tasks

Development of emotion maturity is a primary task
Able to use **deductive** and **hypothetical reasoning**
Can test ideas and change and reform concepts

Can handle **abstract** problems
Logical thought process develops
Sexual attractions develop
Sexual roles are achieved
Accepting the changing body—feeling comfortable in one's body
Achieving emotional independence from parents and other adults
Preparing for adult life—marriage, family life, a career
Developing a set of beliefs, ethics, and morality to use as a guide for behavior
Develops a sense of identity
Needs to be like others in peer group
Difficult period of many adjustments

EARLY ADULTHOOD
— 18 TO 40 YEARS

This period is often referred to as years of "leveling off," and is thought of as a no-growth and/or little development period. This is not true, since many changes take place during adulthood although these may not be as obvious as those that occur during childhood.

EARLY ADULT *18 to 40 years*

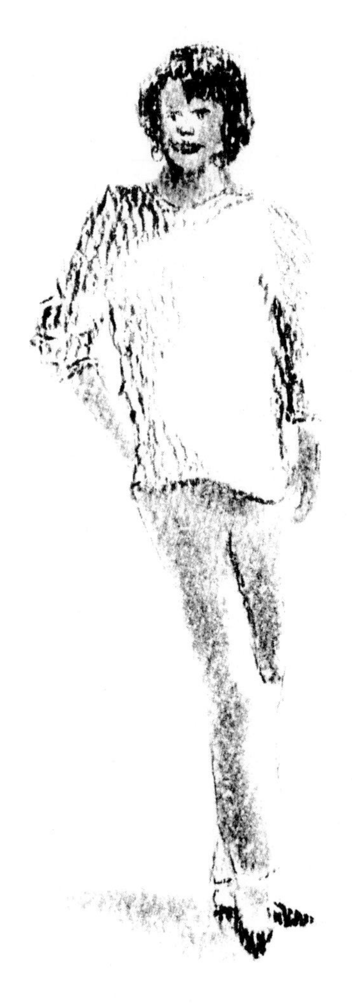

Age	*Physical Changes*
20-30 years	Maximum physiological and intellectual maturity Optimum period for childbearing
30-35 years	Gradual **regression** of approximately 1 percent of organs and body system efficiency
At any point	Hair may turn gray and baldness can occur Wisdom teeth appear
Late in this period	Skin becomes dry, wrinkling begins Intellectual skills are sharpened and peak later

Psychosocial Development/ Developmental Tasks

Selecting a mate
Learning to live with a mate
Starting a family and rearing children
Managing a home
Beginning a career
Becoming involved in the community
Finding a comfortable social group
Establishing intimacy in a lasting, loving relationship
Firming ethical and moral values

MIDDLE ADULTHOOD — 40 TO 65 YEARS

During this period, the biological changes of the aging process become more evident. It has been said that "middle age is a period when you stop growing in length and start growing in the middle." The "battle of the bulge" is only a part of the need to promote wellness that is essential to health in the later years (**Fig. 13–7**).

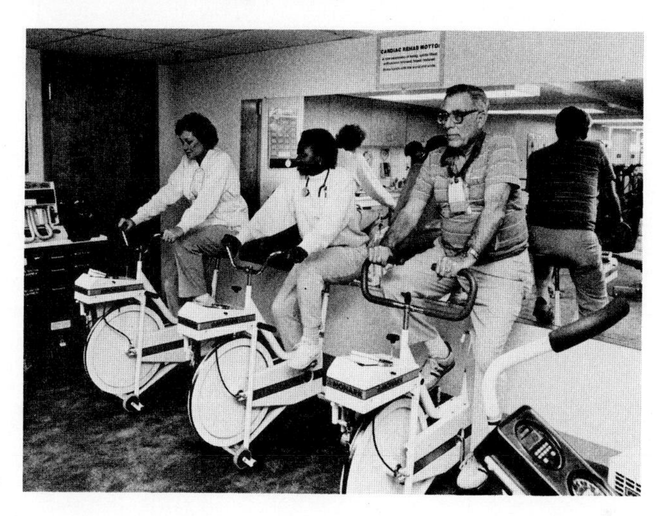

Figure 13–7. People of all ages benefit from daily exercise. (Courtesy of Bridgeton Hospital, Bridgeton, N.J. Photo by Gary Cooper.)

Today, many people have postponed childbearing until middle adulthood, or they have begun a second family (due to divorce or widowhood) during this period. All of the developmental changes expected to occur during both periods will be intertwined and experienced eventually. The later childbearing occurs, the greater the danger to the mother and the infant.

MIDDLE ADULTHOOD *40 to 65 years*

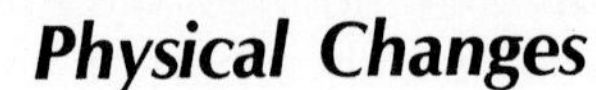

Age	Physical Changes
At any time	Slow decline of physiological processes Eye changes—farsightedness occurs Muscular strength depends upon regular use and exercise Calcium loss begins Skin dryness and wrinkles increase Hair loss and graying continue Hardening of the arteries and enlargement of the ventricles occurs in some persons Loss of teeth usually from periodontal disease Thinking and reasoning skills usually at peak
About age 40	Bone mass decrease begins
Late forties, early fifties	Female reproductive ability generally ceases

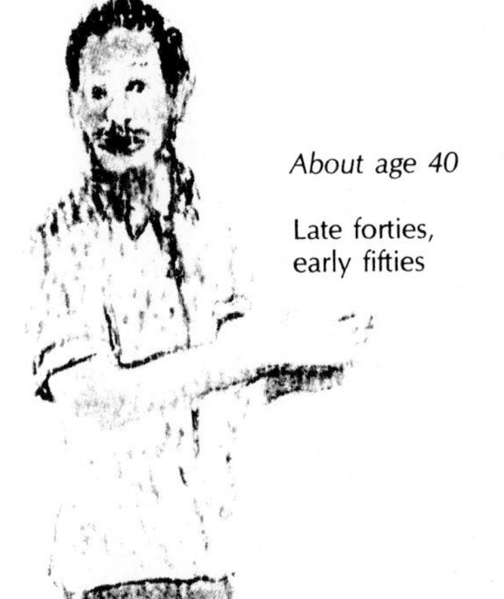

Psychosocial Development/ Developmental Tasks

Helping teenage children to become responsible and happy adults
Assuming social and civic responsibilities
Achieving and maintaining career growth and success
Developing recreational activities
Adjusting to changing relationship with spouse as children leave home
Accepting and adjusting to physical changes of middle age
Adjusting to aging parents
Finding life fulfillment and satisfaction
Guiding and nurturing the next generation
Maintaining a positive self-image

OLDER ADULTHOOD — 65 AND OLDER

The number of older adults in the United States has grown more rapidly than any other age group. In fact, this population is now referred to as the young older adult, from age 65 to age 85, and the old older adult, from age 85 to 100 years plus. The latter group is experiencing the largest increase in growth. Many changes occur during this period, and it is a time when independence is extremely important. Both the adolescent and the older adult share the need to be independent — the adolescent to establish independence and the older adult to maintain independence as long as possible (**Fig. 13–8**).

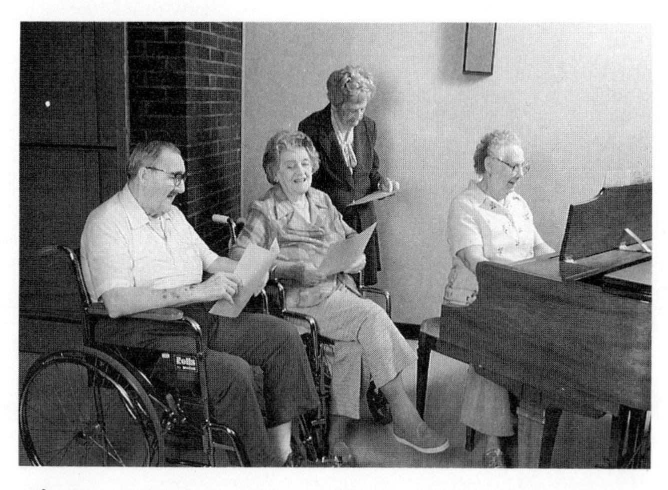

Figure 13–8. Older adults need friendship and companionship just like any age group. (From Sorrentino: Mosby's Textbook for Nursing Assistants, ed. 2, St. Louis, 1987, The C.V. Mosby Co.)

OLDER ADULTHOOD *65 and older*

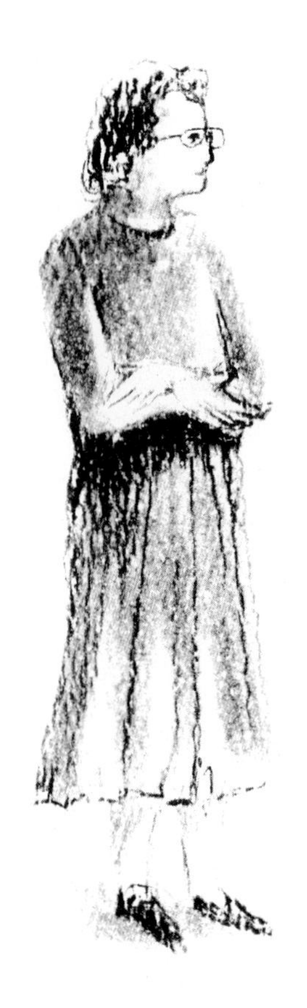

Physical Changes

General slowing and deterioration of all body processes
Difficulty in dealing effectively with stress (emotional, social, physical)
Slow in reacting to stimuli to the nervous system
Poorer balance
Poorer fine motor coordination
Brittle bones, prone to fracture
Stiff joints, loss of flexibility
Hearing loss
Some memory loss
Skin and hair changes continue
Atherosclerosis and arteriosclerosis increases
Decreased heart and lung efficiency
Decreased peristalsis causing indigestion and constipation
Women may loose control of bladder when coughing, sneezing, or laughing
Loss of teeth, poor fitting dentures
Enlargement of prostate gland occurs in 75 percent of men
Able to think and reason unless illness interferes
Learns more slowly

Psychosocial Development/ Developmental Tasks

Adjusting to decreasing physical health and strength
Adjusting to retirement and reduced income
Adjusting to the death of a mate
Developing new friends, interests, relationships
Finding satisfactory living arrangements
Preparing for one's own death
Accepting the past
Coming to terms with one's life and accomplishments
Maintaining a positive self-image, self-identity, and independence

SUMMARY

The charts above give a fraction of the information that is available about human growth and development. There are thousands of books on the subject, and many are devoted to only one developmental period. The process of aging and all that influences aging is just beginning to be studied, and much information is being gathered in this area. As women continue their careers and postpone childbearing, there will be more middle-aged parents with young children and, perhaps, a shifting of developmental tasks to other periods of development.

The material in this chapter can be used to help understand the individuals you will meet in your health career — whether it be the older adult in the physician's office or the toddler who is having a temper tantrum in the dentist's chair. If you have a beginning awareness of normal growth and development, you can be more sensitive to and aware of the typical needs of persons in various age groups.

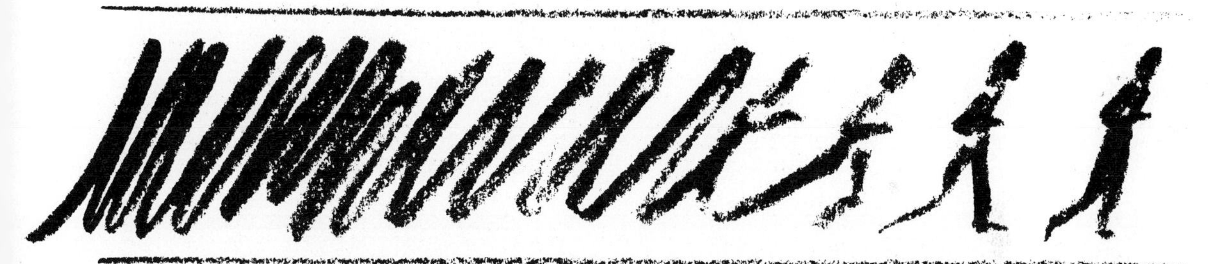

S·T·U·D·E·N·T A·C·T·I·V·I·T·I·E·S

1. Make a collage of magazine pictures showing typical activities of one of the age groups discussed in this chapter.
2. Review the psychosocial development and developmental tasks listed for a person of your age. Which do you think are the most difficult goals? Which do you think are the most important goals that will help you to move on to the next stage of development?
3. Discuss the effects of illness on growth and development?
4. It has been said that "aging begins at birth." Discuss.
5. Interview/observe persons who represent the different age categories. Compare your findings with the information in this chapter.

Chapter 14

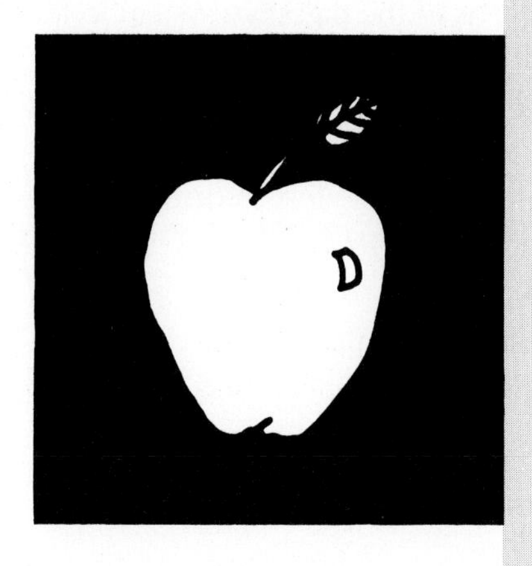

Nutrition For Health

Objectives

After completing this chapter, you should be able to:

- Explain the role each organ of the digestive system plays in the digestion of food.
- Describe the functions of proteins, fats, and carbohydrates in the diet, and name four foods in each category.
- Explain the roles of minerals and vitamins in the diet.
- Describe three key factors that influence our eating habits.
- Plan a balanced menu for one day using the Daily Food Guide.
- Discuss the role that nutrition plays in helping to maintain our health and treating illness.
- Describe four of the principles discussed in *Dietary Guidelines for Americans.*
- Define at least 70 percent of the key terms listed for this chapter.

Key Terms

- **absorption** The process whereby nutrients and water pass from the organs of the digestive system to the bloodstream
- **amino acids** Products of the metabolism of proteins
- **Basal Metabolic Rate (BMR)** Test to determine the rate at which the body uses energy
- **calorie** Unit of heat
- **carbohydrates** Organic compounds of carbon, hydrogen, and oxygen; commonly called sugars, starches, cellulose, and gum
- **cholesterol** The principal animal fat found in all animal tissue
- **digestion** The process by which foods are broken down, both mechanically and chemically in order for nutrients to be used by the body's cells
- **electrolytes** Compounds, when dissolved in water, that are capable of conducting an electrical current. Regulates the functions of the cell
- **fats** Carbon compounds consisting of fatty acids and glycerol
- **glucose** Product of the metabolism of carbohydrates
- **minerals** Nonorganic substances which must be supplied by food
- **nutrients** Substances that nourish or aid in nutrition
- **peristalsis** Wave-like action of the muscle fibers of the esophagus and intestines by which food is propelled along the digestive tract
- **proteins** Derived from the Greek word meaning "of first importance;" compounds containing amino acids
- **Recommended Dietary Allowances (RDA)** Indicates how much of each nutrient is needed each day to maintain health based upon the most recent research

- **therapeutic diet** Special diet prescribed by the physician to treat an illness
- **vitamins** Organic substances found in foods

NUTRITION AND HEALTH

Hardly a day goes by without the topic of nutrition being discussed. Talk show hosts on radio and television interview guests about the latest nutrition theory for keeping healthy, treating overweight, underweight, or other eating disorders such as **bulemia**. Newspapers and magazines contain ads for quick weight loss or gain. "Eat all you want and still lose weight — just take our product along with your regular meals." How many times have we all started a diet on Monday morning, only to abandon it by Wednesday! We are a gullible society. We are convinced that the magical pill or the liquid preparation will lead us to health and happiness with little or no effort on our part and that vitamin preparations, mineral tablets, and crash diets will cure all sorts of problems. Look at the best seller book lists, and you'll find many authors who explain their latest diets. According to the National Council Against Health Fraud, we spend about $25 billion on health fakery of which $5 billion is spent on special diets, foods, and remedies. While some of these scams are just ways of throwing away dollars, others can be very dangerous to our health because they delay us from seeking skilled, effective treatment by bona fide health professionals.

Statistics show that about 35 percent of adults and 20 percent of children in the United States are overweight. Many people have diets which are unhealthy and contain high amounts of salt, fat, and sugar. Despite the abundance of nutritious foods, our lifestyles contribute to eating on the run, snacking, "grazing," or just skipping meals. There are many people who do not realize the importance of good nutrition; unfortunately, those who do often do not put this knowledge into everyday practice.

You, as a future member of the health care team, have a unique opportunity to be a role model to others. Family, friends, neighbors, and acquaintances will look to you for guidance and advice on many matters related to health. You will be, in their eyes, the expert in matters of health and illness. It's important that you know the essentials of good nutrition and practice them as well. The following is a review of the components of the digestive system, basic essentials of nutrition, and a discussion of the role nutrition plays in treating illness and disease.

THE HUMAN MACHINE

The body is often described as an efficiently functioning machine — all parts operating effectively to perform a wide variety of duties. In order for the machine to function, there must be a source of fuel or energy to make all the parts operate. Body fuel comes from the intake of foods and fluids that enter by way of the digestive system. This system then converts the food and liquids into energy, which the cells of the body need to function properly. The remaining materials are either eliminated or stored for future use.

As you know, the digestive system is likened to a tubular canal which begins in the mouth and continues for about 18 to 20 feet (for adults) to its end at the **anus**. The lining of this canal is composed of a moist, mucous membrane. The walls are composed of two layers of smooth (involuntary) muscle. These muscles propel the food and fluids through the various parts of the digestive system. Saliva and digestive juices, which are produced by glands, act on the food to break it down so that absorption of nutrients can take place. The rhythmic action of the muscles (peristalsis) is controlled by the nervous system whose nerve fibers are within the tissue of each organ of the digestive system (**Fig. 14–1**).

The Digestive System — Key Facts

1. Mouth (oral cavity) Food is chewed (masticated) and saliva from adjacent glands mixes with food and fluids. Food is broken down into pieces for swallowing. Partial digestion of sugars begins in the mouth.

2. Pharynx This area extends from the mouth to the esophagus. It provides a passageway for food. Also, it provides a passageway for air from the nose to the lungs. No digestion takes place in this area.

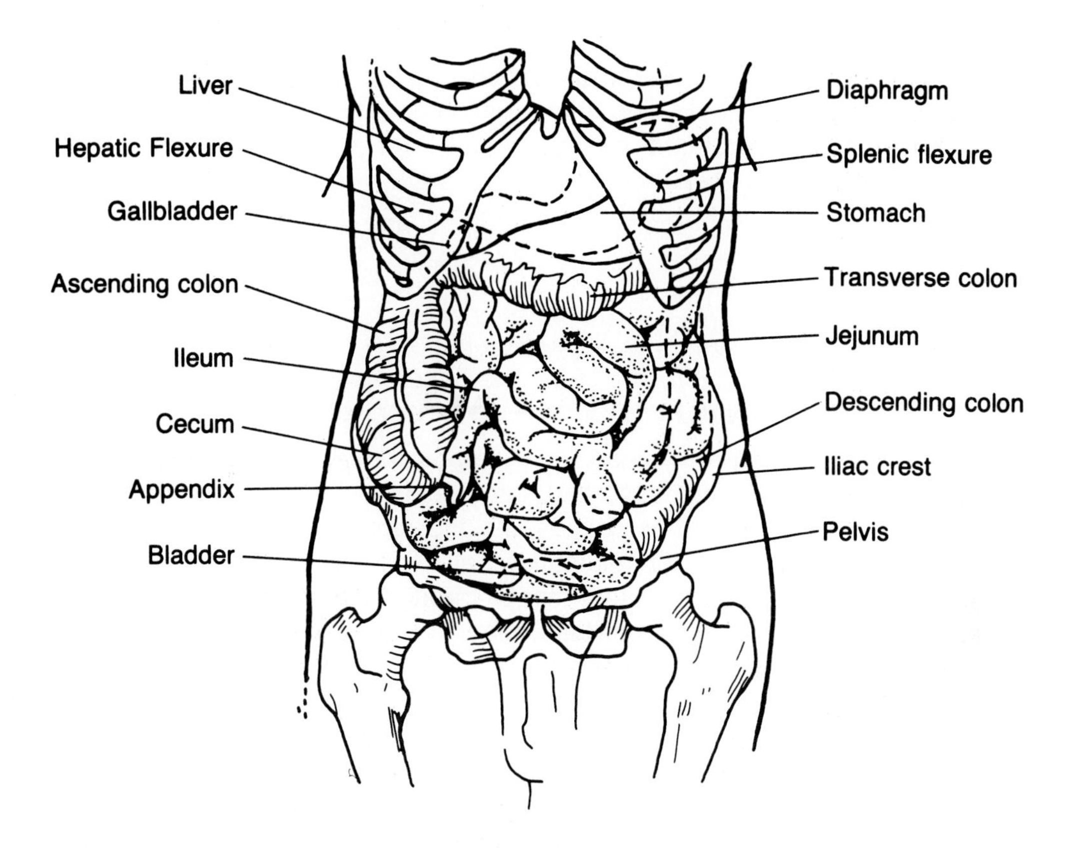

Figure 14–1. Illustration of the digestive system. (From Austrin and Austrin: Young's Learning Medical Terminology, St. Louis, 1987, The C.V. Mosby Co.)

3. Esophagus About 10 inches in length, this tube connects the pharynx to the stomach. It propels food and fluid to the stomach.

4. Stomach The muscular pouch is directly below the diaphragm and when stretched, holds about one-half gallon of food and fluid in an adult. It serves as a storage place for food. Digestive (gastric) juices, which are produced by the stomach, act on the food to break it down into a mass called *chyme.* The peristaltic action continues to propel the chyme from the stomach through the pyloric sphincter (valve-like muscle at the end of the stomach) to the beginning of the small intestine.

5. Liver This is the largest organ of the body and performs many essential functions: manufactures, stores, or changes nutrients and chemicals for the body's use; produces cholesterol; converts glycerol (fat) into glucose (sugar) for storage; when needed, converts glucose back to its original state for absorption into the bloodstream; produces **bile**, and sends it to the gallbladder for storage.

6. Small Intestine In this major organ, food is totally broken down into essential nutrients. The nutrients are absorbed through the walls of the small intestine into the bloodstream. The small intestine has three parts:

Duodenum — Bile from the gallbladder enters the duodenum and begins the breakdown of fats. Enzymes from the pancreas work on the chyme to further break down foods.

Jejunum and Ileum — As food progresses through these areas, it is totally broken down and absorbed into the bloodstream by means of hairlike projections called *villi* which line the small intestine, thereby increasing the surface of the intestinal wall. The villi have a rich blood supply. Through osmosis, nutrients pass through the lining of the villi and are absorbed into the bloodstream. The blood, in turn, transports the nutrients to the cells of the entire body.

7. Large Intestine This organ receives the remaining products not used by the body. Water and electrolytes (sodium, potassium, and other minerals) are absorbed into the bloodstream. Waste products of food breakdown are further propelled through three major parts of the large intestine (ascending, transverse, and descending colon) to the rectum and anal canal for elimination.

The Function of Food

Food, in a variety of sources, provides the nutrients necessary to allow the body systems to function efficiently and effectively 24 hours a day. It gives the body the needed energy for growth and development of cells, tissues, and organs. It also helps us to maintain our physical activity as well. When the body is injured by disease or accidents, food helps to repair the injury. Through a delicate balance of heat production and heat loss, food helps us to maintain a normal temperature.

The amount of food each of us requires depends upon our unique needs and how our bodies use food to produce heat and energy. Older adults require much less food than their teenage grandchildren. Nevertheless, all of us need a combination of foods which include vitamins, minerals, and water for a balanced diet. Energy requirements, then, will vary according to the needs of our bodies at certain stages of physical development and our activity levels.

The test to determine the rate at which the body uses energy is called the Basal Metabolic Rate (BMR). The BMR is defined as the amount of energy needed to maintain basic body processes when the person is at rest. These processes include activities of all the body systems such as breathing, digesting food, circulating blood, and eliminating solid and liquid waste. In order to maintain a proper balance, the intake of food should equal the energy used. If the food intake is *less* than the energy used, a weight *loss* occurs. If the intake of food is *greater* than the energy used, the excess food is stored in the form of fat and a weight *gain* occurs.

Measuring Food Energy

Food energy is measured by means of a unit called the *calorie*. It is a unit of heat and is defined as the amount of heat needed to raise the temperature of one kilogram (a little over four cups) of water one degree centigrade (1°C). The caloric needs of people are as varied as their needs for food. Those needs are determined by:

The size and composition of the body		
	short and thin	tall and muscular
Age of the person		
	older person	teenager
Sex		
	male	female
State of health		
	good health	fractured leg
Activity		
	sedentary	cutting down a tree

Components of Food

Food may be categorized according to its basic composition.

1. Carbohydrates are composed of the chemicals carbon, hydrogen, and oxygen.
2. Proteins are composed of compounds called amino acids which contain carbon, hydrogen, oxygen, and nitrogen. Twenty amino acids have been discovered of which 11 are manufactured by the body. The

remaining nine, called *essential amino acids*, must be provided by the food we eat.

3. Fats are composed of fatty acids which contain carbon, hydrogen, and oxygen.

The following charts provide a review of the characteristics of these nutrients.

CARBOHYDRATES

Function—Provides the body's major source of energy
Supplies fiber which contributes to good digestion and elimination
Enables the body to use proteins and fats effectively
Supplies other nutrients such as vitamins and vegetable proteins

Description—Fruits, vegetables, and grains
Sugars—
Monosaccharides (simple sugars)
.Disaccharides (double sugars)
Starches—the plant's food supply stored in roots, stems, and seeds
Fiber—part of plants which are not digestible. Acts as bulk to help the digestive system function effectively

Examples of Food

Sugars	*Starches*	*Fiber*
Table sugar	Bread	Bran
Honey	Pasta	Nuts
Fruit	Rice	Seeds
Fruit juices	Grits	Popcorn
Dried fruits	Potatoes	Raw fruits with skins

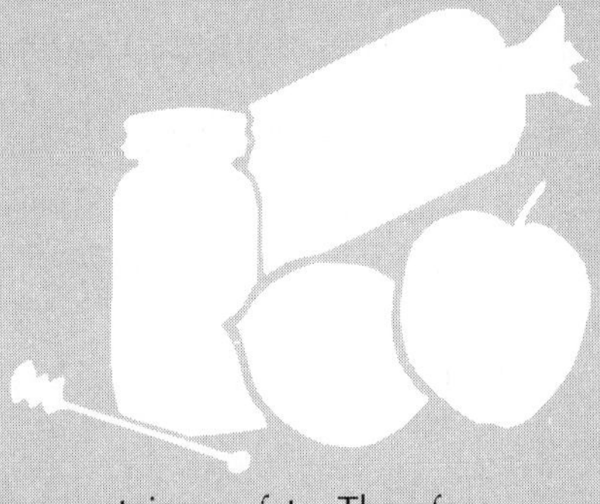

Digestion—Begins in the mouth.
Carbohydrates are broke down more rapidly than proteins or fats. Therefore, carbohydrates are a quicker source of energy.

Amount Needed—Daily intake should be about 55 percent of food consumed.

Energy Produced—Yields four calories per gram.

PROTEINS

Function—Builds and repairs body tissue
Maintains healthy muscle
Helps to produce antibodies to defend the body against disease
Promotes growth

Description—High-quality protein contains all nine essential amino acids.
Lower quality protein does not contain all nine essential amino acids.
Therefore, these foods must be eaten with high-quality proteins to increase their effectiveness.

Examples of Foods

High Quality		*Lower Quality*	
Milk	Yogurt	Cereals	Taco shells
Meat	Cheese	Bread	Spaghetti
Fish	Eggs	Vegetables	Matzos
Poultry	Legumes (dried beans and peas)		

Digestion—Begins in the stomach and is completed in the small intestine. While it is not a quick source of energy, protein intake is essential for energy production.

Amount Needed—Daily intake should be about 15 percent of food consumed.

Energy Produced—Yields four calories per gram.

FATS

Function—Provides a highly concentrated source of energy, more than twice the amount of carbohydrate or protein.

Carries fat-soluble vitamins—A, D, E, and K

Essential for healthy skin and nervous system

Holds vital organs in place and acts as a protection from injury

Provides flavor to food and sense of satisfaction of fullness

Description—Fatty acids are either produced by the body or must come from foods (essential fatty acids). Essential fatty acids are in two categories—saturated and unsaturated.

Saturated fats contain all the hydrogen possible and are solid at room temperature. Note: Cholesterol is a chemical in the blood, digestive juices, and tissue; it is found in saturated fats.

Unsaturated fats contain less hydrogen and become liquid at room temperature.

Examples of Food

Saturated Fat	*Unsaturated Fat*
Butter	Fish
Lard	Vegetable oil
Chocolate	Nuts
Lunch meat	Peanut butter

Digestion—Begins in the small intestine. Fats are broken down slowly by action of bile and other enzymes in the small intestine. A high-fat diet will cause the stomach to empty more slowly.

Amount Needed—Daily intake should be about 30 percent of food consumed.

Energy Produced—Yields 9 calories per gram.

Vitamins

Unlike carbohydrates, proteins, and fats, vitamins do not provide calories in the diet. However, they are essential nutrients which cannot be produced by the body. Therefore, they are provided by the food we eat. Because vitamins occur in very small amounts in food, most vitamins are measured in milligrams (mg-1/1000 of a gram or 0.001G) or micrograms (mcg-1/1000000 of a gram or 0.000001G). Some vitamin quantities are also expressed in international units (IU), which is a specific measurable amount of vitamin activity (Vitamins A, D, and E).

Vitamins are classified into two groups according to **solubility**:

Fat Soluble. Found in the fat portion of cells and food. They are Vitamins A, D, E, and K. These vitamins can be stored in the body. Because they are more stable, these vitamins are not easily lost in cooking or storage of food.

Water Soluble. Found in the watery parts of cells and food. They are Vitamin C and the B Complex vitamins. They are not stored in the body and must be ingested each day. Water-soluble vitamins are more easily lost in cooking water or destroyed by heat.

Table 14–1 describes the major functions and sources of 10 common vitamins. Each vitamin contributes to the effective functioning of one or more parts of the body. Therefore, a deficiency in one or more vitamins results in signs and symptoms of a specific illness.

Minerals

Minerals are chemicals found in water and soil. As plants are nourished from the soil, commercially prepared fertilizer, and water, minerals become a part of the food source. Adequate amounts of minerals are required for proper bone and teeth formation, fluid balance, nerve and muscle function, and other essential body functions (**Table 14–2**).

There are two categories of minerals:

Macrominerals. Those minerals which occur in relatively large quantities and require 100 milligrams or more per day (calcium, potassium, and sodium).

Microminerals. Those minerals which occur in small quantities and require a few milligrams or less per day (iron, iodine, zinc). They are also called trace minerals.

Water

The human body is composed of from 66 to 75 percent water. Therefore, in order to sustain life, we need to replenish our water supply daily. In fact, next to oxygen, it is the most essential substance needed for the continuation of life; we can only live 3 to 4 days without it. Water is found in all body fluids. As part of the blood, water carries nutrients to the cells and carries waste products away.

TABLE 14-1 Major Functions and Sources of Common Vitamins

Vitamin	Major Functions	Sources
Vitamin A	Growth; vision; healthy hair, skin, and mucous membranes; resistance to infection	Liver, spinach, green leafy and yellow vegetables, fruits, fish liver oils, egg yolk, butter, cream, milk
Vitamin B1 (thiamin)	Muscle tone; nerve function; digestion; appetite; normal elimination; utilization of carbohydrates	Pork, liver and other organ meats, breads and cereals, potatoes, peas, beans, and soybeans
Vitamin B2 (riboflavin)	Growth; healthy eyes; protein and carbohydrate metabolism; healthy skin and mucous membranes	Milk and milk products, organ meats, green leafy vegetables, eggs, breads and cereals
Vitamin B3 (niacin)	Protein, fat, and carbohydrate metabolism; functioning of the nervous system; appetite; functioning of the digestive system	Meat, poultry, fish, peanut butter, breads and cereals, peas and beans, eggs, liver
Vitamin B12	Formation of red blood cells; protein metabolism; functioning of the nervous system	Liver and other organ meats, meats, fish, eggs, green leafy vegetables
Folic acid	Formation of red blood cells; functioning of the intestines; protein metabolism	Liver, meats, fish, yeast, green leafy vegetables, eggs, mushrooms
Vitamin C (ascorbic acid)	Formation of substances that hold tissues together; healthy blood vessels, skin, gums, bones, and teeth; wound healing; prevention of bleeding; resistance to infection	Citrus fruits, tomatoes, potatoes, cabbage, strawberries, green vegetables, melons
Vitamin D	Absorption and metabolism of calcium and phosphorus; healthy bones	Fish liver oils, milk, butter, liver, exposure to sunlight
Vitamin E	Normal reproduction; formation of red blood cells; muscle function	Vegetable oils, milk, eggs, meats, fish, cereals, green leafy vegetables
Vitamin K	Blood clotting	Liver, green leafy vegetables, margarine, soybean and vegetable oils, eggs

TABLE 14-2 The Major Functions and Sources of Common Minerals

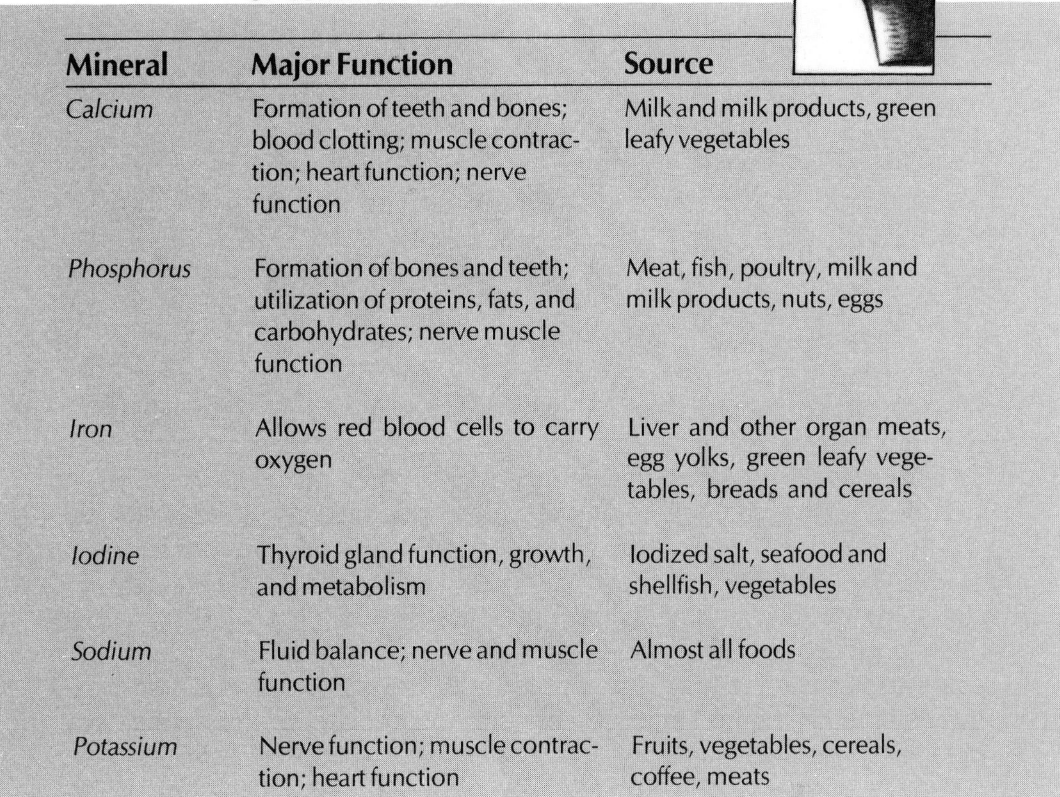

Mineral	Major Function	Source
Calcium	Formation of teeth and bones; blood clotting; muscle contraction; heart function; nerve function	Milk and milk products, green leafy vegetables
Phosphorus	Formation of bones and teeth; utilization of proteins, fats, and carbohydrates; nerve muscle function	Meat, fish, poultry, milk and milk products, nuts, eggs
Iron	Allows red blood cells to carry oxygen	Liver and other organ meats, egg yolks, green leafy vegetables, breads and cereals
Iodine	Thyroid gland function, growth, and metabolism	Iodized salt, seafood and shellfish, vegetables
Sodium	Fluid balance; nerve and muscle function	Almost all foods
Potassium	Nerve function; muscle contraction; heart function	Fruits, vegetables, cereals, coffee, meats

Water is lost from the body through the functions of breathing, perspiring, urinating, and defecating. It is replaced through drinking water itself, beverages, and soups. Most foods contain water — the percentage supplied by food depends upon the type of food itself. It's important that the daily intake of food include adequate amounts of water to assist in regulating body processes and to maintain normal body temperature. Six to eight glasses of water per day should be consumed.

Recommended Dietary Allowances

The Food and Nutrition Board of the National Academy of Sciences — National Research Council lists the amounts of nutrients people should eat every day to maintain health. It is known as RDA or Recommended Dietary Allowances. The list is updated about every five years, according to the latest scientific research. RDA recommends the amount of calories and 17 nutrients. As discussed previously, the caloric and nutrient requirements vary with age, sex, and activity. Therefore, the RDA recommendations are used mainly by dietitians and nutritionists in calculating dietary intake requirements for patients and clients.

In 1975, the federal government instituted a nutrition labeling program to help people in choosing more high-quality, nutritious food. A new set of guidelines, U.S. RDA, was developed based upon the more comprehensive RDA since labels on food containers don't provide enough space for extensive nutrition information. The U.S. RDA combines the sex and age groups of RDA into four groups — infants, children under four years of age, children over four years of age and adults, pregnant women and lactating mothers.

Nutrition Labels

Federal law requires that the manufacturer place a nutrition label on certain foods, including foods that:

are "low calorie," "reduced calorie," "dietetic," or "sugar free"

make a nutrition claim such as "one serving provides the day's supply of Vitamin A"

have nutrients added and claim to be "fortified" or "enriched"

For all other products, labeling is optional.
The label must include:

the size per serving
number of servings in the container
number of calories per serving
amount of nutrients per serving — usually given in percentages

Carbohydrates	Vitamins A and C	Niacin
Proteins	Sodium	Calcium
Fats	Thiamin	Iron
	Riboflavin	

SELECTING THE RIGHT FOODS

In order for the RDA to be put to practical use, food guides were developed to show what kinds of food and amounts are needed each day to meet the recommendations. The USDA Daily Food Guide is comprised of five food groups: milk, meat, fruit-vegetable, grain, and others which includes fats, sweets, and alcohol (**Fig. 14–2**).

Milk Group

Types of food — milk (whole, evaporated, low fat, skim, butter), cheese, ice cream, yogurt

Nutrition provided — calcium, protein, riboflavin

Recommended serving — children under 9: 2 to 3 cups/day (1 cup = 8 oz.); children 9 to 12: 3 or more cups; teenagers: 4 or more cups; adults: 2 or more cups

Meat Group

Types of food — beef, veal, pork, lamb, poultry, fish, shellfish, organ meats (liver, heart, kidney), dry beans or peas, lentils, soybeans, eggs, nuts, peanuts, peanut butter

Nutrition provided — protein, B vitamins, iron, niacin, thiamin, riboflavin

Recommended servings — 2 or more servings totaling 8 to 12 ounces per day of meat, poultry, fish, and organ meats listed above

Fruit-Vegetable Group

Types of food — all fruits and vegetables except dry beans, peas, and lentils (which are included in the Meat Group because of their protein content)

Nutrition provided — citrus fruits (oranges, grapefruit) for Vitamin C; dark green or deep yellow vegetables for Vitamin A

Recommended servings — 4 or more servings to include: 1 citrus fruit or other fruit or vegetable rich in Vitamin C; 1 dark green or deep

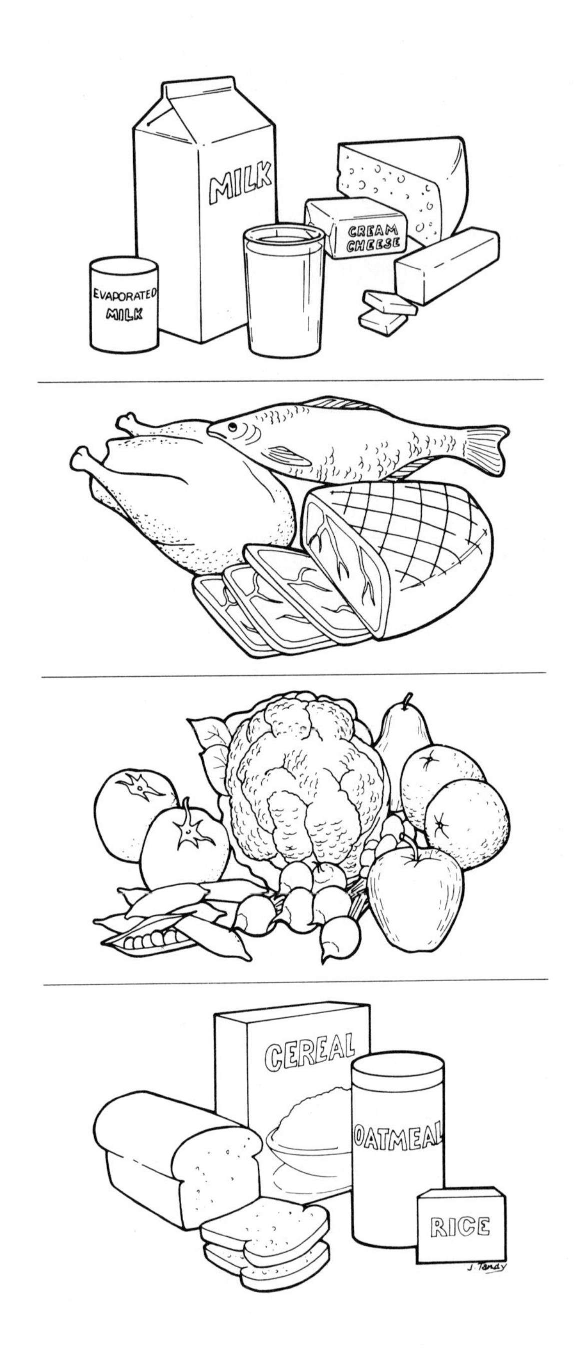

Figure 14–2. Major Food Groups. (From Sorrentino: Mosby's Textbook for Nursing Assistants, ed. 2, St. Louis, 1987, The C.V. Mosby Co.)

yellow vegetable for Vitamin A (every other day but preferably every day). Other vegetables and fruits should be eaten also, including potatoes

Grain Group

Types of food — all breads and cereals including enriched, wholegrain, or restored. Crackers, spaghetti, macaroni, grits and ready-to-eat cooked cereals are also part of this group

Nutrition provided — B Vitamins and iron

Recommended servings — 4 or more per day

Others — Fats, Sweets, and Alcohol Group

Types of food — butter, margarine, mayonnaise, vegetable oil, salad dressings, candy, jelly, jam, syrups, toppings, beer, wine, liquor

Nutrition provided — generally this group is lacking in high-quality nutritional value except for vegetable oils which provide Vitamin E and essential fatty acids

Recommended servings — None

FACTORS AFFECTING THE KINDS OF FOOD WE EAT

The Daily Food Guide provides a great variety of food options. Putting them to practical use by selecting the foods to eat depends on many factors. Food preferences begin during childhood and are developed, changed, or refined during our lifetime. Our eating habits are based upon our cultural background and personal needs.

Cultural Background

Customs and traditions are part of an individual's nationality and race. The types of food we eat and the way the food is prepared and served depend on our cultural heritage. The part of the world that our ancestors came from — its climate and what foods grew in the area — influenced the types of food most often used. Within their country, Orientals tend to use a lot of rice, fish, and vegetables in their diets. Eskimos usually rely on diets rich in fish and caribou meat. Italians seem to enjoy pasta, fruits, and vegetables. We grow up frequently eating the kinds of foods our families have eaten for generations.

Religious Dietary Laws

Some religions have rules on the kinds and amounts of food to be eaten including food for certain religious events and celebrations. Dietary laws indicate the regulations to follow such as fasting, care of cooking and eating utensils, and other rules pertaining to preparing food. The chart below outlines specific dietary requirements according to religious belief (**Table 14–3**).

Costs of Food

Determining what to eat is influenced by what is available and how much it costs. Today, through modern technology and ease of transporting foods, it is possible for the consumer to buy most any kind of food desired regardless of the season. Fresh fruits and vegetables are available at supermarkets all year round. The prices, however, vary widely in relation to the local growing season. The more plentiful the item, the lower the price. Buying in quantity lowers the cost. Large families benefit by taking advantage of this fact whereas the single adult pays the higher price for less food.

For those who do not wish to prepare meals from "scratch," convenience foods, such as commercially prepared frozen dinners, microwave casseroles, and pizzas save time in getting a meal ready to eat but add greatly to the cost. Also, many convenience foods contain excessive amounts of salt and fat which can create serious problems for some people. High-quality protein can be the most expensive item on the food market list. Because of this, families with low incomes, especially older adults, tend to buy less protein and consume more carbohydrates which are generally lower in cost. This can lead to severe nutritional problems over a long period of time. Home economists, from the County Cooperative Extension Service, are available to assist the public in learning how to plan and prepare nutritious meals at low cost. The Extension Service is a part of the United States Department of Agriculture.

TABLE 14-3 Religion and Dietary Practices

Religion	Dietary Practice
Adventist (Seventh Day Adventist)	Coffee, tea, and alcohol are not allowed; beverages with caffeine (colas) are not allowed; some groups forbid the eating of meat
Baptist	Some groups forbid coffee, tea, and alcohol
Christian Scientist	Alcohol and coffee are not allowed
Church of Jesus Christ of Latter Day Saints (Mormon)	Alcohol and hot drinks, such as coffee and tea, are not allowed; meat is not forbidden but members are encouraged to eat meat infrequently
Greek Orthodox Church	Wednesdays, Fridays, and Lent are days of fasting; meat and dairy products are usually avoided during days of fast
Islamic (Muslim or Moslem)	All pork and pork products are forbidden; alcohol is not allowed except for medical reasons
Judaism (Jewish faith)	Foods must be kosher (prepared according to Jewish law); meat of kosher animals (cows, goats, and sheep) can be eaten; chickens, ducks, and geese are kosher fowls; kosher fish have scales and fins, such as tuna, sardines, carp, and salmon; shellfish cannot be eaten; milk, milk products, and eggs from kosher animals and fowl are acceptable; milk and milk products cannot be eaten with or immediately after eating meat; milk and milk products can be eaten 6 hours after eating meat; milk and milk products can be a part of the same meal with meat—they are served separately and before the meat; kosher foods cannot be prepared in utensils used to prepare nonkosher foods; breads, cakes, cookies, noodles, and alcoholic beverages are not consumed during Passover
Roman Catholic	Fasting for 1 hour prior to receiving Holy Communion; fasting from meat on Ash Wednesday and Good Friday—some may continue to fast from meat on Fridays

Lifestyles and Eating Patterns

Lifestyles influence the eating patterns we develop. In the United States, the traditional pattern includes three meals a day — breakfast, lunch, and dinner. Extra calories are consumed by eating snacks between meals or replacing an entire meal through snacking (**Fig. 14–3**).

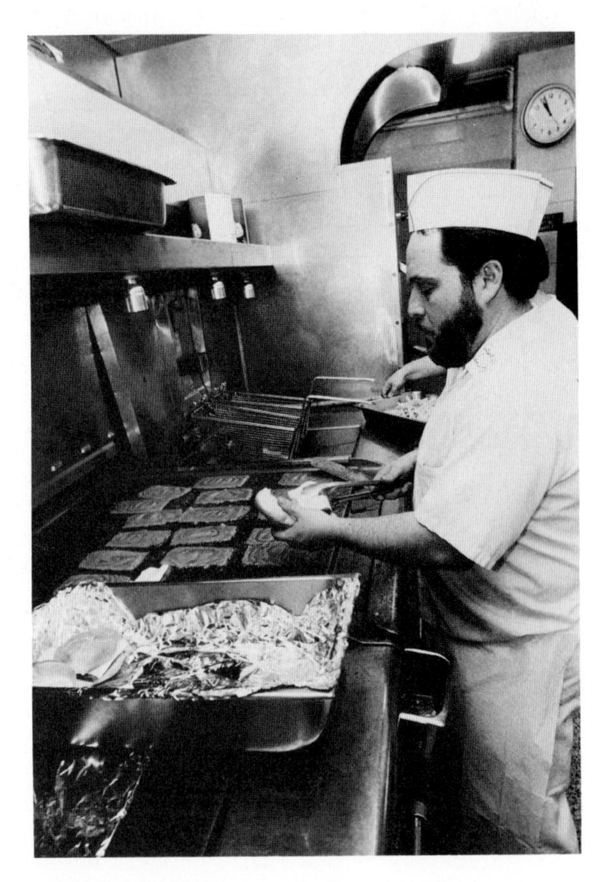

Figure 14–3. The American diet includes many types of fast foods. (Courtesy of Bridgeton Hospital, Bridgeton, N.J.)

When America was primarily an agricultural society, breakfast was an important meal to fortify farm workers for the strenuous activities ahead. Today, in our technological society, workers travel longer distances to get to work. In some instances, it is not unusual to have a person commuting two hours to get to work. Breakfast, then, may consist of a container of coffee and a donut, bought at the train station and eaten on the train.

Some students say they'd rather sleep later in the morning than to get up early enough to eat the traditional breakfast at home. Therefore, students too often arrive at school having had no food since dinner the previous evening. The glucose level in the blood, supplying needed energy to the body, is low. The protein available for building body tissue is diminished. No wonder these students are not able to concentrate and perform at their best — both mentally and physically. By mid morning, some will be so drowsy that they fall asleep in class.

Lunch and dinner may also be eaten "on the run." Many will eat at fast food restaurants or get a snack from street vendors selling hot dogs, pretzels, ice cream, etc. These foods are usually high in fat and salt but low in the required nutrients for a balanced diet. In many instances, dinner at home is eaten later in the evening. It often is the biggest meal of the day. While it is usually more balanced nutritionally than the other meals described, there is not much time for digestion to take place before going to sleep. Digestive problems may result.

Along with an overconsumption of foods with questionable nutritional value, our lifestyles tend to be more sedentary. In this era of information processing and automation, workers are sitting at desks rather than performing physically taxing activities. We drive the car to go around the block instead of walking. Recreational activities include going to the movies, watching television, watching baseball and football games. We passively participate rather than become physically involved in an activity. The overconsumption of food coupled with the sedentary lifestyle contributes of overweight — and overweight is a leading factor in the three major causes of death: heart disease, cancer, and stroke. How does your lifestyle and your family's compare with the above description? Analyze your eating patterns and activities by completing the following chart for one school week.

Time	Activity	Foods Eaten	Nutritional Value

Time	Activity	Foods Eaten	Nutritional Value

THE ROLE OF FOOD IN OUR CULTURE

While food provides the necessary protein, fats, carbohydrates, vitamins, and minerals to sustain life, it serves other important purposes. It provides the opportunity to socialize with others. The evening meal can be a time set aside for the family to discuss the events of the day, share special thoughts, and enjoy each other's company. While the evening meal nourishes the body, the emotional and social aspects are just as important.

Many of our social events revolve around food — church suppers, picnics sponsored by civic organizations, cocktail parties to honor special guests, birthday and anniversary parties, or luncheons for retirees. Also, more and more Americans are eating out, about 44 percent each day. This is not only for the convenience but for the entertainment value of meeting friends and socializing with them.

We have strong feelings when it comes to food. Food brings back memories of childhood or special events in adult life. The reminder of a holiday when a particular type of food was served can provide a feeling of joy or sadness depending on the memories it brings to mind. As we grow older, we accumulate many memories associated with events where food was the central focus.

Nutrition For Wellness

A major public health problem in the United States today is the overconsumption of food along with a sedentary lifestyle as described above. Diets high in sugars, saturated fats, sodium, cholesterol, and alcohol contribute to the development of chronic illness. In 1980, the U.S. Government issued *Dietary Guidelines for Americans* to help us maintain our health. The Guidelines are designed to provide information based upon sound and sensible nutritional principles. While the seven principles listed below pertain to most Americans, they do not apply to those who require special, therapeutic diets because of illness or disease conditions. As stated in the U.S. Department of Agriculture's booklet, *Nutrition and Your Health, Dietary Guidelines for Americans*, "No guidelines can guarantee health and well-being. Health depends on many things, including heredity, lifestyle, personality traits, mental health and attitude, and environment, in addition to diet. Food alone cannot make you healthy. But good eating habits based on moderation and variety can help keep you healthy and even improve your health."

The seven suggestions are as follows:

1. Eat a variety of foods. Select foods each day from each of the five food groups previously discussed. Vary the kinds of food selected in each group. Adjust the number and size of the portions according to your desirable weight.

2. Maintain desirable weight. Balance foods eaten with physical exercise. To lose weight, eat foods that are low in calories and high in nutrients. Eat more fruits and vegetables and less fatty foods, sugar, and sweets. Increase your physical activity.

3. Avoid too much fat, saturated fat, and cholesterol. Use skim milk, low-fat milk, and milk products. Choose lean meat, fish, and poultry. Broil, bake, or boil rather than fry.

4. Eat foods with adequate starch and fiber. Choose whole-grain breads and cereals, fruits, and vegetables. Substitute starchy foods for those with large amounts of fats and sugars.

5. Avoid too much sugar. Limit the intake of cookies, candies, cakes, and soft drinks. Instead, select fresh fruits or canned fruits without syrup. Brush your teeth after eating sweet foods.

6. Avoid too much sodium. Reduce the amount of obviously salty foods such as pretzels, potato chips, pickled foods, and salted nuts. Flavor foods using herbs and spices rather than table salt.

7. If you drink alcoholic beverages, do so in moderation. The effects of alcohol consumption can produce serious consequences to youth and adults. Heavy drinkers can develop nutritional deficiencies, liver diseases, and certain types of cancer. Alcohol consumption by pregnant women may cause birth defects and low birth weight.

Nutrition and Illness

Just as proper nutrition is required to maintain health, nutrition plays an important part in the treatment of illness. Nutritional requirements during illness depend upon the body's need to fight infection, repair tissue, replace lost body fluids or blood cells. Usually, the patient's appetite is decreased. Some medications cause irritation of parts of the digestive system. Nausea, vomiting, sore mouth, or general weakness also affect the patient's ability to eat.

If the patient is admitted to a health care facility, the anxiety of being in unfamiliar surroundings, fear of the unknown, strangeness of sights, sounds, and smells are factors which contribute to a lack of appetite. Loneliness can be a real deterrent. Just eating alone in a unfamiliar area is enough to cause a poor appetite. Also, meals may be served on a different schedule than the person is accustomed. In some cases, meals may be served cold or in an unappetizing way. At a time when nutrition plays such an important part in the treatment of illness, other factors play a key role in suppressing the patient's desire for food. Personnel in the Direct Care careers have a real challenge to provide the kind of atmosphere which encourages patients to eat.

NUTRITIONAL THERAPY

Treatment of disease and illness may include changes in the patient's diet. These changes, in combination with other types of treatment — such as medication, physical therapy, bedrest, and surgery — contribute to the total plan to return the patient to health.

The kind of diet prescribed by the physician depends upon the individual needs of the patient. Perhaps there are problems with the digestion or absorption of food or there is a need to rest an organ or conserve body strength. In the case of burn victims, the amount of protein being lost from the body requires a special diet to replace these nutrients. Nutritional therapy, therefore, is a critical part of the physician's overall treatment plan (**Fig. 14–4**).

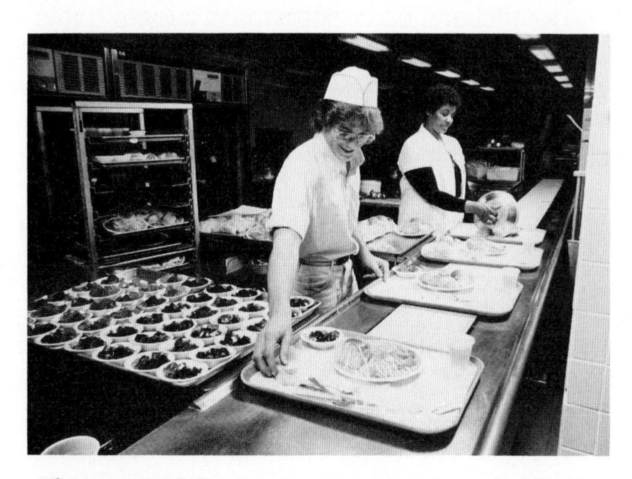

Figure 14–4. Preparing attractive trays is the responsibility of dietary personnel. (Courtesy of St. Lawrence Rehabilitation Center, Lawrenceville, N.J.)

The normal diet is the basis for the modification. In fact, the modified diet should be as similar as possible to the patient's normal diet. Changes may be made in the frequency of meals, the quantity of certain types of foods in the diet, the texture, and the digestibility of the foods consumed.

The following list describes the major types of diets used for treatment of illness.

Regular or House Diet — No restrictions
Clear Liquid Diet — Clear fruit juices, broth, tea, gelatin
Full Liquid Diet — Fruit juices, milk and milk products, strained cream soups, coffee, tea
Soft Diet — Foods that have a soft consistency: no fried or spicy foods, gravy, or pepper; raw fruits and vegetables are restricted
Bland — Similar to Soft Diet described above. No coffee or highly acidic foods permitted

Low-salt Diet (Sodium-restricted Diet) — Salted foods are not allowed: salt may not be added to foods; restrictions on the amounts of certain types of foods such as frozen vegetables, milk and milk products, bread and butter
Low-fat Diet — Restrictions on the types of meats allowed and preparation of foods (no fried foods); restrictions on butter and those foods having hidden fats (nuts, olives, whole milk)
Diabetic Diet — Restrictions on concentrated sugars (table sugar, honey); unsweetened or fresh fruits permitted; types of food used and quantities determined by the use of Exchange Lists
Coronary Diet — Calories are restricted to 1200 per day; low-sodium and low-cholesterol restrictions; fresh fruits and vegetables permitted if tolerated
Low-caloric Diet — Restrictions on fat allowed and on the way food is prepared (no fried foods); skim milk only; restrictions on the amounts of food; raw fruits, and vegetables encouraged.

In order for the therapeutic diet to contribute to the treatment of the patient's disorder or illness, it is important that the food be eaten. Therefore, the health care worker must observe and record the patient's intake of food and fluids. When recording information on the patient's chart, indicate the percentage of food and fluids consumed. For example, "Drank 1/2 glass of milk and ate 3/4 patty of ground beef." Also, record those foods and fluids not consumed. Question the patient before removing the tray concerning the reason why foods were not eaten. This information is essential for the dietitian to know. If the patient dislikes carrots, another vegetable can be substituted.

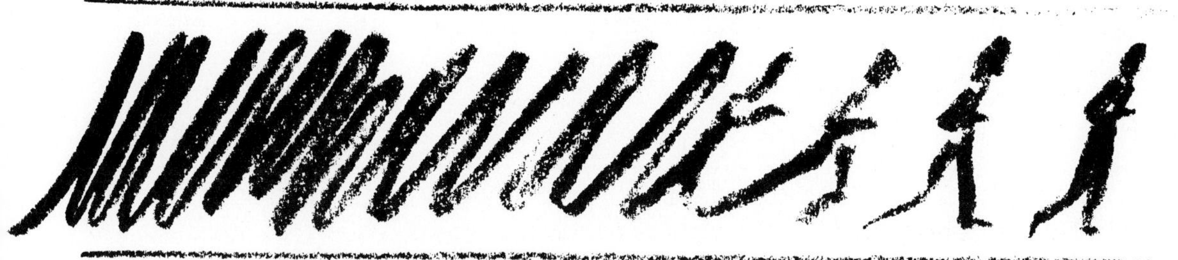

S·T·U·D·E·N·T A·C·T·I·V·I·T·I·E·S

1. Make a chart showing the RDAs listed on three cereal boxes. Which appear to be most nutritious? Why? Compare the cost per serving.
2. Find out the amount of carbohydrates, fats, proteins, and total caloric value of two of your favorite fast foods.
3. Keep a daily record of your food intake for one week. Compare your intake with the RDA for your age group.
4. Evaluate your food intake according to the *Dietary Guidelines for Americans*. What changes, if any, do you need to make in your daily food intake and physical activity?
5. Go to the market and read labels on the following products to determine their fat and sodium content:

   a. Frozen TV dinner
   b. Canned soup
   c. Hot dogs
   d. Potato chips
   e. Unpopped (raw) popcorn.

   Report your findings to the class.

Chapter 15

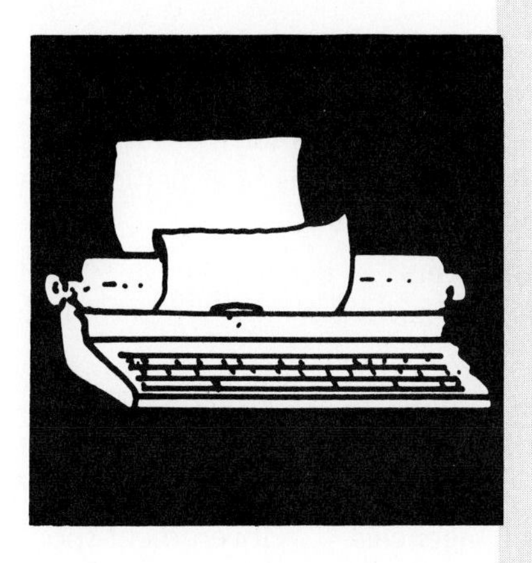

Employment Skills

Objectives

After completing this chapter, you should be able to:

- Discuss four resources available to obtain information about job vacancies in your area.
- Write an appropriate letter of application for a job.
- Prepare your own resume in an acceptable format.
- Discuss six basic principles to follow in preparing for an interview.
- Identify five major "do's" and five major "don'ts" to follow during the interview.
- Identify eight important factors to consider in deciding which job offer to accept.
- Complete a job application form correctly.
- Define at least 70 percent of the key terms listed for this chapter.

Key Terms

- **fringe benefits** In addition to salary, employers pay for a variety of benefits to an employee such as health and dental insurance, sick days, vacation days, etc.
- **networking** The process whereby interaction occurs with others on an informal basis for the purpose of exchanging information which benefits both parties such as career advancement opportunities
- **job placement counselors** Persons in a school who help students to find part-time employment while still in school
- **private employment agencies** Profit-making organizations which charge fees to perform the services listed above
- **public employment agencies** Government-sponsored agencies which match the job seeker with the potential employer
- **references** Persons who can give information to the employer about the applicant's suitability for the job
- **resume** A written summary of information about the employment history of a person including formal education, skills, knowledge, and work experience acquired
- **salary differentials** Additional pay given for working evenings, nights, holidays, etc.
- **salary increments** Pay scale which gives salary increases according to a set schedule
- **want ads/classified job listings** Brief description of a specific job opening which the employer prepares and pays the newspaper to advertise in a specific section of the newspaper called Want Ads or Classifieds

FINDING THE RIGHT JOB

Just as selecting the health career right for you takes time and energy, finding the right job which meets your career objectives and needs takes preparation time and serious thought. It takes time to find out where the potential jobs are located. It also involves the use of certain skills in order for your job search to pay off. Completing the application and preparing for the interview, presenting yourself in the best manner, asking the right questions, and making the final decision are skills needed for you to succeed in finding the right employment. This chapter is designed to give you certain guidelines to follow. Remember that looking for the right job is a process which should be approached systematically and logically. Job-seeking and job-getting skills are extremely important to develop.

Sources of Assistance

The chapters at the beginning of the book not only discussed specific careers but also where health team members work. Through your Health Occupations Education program, you have obtained much information about the variety of job settings available to health workers. Through field trips and perhaps actual experience in a health care agency(ies), you now have a better understanding of where the job opportunities are located and schools for further education. Besides actual experience in a particular agency, there are other sources of information which you can obtain to help you in your job search. There are five major sources of information:

The Newspaper. This source provides a general overview of the local labor market picture. Each paper has a section called Employment Opportunities, Want Ads, or Classified Job Listings, etc. This section is usually divided alphabetically by occupation. Some will list cluster-related occupations (Nursing Personnel, Computer Personnel, Laboratory Personnel) for easy reference. Because there are currently severe shortages in specific health career areas, some newspapers will run expanded sections of ads on a specific day each week for that career field. Contact your local newspaper for details (**Fig. 15–1**).

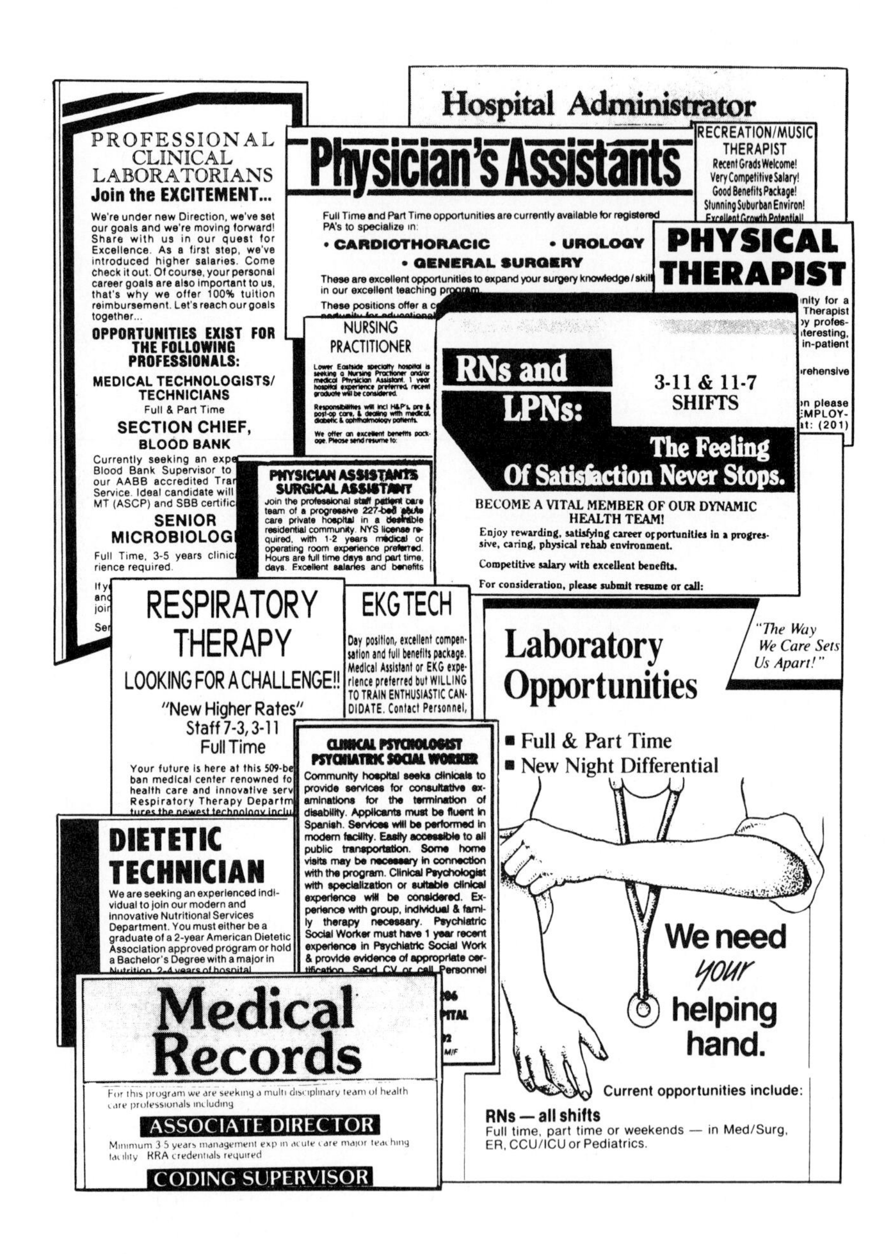

Figure 15–1. Collage of want ads from various newspapers.

There is an art to reading want ads. Acquiring a basic understanding of abbreviations used and reading "between the lines" will help you to use your valuable time in applying for a job for which you qualify (**Fig. 15–2**).

WANT AD
ABBREVIATIONS AND MEANINGS

ABBREVIATION	MEANING
20*K*	K = $1,000 $20,000
CCU	Coronary Care Unit
Certif.	Certification or Certificate
Comp. Bnfts.	Comprehensive Benefits
Depts.	Departments
Diff.	Differential
Eves.	Evenings
Excel. Sal.	Excellent Salary
Exp. Pref'd	Experience Preferred
F/T	Full-time
Gd. Bnfts. Pkg.	Good Benefits Package
ICU	Intensive Care Unit
Lg. med. ofc.	Large medical office
Lic.	License
M-F	Monday through Friday
No Exp. Nec.	No Experience Necessary
P/T	Part-time
Req'd	Required
Wknd.	Week-end
SNF	Skilled Nursing Facility

Figure 15–2. Want ad abbreviations and meanings.

Networking. This is a term which describes contacts with others who are in positions to know where potential jobs are located. Networking takes place by letting people, who are currently working in your field of interest, know what kind of job you're looking for — your special interests.

It's an informal way of obtaining information about the possibility of openings in a particular field.

Professional associations such as the local dental assistants' association or county medical laboratory technicians' association provide the chance for members to "network" during meetings and social events sponsored by the organizations. One of the real benefits of belonging to a professional association is the opportunity to find out from your peers what's happening in your area of interest and where the job openings exist. Many times, jobs are never advertised but vacancies are filled through this informal "networking" system.

Volunteering your time as a judge for a local or state HOSA leadership competitive event following graduation provides an excellent opportunity for you to network with health professionals.

Employment Agencies. The profession of career counselor involves matching the right person to the right job. Career counselors may be employed in *public employment agencies* where clients are assisted in determining the types of skills and knowledge they have in order to qualify for specific jobs available in the area. Each state has an agency responsible for helping business and industry find qualified workers. Usually, both federal and state monies are used to finance the operation of offices throughout the state to serve local needs. The services of the public employment agency are free to anyone seeking help to find a job. Applicants are interviewed by career counselors to determine their interests. Next, the agency will test applicants to find out their aptitudes and capabilities before attempting to match them with existing job vacancies. Because the agency receives state and federal funding, there is no cost to the applicants for these services.

Similar in purpose and responsibility, the *private employment agency* charges a fee for services to the job seeker for counseling and also charges a fee to the employer who is looking for qualified employees. The amount of the fees charged depends upon the services provided and the salary received by the client who obtains a job as a result of the work of the employment agency. The client signs a contract which outlines the fees to be charged and other important information about the rights and responsibilities of both parties. IF YOU DON'T UNDERSTAND THE CONTRACT, DON'T SIGN IT. Also it's important to meet the counselor who will be working with you before you enter into the agreement. Sometimes personality conflicts between client and counselor can delay the process.

Job Placement Counselor. Many schools have counselors whose jobs involve helping students find part-time employment while still in school. Depending upon the student's needs, the employment may or may not be directly related to the occupation that they are pursuing. Nevertheless, the job placement counselor is a vital part of the total guidance and counseling staff of the school and is an excellent resource person to get to know.

Your Instructor. Perhaps the best resources that you have are those who know the strengths and abilities that you've developed in the health field — your instructors. They have excellent sources of contacts in the health care industry. They have had experience working with you in your program and can supply you with leads to your first employment or help you to find a new and more challenging future job. Don't be afraid to ask for their help. Ask them if you can use their name as a reference.

THE LETTER OF APPLICATION

"First impressions are lasting ones" — an old saying that is very true, especially when it comes to the letter you send to the employer requesting an interview for a position. It reveals a lot about the writer and can mean the difference between getting the opportunity to interview for the position or not. It's your chance to "sell" yourself even before you appear in person for the interview (**Fig. 15–3**).

Letter of Application Checklist

Appearance

- Typewritten or computer generated using a letter-quality or near-letter-quality printer, or written legibly on unlined white bond paper, using black or blue ink — no pencil.
- Neat — no strikeovers if typewritten; no crossed out words if handwritten; corrections are made without being obvious.
- Correct punctuation and grammar.
- Business letter format.

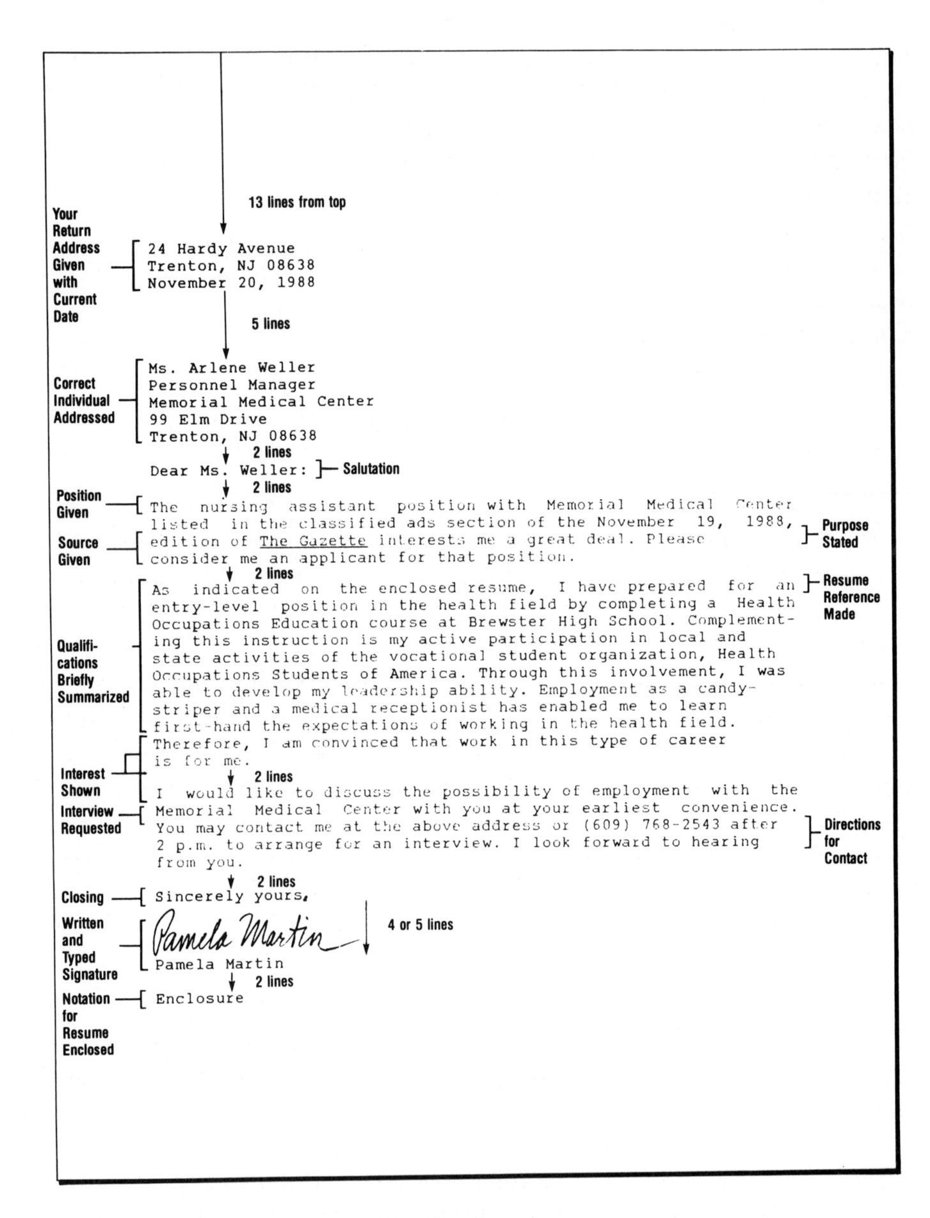

24 Hardy Avenue
Trenton, NJ 08638
November 20, 1988

Ms. Arlene Weller
Personnel Manager
Memorial Medical Center
99 Elm Drive
Trenton, NJ 08638

Dear Ms. Weller:

The nursing assistant position with Memorial Medical Center listed in the classified ads section of the November 19, 1988, edition of The Gazette interests me a great deal. Please consider me an applicant for that position.

As indicated on the enclosed resume, I have prepared for an entry-level position in the health field by completing a Health Occupations Education course at Brewster High School. Complementing this instruction is my active participation in local and state activities of the vocational student organization, Health Occupations Students of America. Through this involvement, I was able to develop my leadership ability. Employment as a candy-striper and a medical receptionist has enabled me to learn first-hand the expectations of working in the health field. Therefore, I am convinced that work in this type of career is for me.

I would like to discuss the possibility of employment with the Memorial Medical Center with you at your earliest convenience. You may contact me at the above address or (609) 768-2543 after 2 p.m. to arrange for an interview. I look forward to hearing from you.

Sincerely yours,

Pamela Martin

Pamela Martin

Enclosure

Figure 15–3. Sample letter of applications.

Content

- Address the letter to the correct individual. Telephone the agency to get the correct spelling of the name and title if unsure.
- State the exact position you are interested in obtaining.
- Give the reason you are interested in working for the employer.
- Briefly discuss your education and any related experiences you've had, particularly involvement with HOSA (if applicable).
- Request an interview and give information on where you can be reached.
- Enclose a copy of your resume.

PREPARING YOUR RESUME

The word resume is a French word meaning a summary of information about an individual. Resumes may be written using several different formats. Regardless of format, the resume should give sufficient information abut your education, work experience, and other pertinent information so that the employer gets an overall picture of your employment potential.

The same principles apply to writing the resume that were discussed under the letter of application. Neatness and accuracy in format and information are essential. While the letter is written in narrative form, the resume is similar to an outline. Both letter and resume should be compatible as to basic information — one should not contradict the other. If you are sending out resumes to several employers, photocopies are acceptable provided they are clear and neat in appearance.

There are many types of format for preparing a resume. Basically, there are seven essential parts as follows:

1. Personal Identification — name, address (including zip code), telephone number (including area code), and social security number.
2. Career Goal (job desired) — the title of and/or statement about the position that you are seeking.
3. Educational Background — name and address of your school, name of the health occupations education program and years enrolled — include any recognition received (honor roll, etc.), other courses or special training such as Red Cross First Aid, CPR training, etc.
4. Employment Background — most recent employment listed first — dates employed, employer's name and address, job title, and duties

performed. List any cooperative education experiences and volunteer work related to the health occupations field.

5. Other Activities — organization memberships. A. Cocurricular: Health Occupations Students of America (no abbreviations, please), years of membership, offices held, recognition received such as First Place in Dental Assisting Skills — State Leadership Conference, 1989. B. School and Community: Other volunteer activities in school and community, hobbies, and special interest.
6. Personal Data (optional) — age, height, weight, condition of health, marital status, number of children. Note: This information is not legally required prior to employment. It needs to be given only if it would be beneficial to you in getting the job; otherwise, leave it off the resume.
7. References — list full name, title, address, and telephone number of reference. Prior approval is *required before* listing the reference's name. It is also acceptable to omit listing references and use a statement like "References furnished upon request." If this is used, a list (typed or written legibly) should be brought to the interview and given to the interviewer.

A resume may be only one page in length or may be two pages long. However, a resume should never exceed two pages, and the most important information should appear on the first page (**Fig. 15–4**).

Resume Checklist

Appearance

Typewritten — preferred
Unlined white bond paper
Free of strikeovers and no smudges
Corrections made but not obvious
Correct punctuation and grammar
Correct margins
Resume proofread by you and checked by another person

Content

Correct names, titles, and addresses
Essential parts included
Educational background includes health occupations education program enrollment

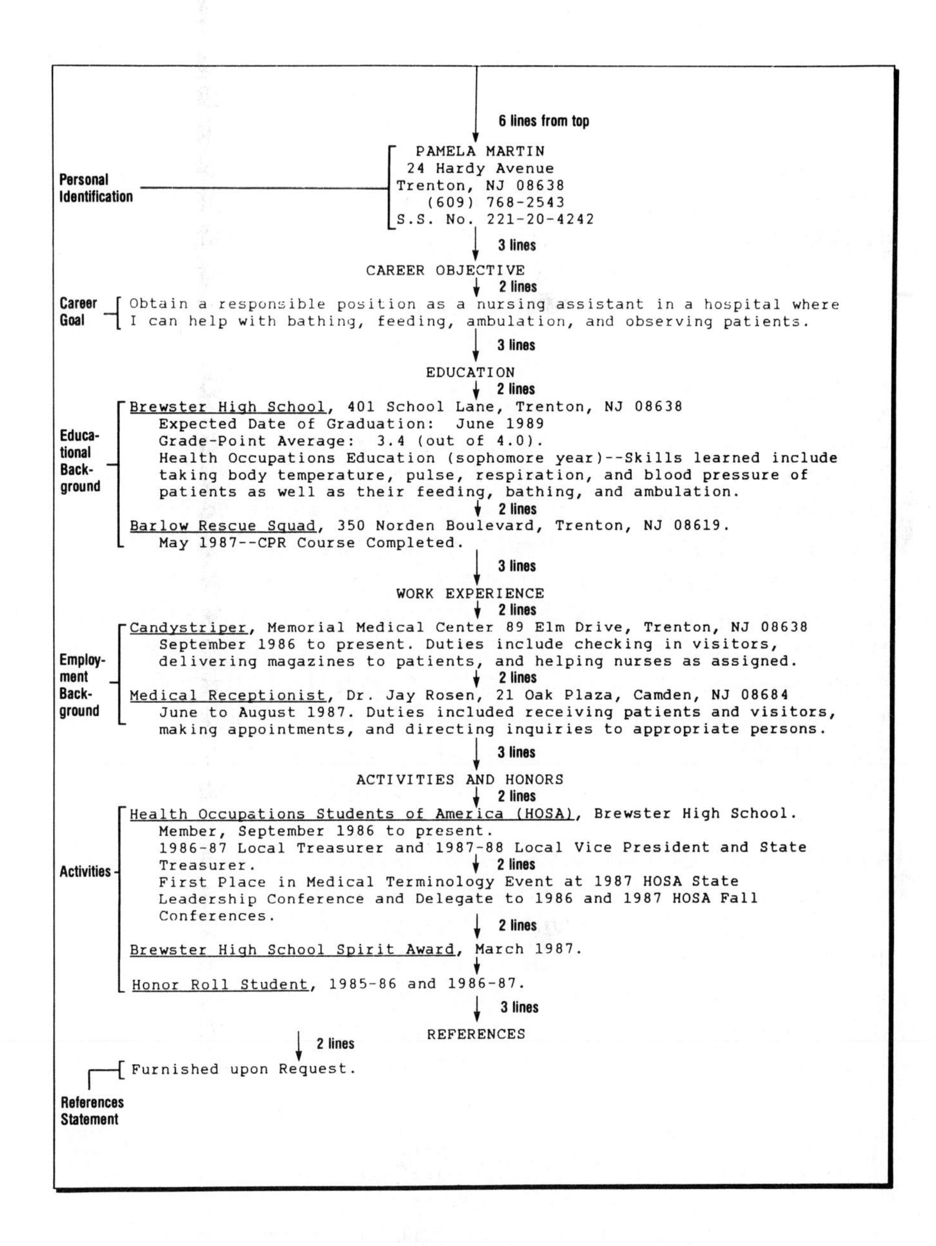

PAMELA MARTIN
24 Hardy Avenue
Trenton, NJ 08638
(609) 768-2543
S.S. No. 221-20-4242

CAREER OBJECTIVE

Obtain a responsible position as a nursing assistant in a hospital where I can help with bathing, feeding, ambulation, and observing patients.

EDUCATION

Brewster High School, 401 School Lane, Trenton, NJ 08638
Expected Date of Graduation: June 1989
Grade-Point Average: 3.4 (out of 4.0).
Health Occupations Education (sophomore year)--Skills learned include taking body temperature, pulse, respiration, and blood pressure of patients as well as their feeding, bathing, and ambulation.

Barlow Rescue Squad, 350 Norden Boulevard, Trenton, NJ 08619.
May 1987--CPR Course Completed.

WORK EXPERIENCE

Candystriper, Memorial Medical Center 89 Elm Drive, Trenton, NJ 08638
September 1986 to present. Duties include checking in visitors, delivering magazines to patients, and helping nurses as assigned.

Medical Receptionist, Dr. Jay Rosen, 21 Oak Plaza, Camden, NJ 08684
June to August 1987. Duties included receiving patients and visitors, making appointments, and directing inquiries to appropriate persons.

ACTIVITIES AND HONORS

Health Occupations Students of America (HOSA), Brewster High School.
Member, September 1986 to present.
1986-87 Local Treasurer and 1987-88 Local Vice President and State Treasurer.
First Place in Medical Terminology Event at 1987 HOSA State Leadership Conference and Delegate to 1986 and 1987 HOSA Fall Conferences.

Brewster High School Spirit Award, March 1987.

Honor Roll Student, 1985-86 and 1986-87.

REFERENCES

Furnished upon Request.

Figure 15–4. Sample resume.

Complete list of employment with accurate descriptions
Other activities, include HOSA participation
References listed were contacted and gave approval

PREPARING FOR THE INTERVIEW

After the letter of application and resume have been sent, it's time to begin preparing for the interview. Allow a few weeks for the employer to contact you regarding the response to your letter of application. If they do not respond to your initial letter of inquiry within a reasonable time, you should contact them again by telephone or letter.

Many employers will call you to set up an appointment for an interview and will confirm the date, time, and place by letter. It is essential that you make every effort to rearrange your schedule, if necessary, so that you are available for the interview at the date and time the employer has set. If it is not possible to come at the time arranged, notify the person *immediately* to explain why you cannot come and set another appointment, if possible. Remember, you are the one who needs employment. Failing to contact a potential employer indicates to them that you are unreliable; you probably won't get another chance for an interview.

This next step is just as important as the actual interview itself. In fact, preparing properly for the interview helps to increase your self-confidence which, in turn, is reflected in your ability to handle the interview with poise and self-assurance.

It is said that interviewers make their decisions about an applicant's suitability within a few minutes after their initial contact. Therefore, initial impressions are extremely important. Your general physical appearance and the way you greet the interviewer are part of these "first impressions."

Next, the actual interview provides the opportunity for the employer to get to know more about you, evaluate your potential as an employee, explain the details of the job, and give you a picture of the health care agency in relation to the position you are seeking. You also have the opportunity to explain more about why you believe you are suitable for the position and to ask specific questions about the job's responsibilities, working conditions, or other questions which will help you to make the right decision. The interview, then, is a "two-way street." It helps both parties to answer the questions: Is this the person for the job? Is this the job for me?

If you are unsure of the exact location of the office where you will be interviewed, a practice run may be helpful. It will give you a better idea of the time you need to arrive.

Preparing for the interview means gathering together the necessary information you will need to complete an application form. Usually, the application form is completed immediately prior to the interview. Bring a copy of your resume so that you can refer to it when filling out the application. Also, it's a good idea to put any additional information, which is not included in the resume, on an index card for easy reference while completing the application form. Always complete an application in ink and print legibly (**Fig. 15–5**).

Get to know some facts about your employer — what the agency is about. What are the positive comments you've heard from others which have caused you to want to be a part of the team? It's to your advantage to use this information during the interview, if the appropriate time presents itself. Preparing ahead of time gives you an added advantage.

Prepare some questions to ask during the interview that pertain to the job responsibilities. Asking questions shows the interviewer that you are interested and inquisitive. Avoid asking questions about sick time, vacations, pay raises, etc., unless the interviewer gives no information about them. Questions that dwell almost exclusively on pay, vacations, and holidays gives the impression that you're more interested in the "off-duty" hours rather than the actual "on-duty" responsibilities.

Most interviewers have a basic set of questions they ask of all applicants. The following questions are examples of those frequently asked. Although it is impossible to anticipate all the questions an interviewer will ask, preparing responses to these may be helpful.

Tell me about yourself.
Why are you interested in working here?
What experiences have you had in the health field?
What makes a good health care worker?
Which school activities have you enjoyed most?
Why did you select work in the health care field?
What personal characteristics are necessary for success?
Why do you believe you are qualified for this position?
What are your strengths — your weaknesses?
If already employed, why do you want to change jobs?
Where do you want to be in your career in five years?
Of all the applicants who have applied, why should I choose you?

APPLICATION FOR EMPLOYMENT

(PRE-EMPLOYMENT QUESTIONNAIRE) (AN EQUAL OPPORTUNITY EMPLOYER)

PERSONAL INFORMATION

DATE: ______________

NAME ______________ LAST FIRST MIDDLE SOCIAL SECURITY NUMBER ______________

PRESENT ADDRESS ______________ STREET CITY STATE

PERMANENT ADDRESS ______________ STREET CITY STATE

PHONE NO. ______________ ARE YOU 18 YEARS OR OLDER Yes ☐ No ☐

SPECIAL QUESTIONS

DO NOT ANSWER **ANY** OF THE QUESTIONS IN THIS FRAMED AREA UNLESS THE EMPLOYER HAS **CHECKED A BOX PRECEDING** A QUESTION, THEREBY INDICATING THAT THE INFORMATION IS REQUIRED FOR A BONA FIDE OCCUPATIONAL QUALIFICATION, OR DICTATED BY NATIONAL SECURITY LAWS, OR IS NEEDED FOR OTHER LEGALLY PERMISSIBLE REASONS.

☐ Height ______ feet ______ inches ☐ Citizen of U.S. ______ Yes ______ No

☐ Weight ______ lbs. ☐ Date of Birth* ______________

☐ What Foreign Languages do you speak fluently? ______________ Read ______________ Write ______________

☐ ______________

*The Age Discrimination in Employment Act of 1967 prohibits discrimination on the basis of age with respect to individuals who are at least 40 but less than 70 years of age.

EMPLOYMENT DESIRED

POSITION ______________ DATE YOU CAN START ______________ SALARY DESIRED ______________

ARE YOU EMPLOYED NOW? ______________ IF SO MAY WE INQUIRE OF YOUR PRESENT EMPLOYER? ______________

EVER APPLIED TO THIS COMPANY BEFORE? ______________ WHERE? ______________ WHEN? ______________

EDUCATION	NAME AND LOCATION OF SCHOOL	*NO OF YEARS ATTENDED	*DID YOU GRADUATE?	SUBJECTS STUDIED
GRAMMAR SCHOOL				
HIGH SCHOOL				
COLLEGE				
TRADE, BUSINESS OR CORRESPONDENCE SCHOOL				

*The Age Discrimination in Employment Act of 1967 prohibits discrimination on the basis of age with respect to individuals who are at least 40 but less than 70 years of age.

GENERAL

SUBJECTS OF SPECIAL STUDY OR RESEARCH WORK ______________

U.S. MILITARY OR NAVAL SERVICE ______________ RANK ______________ PRESENT MEMBERSHIP IN NATIONAL GUARD OR RESERVES ______________

(CONTINUED ON OTHER SIDE)

LAST FIRST MIDDLE

Figure 15–5. Sample employment application.

FORMER EMPLOYERS (LIST BELOW LAST FOUR EMPLOYERS, STARTING WITH LAST ONE FIRST).

DATE MONTH AND YEAR	NAME AND ADDRESS OF EMPLOYER	SALARY	POSITION	REASON FOR LEAVING
FROM				
TO				
FROM				
TO				
FROM				
TO				
FROM				
TO				

REFERENCES: GIVE THE NAMES OF THREE PERSONS NOT RELATED TO YOU, WHOM YOU HAVE KNOWN AT LEAST ONE YEAR.

NAME	ADDRESS	BUSINESS	YEARS ACQUAINTED
1			
2			
3			

PHYSICAL RECORD: DO YOU HAVE ANY PHYSICAL LIMITATIONS THAT PRECLUDE YOU FROM PERFORMING ANY WORK FOR WHICH YOU ARE BEING CONSIDERED? ☐ Yes ☐ No

PLEASE DESCRIBE:

IN CASE OF EMERGENCY NOTIFY

NAME ADDRESS PHONE NO.

"I CERTIFY THAT THE FACTS CONTAINED IN THIS APPLICATION ARE TRUE AND COMPLETE TO THE BEST OF MY KNOWLEDGE AND UNDERSTAND THAT, IF EMPLOYED, FALSIFIED STATEMENTS ON THIS APPLICATION SHALL BE GROUNDS FOR DISMISSAL.

I AUTHORIZE INVESTIGATION OF ALL STATEMENTS CONTAINED HEREIN AND THE REFERENCES LISTED ABOVE TO GIVE YOU ANY AND ALL INFORMATION CONCERNING MY PREVIOUS EMPLOYMENT AND ANY PERTINENT INFORMATION THEY MAY HAVE, PERSONAL OR OTHERWISE, AND RELEASE ALL PARTIES FROM ALL LIABILITY FOR ANY DAMAGE THAT MAY RESULT FROM FURNISHING SAME TO YOU.

I UNDERSTAND AND AGREE THAT, IF HIRED, MY EMPLOYMENT IS FOR NO DEFINITE PERIOD AND MAY, REGARDLESS OF THE DATE OF PAYMENT OF MY WAGES AND SALARY, BE TERMINATED AT ANY TIME WITHOUT ANY PRIOR NOTICE."

DATE SIGNATURE

DO NOT WRITE BELOW THIS LINE

INTERVIEWED BY DATE

HIRED: ☐ Yes ☐ No POSITION DEPT.

SALARY/WAGE DATE REPORTING TO WORK

APPROVED: 1. EMPLOYMENT MANAGER 2. DEPT. HEAD 3. GENERAL MANAGER

This form has been designed to strictly comply with State and Federal fair employment practice laws prohibiting employment discrimination. This Application for Employment Form is sold for general use throughout the United States. We assume no responsibility for the inclusion in said form of any questions which, when asked by the Employer of the Job Applicant, may violate State and/or Federal Law.

Figure 15–5. (Continued.)

There are some questions, however, that are not acceptable for the employer to ask because they are in violation of a person's civil rights. The following questions are discriminatory and should not be asked by the employer prior to one's employment:

Where were you born?
How old are you?
How many children do you have?
Do you plan to have any children?
Do you have a girlfriend/boyfriend?
How much do you weigh?
What type of military discharge do you have?

If the potential employer asks any of these questions, you have the right to refuse to answer the question. This line of questioning by the interviewer may also be an indication to you of the types of biases or principles that exist in the organization.

Preparing for the interview also means getting ready in the physical sense — being well groomed and dressing professionally. Your health occupations education instructor has emphasized the importance good grooming plays in the appearance of the health worker. The interviewer notes carefully the presence or absence of good grooming as an indication of how the potential worker will appear on the job, if hired. Complete the following Good Grooming Do's and Don'ts:

Do's	Don'ts
____________________	____________________
____________________	____________________
____________________	____________________
____________________	____________________
____________________	____________________
____________________	____________________

Health Occupations Students of America members have a unique opportunity to prepare in advance for the job interview. One of the competitive events, Job Seeking Skills, enables students to complete the job-seeking process in a simulated setting.

THE INTERVIEW

Because you have prepared both intellectually and physically for the interview, you now have the confidence to enter the interview with self-assurance. Arrive a little early. It shows your interest and reliability. Also, it gives you a chance to settle down and concentrate on the upcoming interview. Remember: You're prepared, you have the necessary skills the employer is looking for, you're a winner. Go for it! The following outline will guide you through the interview process.

1. Greet the receptionist politely. Give your name and reason for being there.
2. Complete the job application form as requested.
   — Review the form thoroughly before starting to complete it.
   — Complete all areas of the form. If some parts don't apply to you, use **None** or **NA** (Not Applicable).
   — Don't write in spaces labeled "Office Use Only."
3. Take a couple of deep breaths before entering the interview area. It helps to calm and relax you.
4. When introduced to the interviewer, greet the person by name and shake hands firmly.
5. Maintain eye contact during the interview. Be yourself — it's OK to smile! Try not to fidget. Mannerisms may be annoying to the interviewer; they detract from your professional appearance.
6. Speak clearly using correct grammar. Do not chew gum, smoke, or munch on candy during the interview.
7. Be polite. Don't interrupt the interviewer.
8. Maintain good posture. Sit straight in the chair.
9. Answer all questions honestly and to the best of your ability. Emphasize your strong points, not in a bragging manner but with self-assurance.
10. Think about the question and how to answer it before you begin. Don't rush. Answers should be clear and concise.
11. Ask those questions you've prepared in advance. It's OK to refer to a file card for prompting.
12. Give the interviewer your list of references (if not included on the resume).
13. At the conclusion of the interview, thank the person for the opportunity to be interviewed. Again, using a firm handshake, exit the room.

14. Usually, the interviewer will tell you when you can expect to hear from them about the job. On rare occasions, the interviewer will tell you at the end of the interview whether or not you are the successful candidate.

After the interview, send a follow-up letter to the interviewer thanking the person for the opportunity to be interviewed. It's your opportunity to state again, briefly, your interest in the job and why you are the best candidate for the position. Many times the "thank you" letter gives you the competitive edge over the other candidates; it's well worth the time and energy it takes (**Fig. 15–6**).

WHICH JOB SHALL I TAKE?

Now that you've experienced the application process and the job interview, deciding on the right job for you is the next major step. We tend to make decisions about jobs the way we make other important decisions in our lives. Some of us let others control our decision-making — our friends, parents, or relatives. Others make decisions based on only part of a total picture — "I'll take the job that pays the best."

The reasonable approach to decision making, however, is to evaluate all aspects of the issue — in this case — the future job. You must weigh all factors — the positives and negatives, the pros and cons. Putting the facts in writing, then expressing in writing your feelings about each factor, will help you to be more objective in your decision-making. This technique also helps you to decide which of the job offers you should select.

Using the format below, complete the following information.

	Pro	Con
1. Starting wages or salary — Weekly, biweekly, monthly — Can I budget myself to live on the amount being offered?	______	______
2. Salary increments — How frequently, how much — based on length of employment and/or performance?	______	______
3. Salary differentials — Based on time of day — evening or night shift? Special units?	______	______

24 Hardy Avenue
Trenton, NJ 08638
November 30, 1988

Ms. Arlene Weller
Personnel Manager
Memorial Medical Center
99 Elm Drive
Trenton, NJ 08638

Dear Ms. Weller:

Show Appreciation — Thank you for the opportunity to interview for the nursing assistant position on November 28, 1988. I appreciate the time spent with me during the interview and tour of the hospital.

Restate Qualifications — I believe that my Health Occupations Education course at Brewster High School, my active membership in Health Occupations Students of America, and my present and past work experience make me an excellent candidate for this entry-level position in the health field. My leadership ability and desire to succeed will enable me to be an asset to the Memorial Medical Center.

I look forward to hearing from you soon. I am grateful for your consideration.

Sincerely yours,

Pamela Martin

Pamela Martin

Figure 15–6. Sample "Thank You" letter.

4. Fringe benefits —
   Medical insurance, dental insurance, disability insurance, and life insurance? ______ ______
5. Sick Leave —
   How much — Can it be accumulated beyond one year? ______ ______
6. Vacation —
   How much — based on length of employment? ______ ______
7. Pension plan? ______ ______
8. Prescription plan for medications? ______ ______
9. Eye glass prescription plan? ______ ______
10. Tuition reimbursement for participating in programs for advancement? ______ ______
11. Location of employment
    Desirable area?
    Parking provided or available nearby — free, inexpensive, or costly? ______ ______
12. Meals provided or available nearby? ______ ______
13. Other special employee provisions —
    Reduced rates for professional medical/dental services? ______ ______
14. Uniform allowance? ______ ______
15. Continuing education or in-service provided? ______ ______
16. Advancement opportunities available? ______ ______
17. Other — list information which hasn't been included in the categories listed above. ______ ______

Making Your Decision

You've put in writing the information about the job which you have gained from all available sources (interviewer, public relations materials, other employees) and have compared the pros and cons of one job over another. Based upon your career goals, you need to be reasonably confident that your potential employer will provide the kind of job that is compatible with these goals. Is the job one which you will find satisfaction in doing? Is your supervisor the type of person you can work for easily?

Wages and fringe benefits are important factors in deciding about the job. But they are not the only considerations. The job which offers the opportunity for learning experiences which will help you to expand your knowledge and skills may be far more desirable than a job with good benefits which offers little potential for you to grow in your career. The decision is up to you!

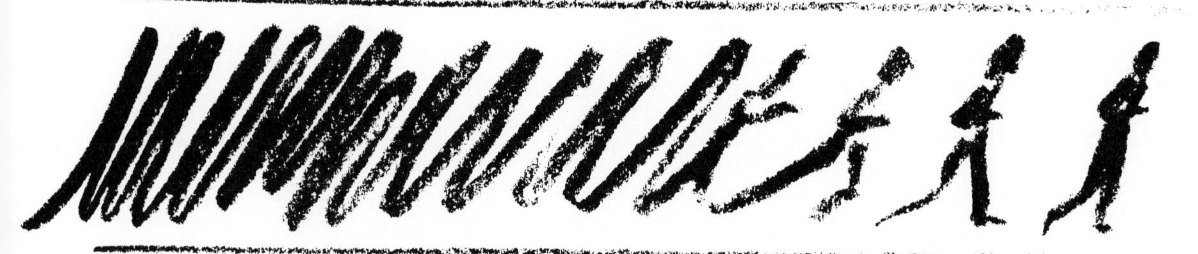

S·T·U·D·E·N·T A·C·T·I·V·I·T·I·E·S

1. Bring to class the Want Ad section of the Sunday newspaper. With two other classmates, remove the ads for health occupations jobs. Read the ads and place each ad in one of three categories: No Experience Required; Requires High School Diploma; and Requires Professional Training.
2. Using the ads, select the three most appealing jobs. Discuss the reasons for your selections.
3. Develop your own resume using the format discussed in the chapter. Bring to class and discuss with classmates and instructor.
4. You are preparing to be interviewed for an entry-level position in the Direct Care Careers cluster at your local hospital. You have minimal experience except for the clinical experience you've received during your health occupations program. How will you respond to the interviewer's questions about the lack of experience? Prepare responses to emphasize the experiences you have had.
5. Prepare your own index card to bring to an interview which lists your essential information. Bring to class and discuss.
6. Prepare a letter of application and a follow-up letter.

Chapter 16

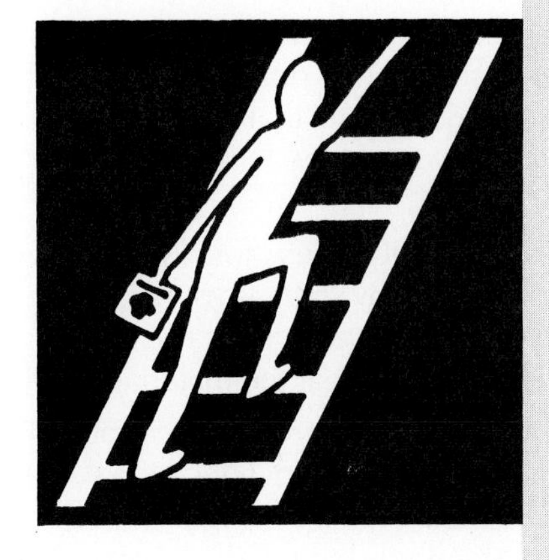

Progressing in Your Health Career

Objectives

After completing this chapter, you should be able to:

- Discuss six reasonable expectations that employers have for their employees.
- Prepare a letter of resignation applying the principles discussed in this chapter.
- Compare the terms "career ladder" and "career lattice."
- Compare three types of educational programs which prepare health workers.
- Explain the difference between program approval and program accreditation.
- Identify four sources of financial assistance and discuss ways in which this assistance can be obtained.
- Define at least 70 percent of the key terms listed for this chapter.

Key Terms

- **accreditation** The process whereby an association or private agency gives public recognition to an educational institution or specialized educational program which meets certain established qualifications and educational standards in addition to that required by a governmental agency, as determined by initial or periodic evaluation
- **advanced standing** Credit given for knowledge and skills previously learned by means of a testing process, usually through written and practical examination, enabling the student not to repeat the material
- **approval** The process whereby a governmental agency gives public recognition to an educational institution or specialized educational program which meets certain minimum standards by initial and periodic evaluations
- **aptitudes** Natural or acquired tendencies; abilities
- **career ladder** Advancement to the next level in a chosen field without having to relearn previously acquired knowledge and skills
- **career lattice** Acquisition of knowledge and skills for a career in a different but related area and being given credit for those related skills and knowledge previously learned
- **challenge examinations** Testing used to determine one's knowledge and skills in order to obtain advanced standing in a program
- **competency examination** Test which demonstrates the person's ability to successfully perform the necessary skills of a specific occupation
- **continuing education units** Credits or units for approved courses or programs assigned by professional associations, licensing, and certification agencies which enable health workers to expand their knowledge and skills in order to keep up with advancements in their field

- **expertise** Having the special skill and knowledge in a particular field
- **external degree** The process whereby college credit is earned for knowledge acquired in other settings than the classroom which leads to a college degree
- **grants** Types of financial assistance to a student which does not require repayment
- **loans** Sums of money advanced for a given period of time, to be paid back
- **marketable** Able to get a job using the knowledge and skills learned
- **proficiency examinations** See definition for competency examination
- **scholarships** Financial assistance to a student which does not require repayment
- **transcript** A written record of grades received for courses taken in school

PUTTING THE PIECES TOGETHER

Congratulations! You have made your decision about taking that position based upon careful review of all the facts. You know why you've made the decision and are eager to start your career. Your employer has made a commitment to you — an agreement to pay you for the duties you will perform. The employer expects you to perform these duties safely and effectively as a part of the health care team. Through your health occupations program, you have developed the beginning skills, knowledge, and positive attitudes that your employer needs. Now you will be putting them into practice in the day-to-day performance of your job.

When you look at the time and energy expended in finding the job best suited to your talents and career objectives, you will be eager to make the job a success as well. Success in any endeavor requires a commitment and hard work by the key players — your employer and you.

Your Employer's Role

During the interview, your employer discussed salary and fringe benefits with you. These are obligations of the employer in return for satisfactory work by the employee. They are obvious. The employer has other responsibilities, too. These include providing a safe and clean environment in which to work, having adequate equipment and supplies for employees to do their jobs, assuring proper supervision of workers, providing any incidental on-the-job training to employees as needed, and providing standards for performance.

Your Role as Employee

Employment is a partnership. If the partnership is a good one, both parties benefit. The employer has agreed to pay you for the services that you will provide. You have made a commitment to perform these services to the best of your ability. This way, both parties benefit. The employer receives monies from the client or patient based upon the services rendered by employees. Because the *employees* perform these services with care and expertise, the *employer is able to pay* the employees from monies received from the client (**Fig. 16–1**).

It is this mutual commitment — employer to employee and employee to employer — that makes the real difference. Unfortunately, there are many employees, in all types of businesses and industries, who do not understand this important fact. The employer *cannot* pay the employee unless the *product or service* being produced is *sold or used*. In the auto industry, the product is the car. In the health care industry, the product is not as tangible. The product is the delivery of health care services of many types to many different clients (infants, children, younger and older adults). Your ability to produce the desired services will affect your employer's ability to have sufficient monies to pay you. Therefore, quality performance on the job is essential.

EVALUATING YOUR PERFORMANCE

From time to time, you will be evaluated by your employer to see how well you are providing the services to the client or patient — how well you are doing on the job. In larger institutions, such as medical centers, the

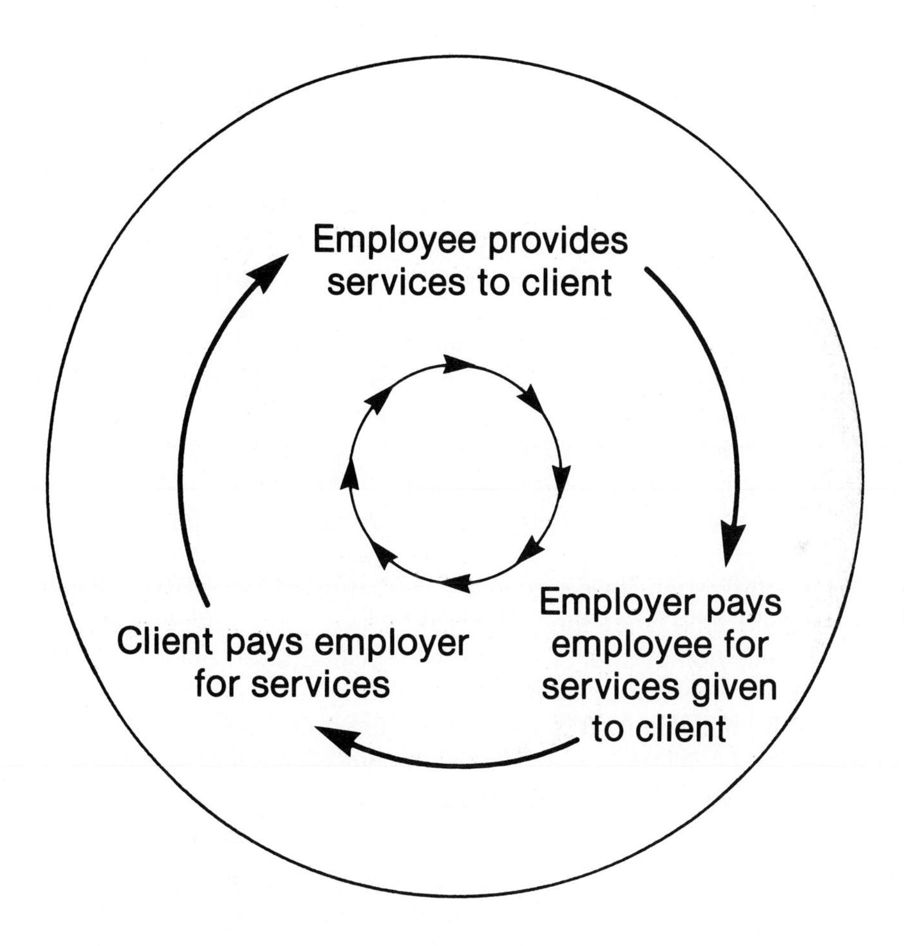

Figure 16–1. Employer/Employee Circle Chart.

evaluation process may be more formal than in a small medical office setting. For example, employee evaluations are given according to a time schedule (every six months or yearly) and follow a specific format which indicates categories to be evaluated (skills, attitude on the job, etc.). Whether the evaluation is formal or informal, the employer will judge your performance to determine your suitability to remain in your job. Let's take a look at the employer's expectations (**Fig. 16–2**).

PERSONAL GROWTH, SATISFACTION, AND FULFILLMENT

This is a pretty big prescription to fill and depends upon how much of yourself you are willing to invest in the career you have chosen. There are many opportunities for personal growth — growth in self-understanding. Health workers touch the lives of many people. With each encounter — sometimes brief, sometimes prolonged — something of each person "rubs off" on the other. Each experience offers a chance to learn more about yourself as well as about others. As one example, the physical therapist who assists an amputee to walk again with the aid of a prosthesis has a special opportunity to learn something about courage, determination, and adaptability. This health worker participates in the patient's physical effort to adjust to the artificial limb. The therapist will see the efforts of both patient and family in handling the activities of daily living, the discouraging days when the rehabilitation program just doesn't seem to work, and, finally, the joyful time when the patient takes those first unaided steps.

The health worker shares moments of discouragement and moments of joy with the patient and family. The knowledge that you played a part in one person's successful struggle to walk again can bring great personal satisfaction and fulfillment. But even an insignificant event — a smile from a patient who never acknowledged you before — can turn a routine day into one of inner joy.

SOME SERIOUS RESPONSIBILITIES

Serious responsibilities go hand in hand with personal satisfaction. This most important responsibility is to be excellent in your chosen career.

Date of Report ____________

TRAINING PROGRESS REPORT

Name: Job Title: Date Hired or Promoted:

Department: Section:

To be completed by the Supervisor and approved by the Department Head for discussion with the staff member and returned to the Personnel Department for filing in the employee's personnel folder.

JOB FACTOR	IMPROVEMENT NECESSARY	SATISFACTORY	VERY GOOD	EXCELLENT
1. RETAINS INSTRUCTION	☐	☐	☐	☐
2. QUALITY	☐	☐	☐	☐
3. QUANTITY	☐	☐	☐	☐
4. CONCENTRATION	☐	☐	☐	☐
5. ATTITUDE	☐	☐	☐	☐
6. COOPERATION	☐	☐	☐	☐
7. INITIATIVE	☐	☐	☐	☐
8. GENERAL PROGRESS	☐	☐	☐	☐

Number of Times Absent ______ Rated By ____________ *(Immediate Supervisor)*

Number of Times Tardy ______ Reviewed By ____________ *(Division or Section Supervisor)*

Approved By ____________ *(Department Head)*

Employee Signature ____________

Explanation, recommendation, and suggested action: ____________

____

____

____

Over for additional remarks

Figure 16–2. Sample employee performance evaluation report.

The program that prepares you to enter the health career of your choice will provide the basic skills and knowledge required. If licensing is required, the school will also prepare you to pass the examination. But learning doesn't stop with receiving a diploma or license. EDUCATION IS AN ONGOING PROCESS! This statement applies especially to the health occupations area because of the rapidity with which advances in treatment result from medical research findings.

CONTINUING EDUCATION

We are living in a time when new knowledge about the world in which we live is coming at an unbelievably fast rate. With it comes new techniques and procedures that may require us to discard or modify the old ones and adjust to necessary change. Therefore, you must keep abreast of changes in your health occupations area so that your skills remain sharp and current through continuing education activities. These activities can be accomplished by participating in meetings and seminars held by your employer or professional associations, reading the professional journals in your chosen field, and participating in workshops sponsored by health care agencies and organizations. Some states consider continuing education to be so important that license renewal depends on proof of the individual's participation in such activities. Those agencies or professional associations wishing to conduct approved continuing education programs must apply to the appropriate agency for approval. They must indicate the objectives and content of the proposed program and show how the participants will be evaluated. A committee reviews the proposal and determines the number of continuing education units (CEUs) to be approved. After successfully completing the approved program, the health worker submits verification to the licensing agency that the required number of CEUs have been obtained.

ADVANCING IN YOUR FIELD

The occupations discussed in this text offer lifetime careers in themselves. Nevertheless, many persons modify their career objectives after being employed for a period of time in one field. They may wish to remain in the same field but want to advance. For example, a physical therapy assistant may wish to resume formal education and study to become a physical therapist. This is called "career ladder advancement." It is sometimes referred to as "vertical mobility" because the individual progresses upward, as in climbing the rungs of a ladder.

Career Ladder Programs

The purpose of the career ladder approach is to enable the health worker to advance in a chosen field without requiring skills and knowledge, already learned, to be relearned. Educational programs are designed so that one level of the program is articulated or connected to the next level. Because of this articulation, there is minimum repetition of subject matter.

Although this is the most logical and economical means of advancement, in many instances it is difficult to design a true career ladder program. Many educational institutions provide parts of a total career ladder in one area but not in others. If you find that, after working for a while in one career, you wish to prepare for the next level of employment in the same field, contact the appropriate school about the availability of a career ladder program. Find out in advance what part of your previous education will be credited toward education for the new career.

Career Lattice Programs

Some persons may decide, after being employed in one health field, to switch to a different but related one. For example, a physical therapy assistant may wish to become an occupational therapist. While both are in similar fields (a part of the Therapeutic/Restorative group), they require different sets of skills. The process of acquiring the knowledge and skills for a career in a different area without having to discard those learned for an earlier career is called "career lattice" or "horizontal mobility." It enables the person to move from one related health career to another and may be thought of as a lattice (similar to a garden trellis). Again, should you be interested in opportunities for career lattice mobility, get all facts before deciding on a program. Find out from the school how much credit you will be given for your previous educational program. You will have to furnish the school with a transcript of the grades you earned during your first educational program. The school will evaluate the transcript and determine how much credit will be transferred toward the new career program.

Advanced Standing

This term means that the applicant has demonstrated mastery of the knowledge and skills taught in certain required courses. In effect, the school gives credit for the course but exempts the student from taking it.

Schools that prepare health workers often use similar course titles to describe what is perhaps very dissimilar course content. No two schools are exactly alike, and no two courses are necessarily alike. For this reason, the applicant who wishes to obtain advanced standing in a Health Occupations Education program must demonstrate proof of previous learning. Many schools administer tests to applicants to determine the extent of advanced standing to be given. These tests are called *competency, proficiency, or challenge examinations*. For example, an LPN/LVN who has graduated from an approved school of practical nursing and now wishes to enroll in a community college's nursing program will take competency examinations to demonstrate knowledge and skill in nursing practice. Successful completion of these tests may mean that the length of the nursing program at the community college will be shortened. However, not every school has provisions for administering this type of examination. It is important to find out from the college what its policy is concerning advanced standing.

MAKING THE DECISION TO LEAVE YOUR JOB

Leaving a job can be a most frustrating, difficult, and stress-producing experience, but it need not be if approached properly. There are many reasons for deciding to leave a job. Perhaps it is no longer challenging, and you wish to move to another position. Or you are planning to continue your education full time. Maybe there are people you work with whose behavior is causing you difficulty in performing your job effectively.

The final decision to leave should be based on careful thought rather than a decision made in haste — on the spur of the moment. Some employees storm the employer's door with the statement "I quit!" This behavior shows that the person's decision is probably based on the immediate problem rather than on the assessment of factors leading to the actual event. At any rate, should you decide that your only alternative is to terminate your employment, it is important that you have a new job *before* leaving your old one. It is much more difficult to obtain a job after you have already left your employer, no matter what the reason. You are much more "marketable" to your potential employer if you already have a job.

Before deciding to leave voluntarily, you need to sort out the reasons for leaving. If a problem situation exists, have you taken the steps necessary to resolve the problem? Can it be solved? Have you talked to your supervisor about it? The best approach to handling the situation may not be to terminate your employment. You need to analyze the problem and come up with possible solutions. Brainstorm the following problems and possible solutions.

The Problem	**Possible Solutions**
The job is no longer challenging.	
My coworker is impossible to work with.	
My supervisor doesn't understand me.	
The pay is too low to live on.	
The routine tasks get me down.	
It's a dead-end job; I see no chance for advancement.	
There is not enough equipment or supplies.	
There is not enough staff to do a good job.	

Leaving the Job Without "Burning Your Bridges"

According to the latest statistics, the average worker in the United States will change jobs at least seven times in the course of one's work life. Therefore, it is important to develop the skills needed to exit the job gracefully. Once you have come to the decision to leave, the following steps need to be taken:

1. Adhere to the organization's policy about notifying superiors about your decision. Make sure that you honor this policy. Let your employer know as soon as possible so that there will be time to hire and train a replacement.
2. If possible, speak to your superior before submitting a letter of resignation to explain why you are leaving. Express your appreciation for their assistance in the past.
3. *Do not* discuss your intentions to leave with coworkers before speaking with your superior. It is poor practice to inform everyone but those who really need to know. Information spreads rapidly through the "grapevine," and you don't want your employer to hear about your leaving from this source.
4. Write the letter of resignation which contains the following:

   When you wish to leave
   Why you are leaving
   Appreciation for the skills you have acquired
   Positive aspects of the job — loyal coworkers, good in-service training programs, understanding superiors, etc.

The same principles of letter writing, previously discussed in Chapter 15, apply to writing the letter of resignation (**Fig. 16–3**).

Taking the time to write a positive resignation letter may pay off by having the employer give you a good recommendation. Some agencies conduct an exit conference with each employee who is leaving. This gives the employer the chance to ask you for information about the job you are leaving. Your honest answers help the employer to improve working conditions in the future. Always leave the interview on a positive note.

ENTERING A HEALTH OCCUPATIONS EDUCATION PROGRAM AFTER HIGH SCHOOL GRADUATION

Deciding to continue your education in a health career following graduation means that you will need some basic information in order to make your decision. What types of schools offer the program that I want?

1088 West Front Street
Baltimore, MD 21202
December 12, 1988

Dr. Lane R. Collins
85 Cathedral Street
Baltimore, MD 21201

Dear Dr. Collins:

As you know, a career in the health care field is one of my goals in life. The experience that I have gained as a medical receptionist in your office during the last six months has made me more sure than ever that a health care career is the right field for me.

Why: In order to pursue this career, I must further my education. I will attend the county college beginning with the spring semester in January **When:** 1989. Therefore, it is necessary for me to resign from my position in your office effective January 7, 1989.

Appre-citation & Positive Aspects

Employment in your office has enabled me to gain on-the-job training while developing my human relations skills by interacting with both patients and health care professionals. I appreciate the opportunity of working with you and the other employees in your office. Thank you for helping me build a foundation of skills and knowledge to use in my future career as a nurse.

Sincerely yours,

Wilma Calvert

Wilma Calvert

Figure 16–3. Sample letter of resignation.

What's the best program for me? Is it approved, accredited? What about clinical experiences? How will I pay for the program? The rest of the chapter will give you basic principles to follow when choosing your program.

Types of Schools

The following four types of schools offer post-high school preparation:

Public educational institutions. City, county, or area vocational/technical schools; community and state colleges; and universities are all examples of public educational institutions. These schools are financed through taxpayers' monies. Educational costs are minimal since the means to finance the institutions are shared by the city, county, or the state. Although tuition fees may be charged, they are lower than those charged by private schools.

Private educational institutions. This group includes community and four-year colleges and universities operated by nonpublic, nonprofit organizations. Operating funds for these institutions are derived from tuition fees, alumni donations, grants, gifts, and other funds, rather than from public sources. Because public monies are not used to finance these schools, the students must assume a large share of financial responsibility for tuition charges and other fees.

Proprietary schools and private trade schools also fall in the category of private educational institutions. They are privately owned by one or more persons and may be incorporated for business purposes. They have a two-fold purpose: (1) to provide an educational program leading to employment and (2) to earn a profit for the owners. Monies for operating expenses are obtained primarily from tuition charges to students.

Health care institutions. Hospitals and medical centers sponsor schools where preparation is provided for specific health occupations. Classes are held in the hospital or medical center and instructors are hired by the institution. Students obtain the major part of their clinical experiences in the hospital or medical center itself. Hospitals may offer stipends (money to defray expenses) to students during the course of their program. Such schools were originally established to serve the special needs of the institutions and their patients. For example, the hospital may have had difficulty in finding qualified radiologic technologists to staff the x-ray department, so it established a school of radiologic technology to assure a continuing group of graduates who would then be employed primarily in that hospital. Today, hospitals and medical centers continue to operate schools; the difference being that the schools serve not only their own needs but also the needs of the larger community. Graduates of these programs may elect to work wherever jobs are available.

Armed forces career schools. These programs are open only to members of the armed forces. Following a period of basic training, a variety of health occupations programs are available to them, according to their aptitudes and interests. Of course, the total education cost is paid by the federal government through taxes.

Choosing the Best Program

Deciding on the right school is important, but just as important is selecting the right program. A wise consumer gets all the facts before buying — and that is what selecting a program is all about. The "buying" is done with money, time, and effort spent in the educational program. In order to make a wise investment and to evaluate the quality of a program, the following questions should be asked.

Is the program approved? Approval of a program means that it has met at least the minimum requirements set by the state agency that oversees it. For example, approval of programs conducted in public secondary schools and private trade schools is the responsibility of the state Department of Education. In programs established within public colleges, the responsibility rests with the state Department of Higher Education or with one of its divisions which approves programs in colleges and universities.

The government agency reviews the following: the qualifications of the teaching staff, the adequacy of the facility and its equipment, and the quality of the curriculum. If these meet at least minimum standards, the program is approved for a given period of time (often, five years). Renewal of the approval is granted after a second review.

If the career you seek is one requiring a license to practice, then the state licensing agency must also approve the program to ensure that graduates meet the necessary requirements for the licensing examination. Usually two agencies of state government, Education/Higher Education and the licensing agency (state Board of Optometry, Dentistry, Nursing, etc.) review the program and, if it is acceptable, issue a joint approval.

These agencies are the ones that you should write to for information about approved programs: (1) state Department of Education or Public Instruction, state capital; (2) state Department of Higher Education, state capital; (3) state Board of Optometry, Dentistry, Medicine, etc., state capital.

Most state education departments employ one or more professional staff members whose primary responsibility is in the area of health occupations education. These persons are excellent resources for information about approval of health occupations education programs in the state.

Is the program accredited? For some careers, it is important that you enroll in a program that not only is approved by the appropriate state agency but that also undergoes additional scrutiny by a professional organization (usually a national association) in the designated field. Accreditation allows you, upon graduation, to "sit for" (be tested in) the association's examination to determine your competency. An accredited school is one that has applied to the professional organization to have its program evaluated and has met the criteria for educational superiority. The program is accredited for a given period of time, after which it is re-evaluated.

Keep in mind, however, that because a program is not accredited, it is not necessarily inferior to an accredited one. There may be a good reason for a school's not wishing to apply for accreditation, such as the cost involved. The accrediting agency charges an application fee to the institution. Then there are additional expenses to the institution related to preparing the necessary forms, information, and requested materials. The entire process of applying for accreditation, then, is a costly one. For this reason, a school may choose not to apply.

The true test of the excellence of a program is the outcome for its graduates. Are they successful in their field? Are they respected members in their occupational area? It is a good idea to speak with graduates or students currently enrolled in given programs about their experiences.

The Committee on Allied Health Education and Accreditation of the American Medical Association is a coordinating agency for accrediting allied health occupations programs in 18 health careers areas. Its publication, *Allied Health Education Directory*, lists by state the accredited schools in each occupational area. If you are interested, you may purchase the most recent directory by writing to:

American Medical Association
Order Department
535 N. Dearborn Street
Chicago, Illinois 60610

Does the program offer clinical experiences? A program that promises to teach you to swim but never allows you in the water is a farce. This is also true of a few programs in health careers which allow almost no time for learning in the actual work setting. In the health occupations, such experience is called a *clinical experience or practicum.* It may take place in a private dental office, a large medical center, a nursing home, a city public health agency — any place where the student is actually putting into practice the skills and principles learned in the classroom. These experiences should be supervised and directed by the school faculty. A program that does not include clinical experience is of questionable value.

A WORD OF CAUTION. Beware of correspondence course advertisements implying that you will have the necessary skills for entry-level employment while offering no clinical experiences supervised by their teaching staffs. However, there are some correspondence courses that **are** accredited by professional organizations for the purpose of *upgrading the knowledge of practicing health workers* who already have the necessary skills.

Before you enroll. Check with your state Department of Education for information on approved correspondence courses. Just because the advertisement says "Approved by ________ state," doesn't mean that *your* state necessarily has given its approval.

Check with the professional association in your state about the correspondence course.

Check with the Better Business Bureau or local consumer protection office about the course.

What is the cost of the program? Depending upon the program and the school that you choose, the costs will vary, even though the type of program is the same. For example, you may choose to commute to a public vocational/technical school in your area which offers a practical nursing program. Another student may select a similar program operated by a hospital in another part of the state which has residential facilities. The difference in cost between the two programs may be considerable. The vocational/technical school offers low tuition and fees to the residents of the area it serves. The hospital-based school must charge higher tuition and fees to meet its expenses. Add the cost of residential living, and the total bill for education rises dramatically!

How do I pay for it? Most students choose to finance their education partially by part-time employment during the school year and full-time jobs during the summer. However, jobs are not always easy to find, and usually the money saved does not cover the total cost of education. If your family is unable to make up the difference, other sources of help need to be tapped. The information provided below may be of assistance in identifying financial resources.

To be eligible for most kinds of financial assistance, you must either be enrolled in the school or be accepted for enrollment. The school's counseling department or financial aid officer is a good source of advice about financial aid. It is wise to explain your financial situation at the time of your preadmission interview. You can also apply for assistance at this time. Remember that financial aid is not usually given until you are actually accepted into the program. The most common types of assistance fall into three major categories: scholarships, grants, and loans.

Scholarships and Grants

These forms of financial aid are gifts that do not have to be repaid. Scholarships are provided by many sources: the state, and private organizations such as churches and fraternal organizations, professional health career associations, health agencies, veterans' groups, labor unions, and business firms. See your guidance counselor for information about scholarships available in your community. For information about state scholarship programs, contact your school guidance counselor, the state Department of Education, or the Department of Higher Education's Office of Student Scholarships in the state capital.

Scholarships may also be available from state associations of Health Occupations Students of America for members who plan to continue their education in a health occupations education program at the postsecondary level. Contact your state association of HOSA for details.

Loans

A loan is a sum of money advanced for a given period of time; interest (the amount charged varies according to the lender) is added to the loan (which is called the principal). Under the federal government-sponsored Guaranteed Student Loan Program, the student must be enrolled at least half-time in an eligible vocational/technical school, school of nursing, college, or university. The student may then borrow directly from a bank, credit union, or any other participating lender. The loan is guaranteed by a state or nonprofit private agency, or it is insured by the federal government. Payments on the loan begin within six months after the student terminates the program.

Further information about student loans can be obtained from the school itself or the state Department of Education or Higher Education, Office of Student Loans.

Special Aid

The following agencies will provide further information about financial aid:

Local Social Security Administration Office	Students whose parent(s) is/are disabled, retired, or deceased
Nearest Veterans Administration Office	Students whose parent(s) has/have died or who is/are permanently or totally disabled from disease or injury incurred while in the U.S. Armed Forces
Nearest Veterans Administration Office	Veterans of armed forces with honorable discharges
U.S. Department of Education	Catalog of Federal Assistance Programs available by writing to: Superintendent of Documents, U.S. Government Printing Office, Washington, DC 20402

When should I apply? This question is not an easy one to answer, and the answer in many cases depends on the number of people applying for admission. Some programs admit only a small group of students to each class and have long waiting lists. The student who waits until the last minute to apply for admission will probably be disappointed. However, although some programs have two-year waiting lists, others do not. Therefore, it is advisable to write to the school to which you wish to apply as early as possible (a year or two in advance is not too early) to ask about application deadlines. Also, some programs have preadmission requirements or prerequisites that may determine the preparatory courses you need to take in high school. If you have not taken the prerequisite courses, admission to the program can be delayed until you have successfully completed them.

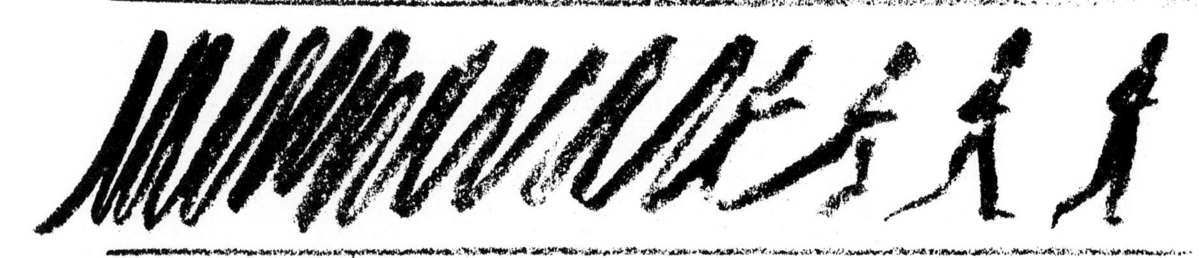

S·T·U·D·E·N·T A·C·T·I·V·I·T·I·E·S

1. Interview an employer of health care workers. During the interview, identify six key points that the employer has stated are essential characteristics of a productive employee. Compare your list with your classmates' lists.
2. Survey your community to find out what continuing education programs are available for health workers. Who sponsors the programs? What are the costs? Who is eligible to enroll? When are the programs given? Bring information to class and discuss.
3. Prepare a letter of resignation. Critique your letter with others in class. Participate in a mock exit interview and critique the process.
4. Obtain a catalog from a school that offers an educational program in a health career of interest to you. Answer the questions outlined in this chapter regarding program approval and accreditation.
5. Research the availability of scholarships or loans for a health career program of your choice. How many are available? What are the requirements, conditions, and application procedures for each?

Glossary

Abstract Hard to understand; expressing a quality without reference to actual person or thing that possesses it.

Acute stage of an illness As an illness progresses, the acute stage is the one where the symptoms are the most severe and proper care is necessary for a person to recover.

Analysis To examine something in order to determine its parts.

Anatomy A science that deals with the structure of the body.

Antibodies Substances produced by the body that counteracts the effects of a disease germ or its poisons.

Antitoxins Substances that form in the blood of someone who has been exposed to a toxin that usually counteracts the toxin.

Anus The opening at the end of the anal canal.

Artesian well A deep bored well.

Autism Mental disorder where the child/person is abnormally absorbed in a fantasy world and is often completely withdrawn.

Baccalaureate degree Degree given by a college or university for successful completion of four years of study.

Biases To like or dislike someone or something without a good reason; prejudices.

Bile Yellowish, bitter fluid produced by the liver to help the digestion of fat.

Biochemistry Science that deals with the chemistry of living things.

Biomedical engineer Person who uses the knowledge of biologic processes to help solve medical problems or questions.

Blood values The measurement of substances found in the blood.

Bowel Another word for intestines.

Bulimia An eating disorder where the person will crave and eat a tremendous amount of food. Afterward the person may force him/herself to vomit.

Cancer A spreading growth of cells on or in the body that destroys other healthy tissues and organs; malignancy.

Cardiac Having to do with the heart.

Cardiac diagnostician Person who specializes in identifying heart ailments.

Cholera Disease caused by a bacterial infection in the small intestine. Symptoms include vomiting and diarrhea.

Chronic Something that continues for a long time or reoccurs often.

Cleft lip An abnormal split, or division, of the upper lip present at birth.

Cleft palate An abnormal split, or division, of the roof of the mouth present at birth.

Compression fracture A bone break that compresses the bone. Vertebrae are often broken by a compression fracture.

Concrete conduit Pipe or channel in which water or other fluids travel.

Controlled substances Drugs regulated by federal law that require prescriptions from a doctor and are illegal to use except when authorized by a doctor.

Credentialing To be given written approval of your qualification.

Critical Having to do with a crisis or turning point; severe condition.

Culture medium A sterile, nutritious substance that gives microorganisms an environment to multiply.

Deductive reasoning The ability to come up with answers or make decisions based on various information or facts available.

Defecation To eliminate feces from the bowels.

Dentifrice Tooth-cleaning paste, powder, or other agent.

Deterrent Something that discourages.

Diabetes A disease where the body fails to produce insulin and use carbohydrates efficiently.

Dietitian A person who is a specialist in nutritional diets and the preparation of food.

Document Written material having to do with a computer or a computer program, to record information on a patient's record.

Electrocardiogram The graph produced during an electrocardiograph that shows and records the activity of the heartbeat.

Emotional trauma Any experience or event that causes a person to become very upset. The effects of this upset may last a long time.

Epidemic A widely spreading disease that attacks many people at the same time.

Extremities The end parts of a body's limbs, such as feet, hands, and fingers.

Glaucoma An eye disease caused by increased pressure within the eyeball. This condition causes blurred vision, redness, and if untreated, eventual loss of eyesight.

Hypertension High blood pressure.

Hypothetical reasoning A decision or conclusion based on established, supposed facts.

Immunization Medical treatment, such as a vaccine, that enables the body to produce antibodies against specific diseases.

Influenza Respiratory infection caused by a highly spreadable virus.

Institutionalization To confine a person in a protective area, such as a hospital, to receive physical or mental treatment.

Inoculate To inject by needle (or other method) a substance that protects against a disease.

Intravenous To inject or go inside of a vein.

Laceration A wound or injury caused by tearing of the skin.

Lay person Person who is not a member of a particular profession.

Lumbar vertebrae Bones of the spinal column located in the small of the back.

Malnutrition Poor nourishment due to lack of proper food, or faulty use of food.

Manipulative therapy Skillful, therapeutic use of the hands intended to correct or relieve a medical problem.

Medicolegal Combining the use of medicine and law. Treatment of many patients takes into consideration not only medical care, but the legal rights of patients as well.

Microbiology Science that studies microorganisms.

Noninvasive To examine a person without breaking the skin or entering the body.

Nosocomial infection A sickness or infection acquired while in a hospital.

Ophthalmoscope A medical tool used to examine the inside of the eyes.

Orthotist A person who makes and fits braces and other appliances that help correct the skeletal system (bones in body).

Paralysis To lose one's ability to move the body or to feel anything. Usually caused by an accident, disease, or poison.

Pathological Due to or involving disease.

Pediatric Branch of medicine that handles the care of children and their diseases.

Perspectives When a person is able to look at ideas or events with a broad viewpoint.

Pharmacology Science that deals with the uses and effects of drugs.

Physical therapist Person who treats the physical effects of disease or injury with massage, heat, and exercise.

Physiologist A doctor who studies the functions of the human body.

Physiology Study of the way the different systems of the body operates.

Poliomyelitis An infectious disease of the nervous system that usually affects children.

Potable A substance that is drinkable.

Practitioner A person who is qualified to practice in an area or profession, such as a nurse.

Prejudice Having or forming an opinion without fair reasons.

Prosthetist Person who makes and fits artificial arms, legs, etc.

Rabies An infectious, often fatal disease carried by certain wild animals. The disease is transmitted to humans through animal bites and can be treated if diagnosed immediately.

Rectum A part of the large intestine connected to the anus; an opening where waste products are removed.

Regression To go backward or start at the original point.

Respiratory therapist Person who specializes in treating patients with breathing difficulties.

Saliva A clear fluid present in the mouth which aids in the chewing and digestion of foods.

Sanitarian Person who is a specialist in public sanitation and health.

Scrutiny To examine with close detail.

Silicosis Lung disease caused by inhaling silicon (a chemical element).

Smallpox A highly contagious disease whose symptoms include fever and skin rashes.

Solubility A substance that can be dissolved in liquid.

Spinal Cord A major part of the human central nervous system. This system is the main network of coordination and control. The spinal cord starts at the brain and extends down the back. It plays a dual role with the brain in connecting nerve fibers.

Spinal fluid A protective fluid that cushions the brain and spinal cord from shock.

Spreadsheet A computer-created worksheet used to enter figures and other data in order to prepare a final document.

Statistician Person who collects and interprets statistics.

Sterile technique Process by which sterility is maintained.

Stool Waste discharged through the rectum; feces.

Subpoenaed To be served a written summons that requires your appearance in a court of law.

Synovial fluid A transparent fluid secreted by membranes that lubricate joints and tendons.

Systemic diseases Diseases or illnesses that affect the whole body.

Tetanus An infectious, often fatal disease, caused by bacteria that can enter the body through wounds, abrasions, burns, etc. It can be fatal but is preventable through vaccine.

Therapeutic Pertaining to treating or curing of disease.

Treatment protocol Written plan that outlines the procedures to be followed to treat a particular patient's disease or illness.

Tuberculosis A contagious lung disease caused by rod-shaped bacteria, known as bacillus.

Typhoid fever Infection caused by bacteria found in food or liquid. Symptoms include diarrhea, headache, and fever.

Typhoid Mary A notorious woman who never exhibited the disease whose causative agent (typhoid) she carried.

Typhus A group of infectious diseases usually transmitted by bites from lice, ticks, or infected rodents.

Uterus Womb; an internal female organ of reproduction. It is the place where babies develop until they are ready to be born.

Vaccine Substance used to produce immunity.

Vulnerable Position where a person is exposed to possible attack or injury.

Work simplification techniques New—or different—ways a handicapped or ill person learns to simplify and perform everyday living tasks.

Index

(Page numbers in italics indicate figures and boxed material. Page numbers followed by a *t* indicate tables.)